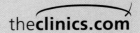
theclinics.com

CLINICS IN PLASTIC SURGERY

Challenges in Hand Surgery

Guest Editor
NANCY McKEE, MD, FRCS(C), FACS

Ocotber 2005 • Volume 32 • Number 4

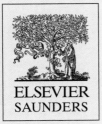

**ELSEVIER
SAUNDERS**

An imprint of Elsevier, Inc
PHILADELPHIA LONDON TORONTO MONTREAL SYDNEY TOKYO

W.B. SAUNDERS COMPANY
A Division of Elsevier Inc.

1600 John F. Kennedy Blvd., Suite 1800, Philadelphia, PA 19103-2899

http://www.theclinics.com

CLINICS IN PLASTIC SURGERY Volume 32, Number 4
October 2005 ISSN 0094-1298, ISBN 1-4160-2697-5

Editor: Joe Rusko

Reprints. For copies of 100 or more, of articles in this publication, please contact the Commercial Reprints Department, Elsevier Inc., 360 Park Avenue South, New York, New York 10010-1710. Tel. (212) 633-3813 Fax: (212) 462-1935 email: reprints@elsevier.com

The ideas and opinions expressed in *Clinics in Plastic Surgery* do not necessarily reflect those of the Publisher. The Publisher does not assume any responsibility for any injury and/or damage to persons or property arising out of or related to any use of the material contained in this periodical. The reader is advised to check the appropriate medical literature and the product information currently provided by the manufacturer of each drug to be administered to verify the dosage, the method and duration of administration, or contraindications. It is the responsibility of the treating physician or other health care professional, relying on independent experience and knowledge of the patient, to determine drug dosages and the best treatment for the patient. Mention of any product in this issue should not be construed as endorsement by the contributors, editors, or the Publisher of the product or manufacturers' claims.

Clinics in Plastic Surgery (ISSN 0094-1298) is published quarterly by W.B. Saunders Company. Corporate and editorial offices: Elsevier Inc., 1600 John F. Kennedy Blvd., Suite 1800, Philadelphia, PA 19103-2899. Accounting and circulation offices: 6277 Sea Harbor Drive, Orlando, FL 32887-4800. Periodicals postage paid at Orlando, FL 32862, and additional mailing offices. Subscription prices are $260.00 per year for US individuals, $390.00 per year for US institutions, $130.00 per year for US students and residents, $295.00 per year for Canadian individuals, $445.00 per year for Canadian institutions, $315.00 per year for international individuals, $445.00 per year for international institutions, and $155.00 per year for Canadian and foreign students/residents. To receive student/resident rate, orders must be accompanied by name of affiliated institution, date of term, and the *signature* of program/residency coordinator on institution letterhead. Orders will be billed at individual rate until proof of status is received. Foreign air speed delivery is included in all *Clinics* subscription prices. All prices are subject to change without notice. POSTMASTER: Send address changes to *Clinics in Plastic Surgery*, W.B. Saunders Company, Periodicals Fulfillment, Orlando, FL 32887-4800. **Customer Service: 1-800-654-2452 (US). From outside of the US, call 1-407-345-4000.**

Clinics in Plastic Surgery is covered in *Current Contents, EMBASE/Excerpta Medica, Science Citation Index, Index Medicus, ASCA,* and *ISI/BIOMED.*

Printed in the United States of America.

CHALLENGES IN HAND SURGERY

GUEST EDITOR

NANCY McKEE, MD, FRCS(C), FACS
Professor, Department of Surgery, University of
Toronto, Toronto, Ontario, Canada

CONTRIBUTORS

ANNE M.R. AGUR, PhD
Department of Surgery, University of Toronto,
Toronto, Ontario, Canada

DIMITRI J. ANASTAKIS, MD
Associate Professor of Surgery, Divisions of Plastic
and Orthopaedic Surgery, University of Toronto,
Toronto, Ontario, Canada

WARREN CARTOTTO, MD, FRCS(C)
Attending Staff, Ross Tilley Burn Centre; and
Associate Professor of Surgery, University of
Toronto, Toronto, Ontario, Canada

ROBERT CHEN, MD
Associate Professor of Medicine, Division of
Neurology, University of Toronto, Toronto,
Ontario, Canada

**HOWARD M. CLARKE, MD, PhD, FRCS(C),
FACS, FAAP**
Professor of Surgery, Department of Surgery,
University of Toronto; and Division of Plastic
Surgery, The Hospital for Sick Children, Toronto,
Ontario, Canada

KAREN D. DAVIS, PhD
Professor of Surgery, Division of Neurosurgery,
University of Toronto, Toronto Western Research
Institute, Toronto, Ontario, Canada

ALAN E. FREELAND, MD
Professor, Department of Orthopaedic Surgery
and Rehabilitation, University of Mississippi
Medical Center, Jackson, Mississippi

BRENT GRAHAM, MD, MSc, FRCSC
Director, University of Toronto/University Health
Network Hand Program, Banting Institute,
Toronto, Ontario, Canada

EMILY S. HO, MEd, OT
Division of Occupational Therapy, University of
Toronto; and Department of Rehabilitation
Services, The Hospital for Sick Children,
Toronto, Ontario, Canada

LOREE K. KALLIAINEN, MD
Department of Plastic and Hand Surgery,
Regions Hospital; and Division of Plastic and
Reconstructive Surgery, The University of
Minnesota, St. Paul, Minnesota

YASMIN KHALIQ, PharmD
Department of Pharmacy, Ottawa Hospital
General Campus; and Faculty of Medicine,
University of Ottawa, Ottawa,
Ontario, Canada

W.P. ANDREW LEE, MD
Division of Plastic Surgery, University of
Pittsburgh School of Medicine, Pittsburgh,
Pennsylvania

SUSAN E. MACKINNON, MD
Shoenberg Professor and Chief, Division of
Plastic and Reconstructive Surgery,
Washington University School of Medicine,
St. Louis, Missouri

STEVEN J. McCABE, MD, MSc
Associate Clinical Professor of Surgery,
University of Louisville, School of Medicine;
and Director of Decision Science,
University of Louisville, School of Public
Health and Information Sciences,
Louisville, Kentucky

NANCY McKEE, MD, FRCS(C), FACS
Professor, Department of Surgery, University of
Toronto, Toronto, Ontario, Canada

WYNDELL H. MERRITT, MD
Clinical Professor of Surgery, Virginia
Commonwealth University School of Medicine,
Richmond, Virginia

DAVID MIKULIS, MD
Associate Professor of Medical Imaging, University
of Toronto, Toronto, Ontario, Canada

JOHN MYERS, MSPH, PhD
Postdoctoral Fellow, Department of Epidemiology
and Public Health, Division of Biostatistics, Yale
University School of Medicine, New Haven,
Connecticut

VU T. NGUYEN, MD
Division of Plastic Surgery, University of Pittsburgh
School of Medicine, Pittsburgh, Pennsylvania

MICHEL M.E. SCHOFIELD, MD, MSc
Physician Coordinator of the Specialty Programs,
Workplace Safety and Insurance Board of Ontario;
and Medical Consultant to the University of
Toronto Hand Program, University Health
Network, Toronto, Ontario, Canada

WARREN SCHUBERT, MD
Department of Plastic and Hand Surgery, Regions
Hospital; and Division of Plastic and
Reconstructive Surgery, The University of
Minnesota, St. Paul, Minnesota

KARAN S. SINGH, PhD
Department of Computer Science, University of
Toronto, Toronto, Ontario, Canada

ACHILLEAS THOMA, MD, MSc, FRCSC, FACS
Clinical Professor, Department of Surgery and
Head, Division of Plastic Surgery, McMaster
University; and Surgical Outcomes Research
Centre, St. Joseph's Healthcare, Hamilton,
Ontario, Canada

WINNIE TSANG, MSc
Department of Computer Science, University of
Toronto, Toronto, Ontario, Canada

**HERBERT P. VON SCHROEDER, MD,
MSc, FRCSC**
University of Toronto Hand Program and Bone
Laboratory, Faculty of Dentistry, University Health
Network and University of Toronto, Toronto,
Ontario, Canada

RENATA V. WEBER, MD
Instructor of Surgery, Division of Plastic and
Reconstructive Surgery, Washington University
School of Medicine, St. Louis, Missouri

BIRGIT WEYAND, MD
University of Toronto Hand Program and Bone
Laboratory, Faculty of Dentistry, University Health
Network and University of Toronto, Toronto,
Ontario, Canada

GEORGE G. ZHANEL, PhD
Faculty of Medicine, Department of Medical
Microbiology, University of Manitoba; and
Departments of Medicine and Clinical
Microbiology, Health Sciences Centre, Winnipeg,
Manitoba, Canada

CHALLENGES IN HAND SURGERY

Volume 32 • Number 4 • October 2005

Contents

John Myers and Steven J. McCabe

> The practice of medicine takes place in an environment of uncertainty. Expected value decision making, prospect theory, and regret theory are three theories of decision making under uncertainty that may be used to help us learn how patients and physicians make decisions. These theories form the underpinnings of decision analysis and provide the opportunity to introduce the broad discipline of decision science. Because decision analysis and economic analysis are underrepresented in upper extremity surgery, the authors believe these are important areas for future research.

W.P. Andrew Lee and Vu T. Nguyen

> The early experience of hand transplantation has yielded a mixture of successes and failures. No life-threatening adverse effects have been encountered from immunosuppression, yet additional medications were required in some cases with unknown long-term efficacy or side effects. Limited functional returns have been observed, but any effect of chronic rejection is too early to determine. Although the experience has confirmed the benefits of hand transplantation to patients and their families, the future of hand transplantation on a wide scale is dependent on further research to alter its risk-benefit balance.

Emily S. Ho and Howard M. Clarke

> Achieving optimal upper limb function is a priority in the management of children with congenital hand malformations. Professionals need to be well equipped to help families understand the best surgical and rehabilitative options available for their child. Our ability as professionals clearly to define and evaluate the child's optimal function will assist in achieving this balance. This article examines the existing literature to evaluate critically functional outcome studies of children with congenital upper extremity malformations and to address the challenges of defining and measuring functional outcome in this patient population.

trial. Although the level of evidence associated with nonrandomized designs is always lower than that of a randomized trial there are many instances in which the inferences based on these designs are sufficiently strong that important and meaningful conclusions can be made. The key considerations in using nonrandomized designs are to frame the research question appropriately and to recognize and anticipate the limitations and biases that are inherent to each one of these approaches.

Bone Challenges for the Hand Surgeon: From Basic Bone Biology to Future Clinical Applications 537

Birgit Weyand and Herbert P. von Schroeder

Bone is a complex tissue composed of a calcified extracellular matrix with specialized cells that produce, maintain, and resorb the bone. Bone also has a rich vascular and neural supply. Bone has a great capability of regeneration, healing, and remodeling that is influenced by external factors, such as stress forces, and internal regulators that include hormones, vitamins, and growth factors. These factors dictate bone biology, and variations result in pathophysiologic conditions that have clinical implications in hand surgery. Solutions to the challenges in hand surgery rely on a thorough understanding of the biology of bone.

Closed Reduction of Hand Fractures 549

Alan E. Freeland

Stiffness is the most frequent consequence of open hand fracture treatment. Although initial injury severity and occurrence adjacent to the flexor tendon sheath are the most highly correlated determinants of hand fracture outcome, operative intervention accentuates the ultimate risk of stiffness. Closed treatment may minimize this risk. Articular fractures are at greater risk for stiffness than extra-articular fractures. Functional tolerance for small amounts of variation from perfect anatomic restoration gives us increased latitude for closed hand fracture management. Operative treatment may be justified for simple closed fractures when they are unstable, irreducible, or open, or when the surgeon believes that the risk-to-benefit ratio is favorable.

Challenges in Creating a Good Randomized Controlled Trial in Hand Surgery 563

Achilleas Thoma

The goal of this article is to inform readers of hand surgery literature and, more importantly, investigators about key design issues in randomized trials in hand surgery. Specifically, it describes the application of the Consolidated Standards of Reporting Trials in hand surgery trials and provides tips for reading the hand surgery literature. Unique challenges in the execution of a randomized controlled trial in hand surgery are explained, including the surgical learning curve, randomization, concealment and blinding, loss to follow-up, intention to treat analysis, surgical equipoise, differential care, and treatment effect and its implications for sample size. Additionally, the relevance of incorporating economic analyses into hand surgery trials and the importance of changing the hand surgeons' research culture are addressed.

The Challenge to Manage Reflex Sympathetic Dystrophy/Complex Regional Pain Syndrome 575

Wyndell H. Merritt

The challenge to understand reflex sympathetic dystrophy/complex regional pain syndrome may require a better understanding of the complex relationship between the central and peripheral nervous systems. There is no comprehensive hypothesis that clearly explains the etiology and no uniformly successful treatment method. This brief summary of the challenge reviews some of what is known, hypothesizes a possible etiologic mechanism, and proposes 10 common-sense principles for management that recognize the handicap of limited knowledge.

A major limitation to overall success in peripheral nerve surgery is time for regeneration. Although one can help speed up the regenerative process to some extent, success is hindered by issues such as number of coaptation sites, supply of donor nerves, and the limitations of nerve substitutes. In the case of a large gap, a nerve graft is often used to fill in the deficit. Autogenous nerve grafts are in limited supply, with sural nerve grafts being the primary source. Alternatives to the standard treatment include vein grafts, synthetic nerve conduits, nerve transfers, and nerve transplantation. Schwann cell–lined nerve conduits and tissue-engineered substitutions are still in their infancy and have some limited clinical application.

Today's view of the adult central nervous system is that of an adaptive and responsive system. Plastic surgeons, because of the motor and sensory reconstructions they perform, need to have an understanding of brain plasticity following upper extremity injury, reconstruction, and rehabilitation. Functional MRI and transcranial magnetic stimulation can identify cortical plasticity in humans. For instance, these techniques have identified changes in excitability and body site representation in the motor cortex in patients following motor reconstruction and motor relearning. Therefore, cortical plasticity and its manipulation may be an important contributor to functional outcome following reconstruction. In the future, cortical plasticity may have implications for reconstruction and rehabilitation.

This article includes a brief description of an approach to functional limb modeling including a summary of "helping hand," a computer model created by the authors. Potential uses of three-dimensional computer modeling of hand function are presented with some illustrations relevant to clinicians.

ELSEVIER
SAUNDERS

CLINICS IN
PLASTIC
SURGERY

Clin Plastic Surg 32 (2005) xi

Preface
Challenges in Hand Surgery

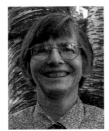

Nancy McKee, MD, FRCS(C), FACS
Department of Surgery
University of Toronto
Toronto, Ontario
Canada

E-mail address:
n.mckee@utoronto.edu

Nancy McKee, MD, FRCS(C), FACS
Guest Editor

Hand challenges! This issue of the *Clinics in Plastic Surgery* illustrates some of the thoughts that are part of our creative work, both in what we do and why we do it. It includes articles that examine outcomes, patient values and decisions, evaluation tools, and clinical research tools.

Other articles address specific understanding of a spectrum of surgical hand practice. Functional MRI is shedding new light on cortical plasticity. Closed reductions of hand fractures are still a useful option. Exciting advances are being made in our understanding of bone degeneration and regeneration. Alterations in tendons have been documented with the fluoroquinolone antibiotics. Some hand transplantations have survived long periods with currently available immunosuppressive approaches. Judicious use of skin grafts and skin flaps contribute to burned hand rehabilitation and to challenging web contractures from any cause. Nerve injuries continue to challenge us with nerve gap bridging opportunities and chronic regional pain syndrome. Work-related hand injury trends are viewed from the perspective of Ontario's Workplace Safety and Insurance Board.

There is not a specific article on the art of medicine, but it is clear from these articles that progress has been made in studying and quantifying some of the aspects of care that contribute to the "art." Surgeons have the wonderful possibility of tailoring their treatment to the whole individual. These articles help illuminate how far we have come along that path, yet some of the challenges remain open for solutions. Surgeons are well aware that is not enough to graft a burned hand or minimize deformity of a congenital malformation. It can also be important that the hand not be kept in a pocket and that it be useful.

It is hoped that these articles will motivate others to be innovative in advancing our understanding of the results of hand surgery and care.

plasticsurgery.theclinics.com

doi:10.1016/j.cps.2005.06.004

CLINICS IN
PLASTIC
SURGERY

Clin Plastic Surg 32 (2005) 453–461

Understanding Medical Decision Making in Hand Surgery

John Myers, MSPH, PhD[a], Steven J. McCabe, MD, MSc[b,c],*

- Glossary of terms
- Abbreviations
- Introduction
- Normative versus descriptive decision making
- Expected utility decision making
  Utility
  Quality-adjusted life years
- *Decision analysis*
- *Risk attitudes*
- *Problems with expected utility decision making*
- Prospect theory
- Regret theory
- Summary
- References

Glossary of terms

Certainty effect—the preference for a sure outcome over a lottery, although the lottery has a higher *expected utility*.

Decision analysis—an unambiguous, quantitative, systematic approach to decision making under conditions of uncertainty in which probabilities and *utilities* are assigned to all plausible outcomes.

Decision tree—a graphical depiction of a decision that involves alternative choices, uncertain events, and plausible outcomes.

Descriptive decision making—a group of principles whose objective is to explain how people actually make decisions under uncertainty.

Effectiveness—the extent to which health interventions improve health.

Expected utility—a quantity used to represent the value of a course of action where the outcome of the action is uncertain. Each outcome is assigned a probability of occurrence as well as a *utility*. The expected utility is a probability weighted average of the utilities.

Health state—the health experience of an individual at a particular time point.

Normative decision making—a group of principles whose objective is to explain how people should make decisions under uncertainty.

Quality-adjusted life years—a measure that aggregates quality of life across time periods.

Quality of life—a measurement, subjective or objective, that reflects judgment of all aspects of an individual's existence (eg, health-related, economic, political, cultural, spiritual).

Reference point—term used in *prospect theory* to represent the current state of health.

Sensitivity analysis—mathematical calculations in which factors involved in a *decision analysis* are isolated to investigate the influence each factor has on the entire analysis.

Standard gamble—a scenario in which raters are asked to compare life in their current state (ie, a

[a] Yale University School of Medicine, Department of Epidemiology and Public Health, Division of Biostatistics, New Haven, CT, USA
[b] University of Louisville, School of Medicine, Louisville, KY, USA
[c] University of Louisville, School of Public Health and Information Sciences, 555 South Floyd Street, Louisville, KY 40202, USA
* Corresponding author. University of Louisville, School of Public Health and Information Sciences, 555 South Floyd Street, Louisville, KY 40202.
E-mail address: steven.mccabe@louisville.edu (S.J. McCabe).

doi:10.1016/j.cps.2005.05.001

"sure thing") to a gamble with probabilities assigned to perfect health (P) and death ($1-P$). The probability P is changed until the rater is indifferent between the "sure thing" and the gamble. The probability P that makes raters indifferent between the sure thing and the gamble is their preference for their current state of health.

Time trade-off technique—a scenario in which raters are asked to trade life years in a health state that is less than perfect for a shorter time in a state of perfect health. The ratio of years of perfect health that is equal to the longer years in less than perfect health provides a measure of preference for the less than perfect health state.

Utility—the preference an individual has for a particular health state.

Value—a judgment of the desirability of a health state.

Visual analogue scale—a scenario in which raters place a mark at some point between two anchor states appearing at the ends of a line whose distance is known.

Abbreviations

CEA, cost effectiveness analysis
CTS, carpal tunnel syndrome
CUA, cost utility analysis
HUI, health utilities index
MAUT, multi-attribute utility theory
QALY, quality-adjusted life year
SG, standard gamble technique
TTO, time trade-off technique
UCL, ulnar collateral ligament
VAS, visual analogue scale

Introduction

In the practice of medicine, clinicians encounter many uncertainties. The probability that the patient has the disease of interest, the likelihood of successful surgery, and the risk of infection are all examples of uncertainties that may confront a surgeon.

This article reviews modern concepts and methodologies that guide decision making under uncertainty. Hand and reconstructive surgery examples are used to illustrate important points. The three theories of decision making discussed in this chapter are (1) expected value decision making, (2) prospect theory, and (3) regret theory.

Normative versus descriptive decision making

A distinction is made between understanding how people *should* make decisions, called normative decision making, and how they actually *do* make decisions, termed descriptive decision making [1]. It is traditionally thought that a rational person will seek to maximize quality of life. To do this, it is believed that an individual should make decisions consistent with normative decision making. However, it is observed that people will violate normative rules in their decision making in predictable manners and situations [2]. Understanding both normative and descriptive decision making offers insight into increasing patient satisfaction and health-related quality of life. Both are valuable and active research areas in health care.

The characteristics of a decision can be described with the aid of a simple 2-by-2 table [Table 1]. A decision is needed when there is more than one alternative. One characteristic of a decision is whether the outcome of an alternative is achieved with certainty [see first row of Table 1]. If the result of the decision is certain and the outcome of interest is simple and understood, then the decision maker need only choose the alternative with the highest value. However, if the value of the outcome is complex or difficult to compare with outcomes of other competing alternatives, then the decision maker will need to create a common currency in which to compare the alternatives. In health care, this common currency is *utility*, the strength of preference for a state of health [3].

The more common situation in medicine is one where the results of a decision are uncertain [see second row of Table 1]. If the values of the outcomes are the same, the alternative with the highest probability of occurrence should be chosen. When there is uncertainty and the values of outcomes are complex, then a mechanism must be employed that evaluates the value of an outcome modified by the probability of actually receiving that outcome. Typically, the probability of occurrence of an outcome is multiplied by the value of that outcome, providing a weighted value, the "expected value." Many medical decisions take this form, and this type of decision forms the subject of this article. In keeping with expected value decision making, individuals should choose alternatives that maximize expected value and utility.

Table 1: **Characteristics of a decision**

	Outcomes are simple	Outcomes are complex
Results of alternatives are known with certainty	Certain/ Simple	Certain/ Complex
Results of alternatives are uncertain	Uncertain/ Simple	Uncertain/ Complex

Expected utility decision making

"von Neumann–Morgenstern utility theory, first postulated in the 1940s, continues to be the dominant normative paradigm for decision making under uncertainty" [4]. These rules form the basis of medical decision analysis as it is typically used today. Each plausible outcome in a decision is given a value (its utility). The value assigned to each outcome is weighted by the probability that it will occur if the alternative is chosen (its expected utility). Complex and conditional probabilities are handled with simple arithmetic, producing a simple method for making the best decision in the face of uncertainty.

Medical decision analysis uses these principles. The decision to be analyzed is modeled, often as a tree structure. Other, more complex forms of modeling are possible and widely used for medical decision analysis but are not well represented in the reconstructive literature. Probabilities of outcomes occurring are estimated by referencing data in the literature or by recruiting expert opinion. Values may be assigned to outcomes by numerous mechanisms that are reviewed later in this discussion.

Utility

Utility is the term assigned to the strength of the preference a decision maker or individual has for an outcome. Preference for a state of health is called a *value* when the preference is expressed without uncertainty and is called a utility when the preference is expressed under conditions of uncertainty [4]. In addition, a health state that is more highly preferred has been traditionally accepted as providing an individual with a higher health-related quality of life than do health states that are less highly preferred. Utility is a measurement of the strength of preference for a particular state of health and has been recognized and widely used to compare states of health and their associated values across broad interventions and medical conditions. As a common measure of the value of a state of health, utility is often used as the measure of effectiveness in cost-effectiveness analysis [5,6]. Such an analysis has been given a distinctive name: "cost-utility analysis."

Measurement of utility

Three common methods are used to measure an individual's strength of preference for health states [7]. The visual analogue scale (VAS) is an easily administered method to rate the value of a health state. The values 0 and 1 are anchored at each end of a straight line whose length in known (typically 10 cm). Raters mark on a straight line where their preference for a given health state lies.

The time trade-off (TTO) is a technique in which raters are asked how many future years of life in their current state of health they would give up in exchange for instantaneously receiving perfect health. The value an individual assigns to the health state is estimated by the proportion of life the individual is not willing to sacrifice in the exchange.

The VAS and TTO are not measured with probabilities, so these methods result in a value score for a state of health. The standard gamble (SG) asks raters to choose between maintaining their current state of health (the state to be measured) and some alternative with probabilities of obtaining perfect health or death. The probabilities are methodically changed until the individual is indifferent between the two choices. The probability of perfect health that makes the individual indifferent between the two choices is estimated as the individual's utility for the health state being measured. The SG is the only one of the three methods that results in utilities in the true sense of the word. In clinical research, the SG is usually combined with one of the other measurement methods to elicit utilities. Unfortunately, the three methods are not yet interchangeable: the VAS yields a lower score than the TTO, which is lower than the SG [7].

Utility function

A utility function is the relationship between the utility for an attribute and the quantity of the attribute present [8]. For example, as a disease becomes more severe (the attribute), the utility or preference for that attribute will likely decrease. It appears reasonable that the utility of a disease would correlate with disease severity. This result has been shown in several diseases, and we have shown it to be the case in carpal tunnel syndrome (CTS) [9,10].

Multi-attribute utility theory

A utility should encompass all important aspects of a health state (eg, morbidities, mortality, costs). This process of assigning utilities is complicated for many complex health states because a patient or surrogate may not be able to incorporate all the relevant aspects of the health state. An emerging method of representing the complexity of a group of related health states is to define attributes of the health state and then combine those attributes using multi-attribute utility theory (MAUT) [4,8]. Using MAUT, raters can focus on each important attribute of a complex health state and provide a rating through the combination of attributes.

In the simplest case, the utilities assigned for all the attributes will add up to form a multi-attribute utility score. However, one attribute may influence the rating of others. More complicated methodologic and mathematical methods of combining the scores of attributes have been published and are widely used [8].

MAUT has been used extensively in health care measurement in fields other than hand surgery. The Health Utilities Index has been developed in several versions using the principles of MAUT [4,11]. Preferences for problems of the prostate [12], periodontal health [13], and laboratory testing [14] are examples where MAUT has been used to combine attributes to create a utility measure for health states.

Despite the important role of utility measurement in health care research, there has been a paucity of literature focused on measuring utilities in upper-extremity disorders and reconstructive problems. In a previous study using the TTO, the authors measured the utility of amputation of the hand at 0.93, which could be viewed as establishing the lower limit for all hand problems [15]. The authors have measured the utility for CTS as 0.97 in patients using the SG. The utilities for postoperative states following carpal tunnel release were measured by Chung and colleagues [16] using a rating scale and a sample of health care practitioners. The score for open carpal tunnel release without complications was 0.798. This score is lower than the authors' measurements of CTS with the SG and, more interestingly, lower than that of amputation of the hand using the TTO. This finding illustrates the need for further research to evaluate the comparability and interchangeability of methods for assessing utilities from patients and surrogates.

Quality-adjusted life years

Quality-adjusted life years (QALYs) is a measurement that combines both the length of life and the quality of life in a health state [5–7]. Typically, each year of life is multiplied by the quality (utility) of that year. QALYs are often used in decision analysis because they incorporate quantity and quality of life in a single measure. The benefits of a treatment can be measured as the number of QALYs gained. In economic evaluations that help frame medical guidelines, the results are often reported as the cost per QALY gained.

Decision analysis

Decision analysis is an explicit process of analyzing the potential alternatives of a decision and determining which alternative is optimal in the face of uncertainty [7]. The first step in a formal decision analysis is to model the decision to be made, including all the plausible choices (alternatives); the modeling technique usually employed is a decision tree. The likelihood that an uncertain event will occur is estimated by its probability. Probabilities can be obtained from the literature, estimated, or measured. The utilities for each outcome may be assigned by the decision maker, collected from the literature, or measured by utility measurement techniques. The tree is then analyzed by a process called folding back, in which the utility of each outcome is multiplied by the probability of its occurrence. These values are added across subtrees for each branch. The alternative with the highest expected value is the optimal decision and should be supported by the decision maker. To evaluate the robustness of the optimal decision—that is, the degree to which the preferred decision does not change with variation in probability or utility estimates—each baseline utility and probability can be systematically changed in a process called sensitivity analysis. The tree is reanalyzed on an iterative basis to determine whether the recommended decision remains optimal when any baseline probabilities or utilities singly or in combination are changed within a plausible range of clinical possibility.

The authors performed a simple decision analysis to evaluate the decision whether to perform hand transplantation [15]. The clinical decision was modeled as a decision tree [Fig. 1].

If the decision is made not to have surgery, the patient is left with an amputation. Because there is no uncertainty, the expected value of this decision is the utility of an amputation. The authors mea-

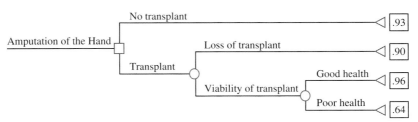

Fig. 1. Decision tree modeling the decision for transplantation of the hand. (*Modified from* McCabe S, Rodocker G, Julliard K, et al. Using decision analysis to aid in the introduction of upper-extremity transplantation. Transplant Proc 1998;30(6):2784; with permission.)

sured the utility of an amputation in a group of surrogate patients using the TTO technique at 0.93. The possible subsequent events for this example if transplantation is chosen are depicted in the tree. The hand could survive or be lost because of rejection. If the hand survives, the patient could become ill owing to the immunosuppressant medication or could stay healthy.

In addition to measuring the utility of an amputation of a single hand, the authors measured the utility of a transplanted hand and the ill state in a group of undergraduates by means of the TTO technique. Probabilities were estimated for the base case analysis. The authors initially estimated the probability of survival of the hand at 0.5 (50%) and the probability of good health if the hand survived at 0.8. To analyze the tree, the expected utility of each branch is calculated. The expected utility of the "no transplant" branch is 0.93. This is a probability of 1.0 multiplied by 0.93, the utility of an amputation. To calculate the expected utility of the "transplant branch," the authors first calculated the expected utility of the "success branch" and added it to the expected utility of the "loss branch." To calculate the expected utility of the "success branch," the product of 0.96 multiplied by 0.8 and the product of 0.64 multiplied by 0.2 are added. This sum is the expected utility of the "success branch." It is multiplied by 0.5, the probability of success, and added to the expected utility of the "loss branch" (the product of 0.5 multiplied by 0.9). Thus the expected value for transplantation is estimated at 0.90, whereas the expected value of the "no transplantation" branch is estimated at 0.93. In this example, no transplantation is recommended. More importantly, through sensitivity analysis, it was found that the decision is sensitive to the utility assigned to the ill state of health on immunosuppression. This result interested the authors, who had hypothesized before analysis that the decision would hinge on the probability and utility assigned to loss of the transplanted hand.

The decision to operate for ski-pole injury of the ulnar collateral ligament (UCL) of the thumb illustrates several points. In ski-pole injury to the UCL of the thumb, the presence of a Stener lesion is thought to reduce the probability of strong healing in the absence of ligament repair [17]. Surgery can be used to repair the ligament. If no Stener lesion is present, then splinting alone without surgery is thought to be an effective treatment. If a Stener lesion is common, then surgery may be preferred for all patients with a complete ligament injury, even when there is uncertainty about the presence of a Stener lesion in an individual. However, if the Stener lesion is rare, then surgery will not add

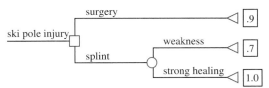

Fig. 2. Hypothetical decision tree modeling the decision to perform surgery or to splint a UCL injury. The utility of strong healing with splint wear is rated at 1.0, the utility of surgery at 0.9, and the utility of failed splinting at 0.7. For the base case, the probability of a Stener lesion's resulting in weak healing was estimated at 0.3. The expected value (EV) of surgery is the product of 0.9 and 1.0, which is 0.9. The EV of splinting is the product of the probability of strong healing in a splint (0.7) and the utility of splinting with strong healing (1.0) added to the product of the probability of weak healing (0.3) and the utility of weak healing (0.7). EV (surgery) = 1.0 × 0.9 = 0.9. EV (splint) = (0.7 × 1.0) + (0.3 × 0.7) = 0.91. In the base case the splinting alternative has the highest EV.

benefit for most patients but could add morbidity, supporting splinting as the preferred treatment for all. Currently many surgeons advocate surgery for all patients with a complete UCL injury on the basis of the probability of a Stener lesion. If there were a good diagnostic test, perhaps MRI, patients with a proven Stener lesion could be directed to surgery and those without a lesion could be treated without surgery. The value of a test depends on the qualities and morbidity of the test. A more sophisticated analysis may include costs as well.

A simple tree for complete UCL injuries is illustrated in **Fig. 2**. The decision model includes surgical and nonsurgical treatment. A potential third branch in the tree would be a diagnostic test, but this is omitted for simplicity. If the thumb is splinted, the probability of a good result is related to the probability of a Stener lesion. If the patient has surgery, the probability of a good result is high, although the patient has been exposed to some morbidity and the surgical risk. If a test can accurately direct patients with a Stener lesion to surgery and those without a lesion to splinting, it will reduce the risk of unneeded surgery and assure most patients a good result. The probabilities and utilities are hypothetical but illustrate how the calculations for expected value are performed.

Fig. 3 shows a hypothetical tree analyzing the decision to replant amputated digits. If revision amputation is performed, the expected value is the utility of the amputated state. If replantation is attempted and fails, the utility will be lower because of the morbidity of the surgical intervention. If the replantation is successful, the utility should be higher. The utilities and probabilities

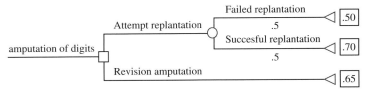

Fig. 3. Hypothetical decision tree modeling the decision to replant digits or revise the amputations. The utility of successful replantation is 0.7, failed replantation, 0.5, and revision amputation, 0.65. The probability of success is arbitrarily set at 0.5. Expected value (EV) (revision amputation) = 1.0 × 0.65 = 0.65. EV (attempted replantation) = (0.5 × 0.5) + (0.5 × 0.7) = 0.6. In the base case the decision to revise the amputation has the highest EV.

have been arbitrarily set in this example to yield a higher expected value for revision amputation.

Risk attitudes

A lottery or gamble with a 50/50 chance of winning $100 or $0 has the same expected value as a sure gift of $50. When given a choice to receive a sum of money or choose a "risky" alternative that may give them more or less money with the same overall expected value, most people will take the "sure thing." Even though the expected value of both alternatives is the same, most people will choose the sure thing in this kind of lottery involving money, a phenomenon that is called risk aversion. In other words, people will choose a sure thing over a gamble with the same expected utility. Fig. 4 shows this characteristic. The oblique line is the expected value of the lottery. The curved line above reveals that the decision maker requires a higher value than the expected value to choose the lottery. This concept of risk aversion shows that people do not always make decisions in keeping with the well-formulated logic of expected value decision making.

Problems with expected utility decision making

Expected utility decision making is grounded in firm rules or axioms. These rules suggest how people should make decisions to maximize their ability to get the highest expected value in the long run. Interestingly, it has been shown that there are circumstances where people break these rules on a regular basis.

Certainty effect

A well-known violation of the expected utility theory of decision making is known as Allais' paradox. Individuals will violate the tenets of expected utility theory when one of the alternatives of the decision occurs with certainty. The following examples are used by Kahneman and Tversky [18] to illustrate this point. If an individual is given the choice between alternatives A and B shown in Box 1, expected utility theory predicts that rational individuals would choose alternative A (with an expected utility of $2442). In Allais' experiments, 82% of individuals choose alternative B. The underlying principle behind this observation is known as the certainty effect, in which individuals violate expected utility theory by choosing alternatives that give a certain gain even when they mathematically have lower expected utilities.

Mirror effect

In the Allais' paradox already shown, all outcomes are gains. When a similar lottery is created with outcomes as losses, once again individuals fail to follow expected utility theory. Nearly 92% of individuals will choose the alternative A shown in Box 2, demonstrating that people will take a gamble to avoid a sure loss even when the expected value of the gamble is less (ie, they lose more).

This trend is known as the mirror effect, in which individuals are risk seeking when faced with a decision involving losses and are risk averse when faced with a decision involving gains.

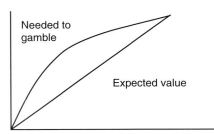

Fig. 4. A person will typically require a higher reward than the expected value to gamble.

Box 1: Certainty effect

Choose between the two alternatives, A or B, below:

Alternative A

    Receive $2500 with a probability of 66%
    Receive $2400 with a probability of 33%
    Receive $0 with a probability of 1%

Alternative B

    Receive $2400 for certain

Low probabilities

A second common violation of expected utility theory involves alternatives that have low probabilities of occurrence. Evidence suggests that, when alternatives have a low probability of occurrence, individuals will overweight the low probability [18].

Prospect theory

People are known not to make decisions in complete agreement with expected value decision making. After studying how people actually make choices between simple monetary gambles, Kahneman and Tversky [19] introduced prospect theory as a descriptive theory of how people actually make decisions. By contrast, methods such as the standard gamble and decision analysis are based on expected utility theory and may not accurately represent the way people make decisions.

In expected utility theory, the value of an outcome is weighted by the probability that it will be achieved. Prospect theory suggests that the decision maker considers the weighted value of the outcome but also considers whether the outcome represents a gain or a loss when compared with the status quo [18,19]. Decision makers are believed to be risk averse in the direction of gains and risk seeking in the direction of losses. Hence the decision maker will choose a sure gain as opposed to an alternative gamble even when the expected value of the gamble is higher. Alternatively, the decision maker will gamble to avoid a sure loss even when the gamble has a lower expected value.

Moreover, close to the reference point or status quo, a small change in health status will have a greater difference in value compared with changes of the same magnitude at some distance from the reference point.

To explain their findings, Kahneman and Tversky suggested that we have an S-shaped value function [Fig. 5] that is risk averse in the realm of reward and risk seeking in the realm of loss. In addition, they noted that the curve is steeper for a loss than for a reward. Finally, they proposed a weighting function for probabilities that suggests that people overweight low probabilities and underweight others.

Treadwell and Lenert [20] have explored how prospect theory may be applied to understanding medical decisions, observing that phenomena in health and medicine are consistent with this theory.

If we revisit the decision tree for UCL repair of the thumb [see **Fig. 2**], we may conclude that, although surgery typically has more morbidity than splinting, surgery should result in repair and strong healing of the ligament. For the sake of illustration, we can consider surgery as a "sure thing," whereas splinting would be viewed as a "risky choice." Because the patient is injured and we are planning to improve the situation, we are deciding on management in the realm of a gain. According to prospect theory, the decision maker may choose surgery over splinting even if splinting results in a higher expected value.

As an example of the influence of prospect theory when considering a loss, consider the decision tree for replantation of the fingers [see **Fig. 3**]. The tree has been simplified and hypothetically constructed so that revision amputation has a lower expected value. In this decision, revision amputation of the digits is a "sure thing" and can be construed as a loss. Replantation is a "risky" alternative that may have a lower expected value. Nonetheless, many patients strongly desire replantation even when it is not advised by the surgeon, violating expected utility theory. Although this result may be related to altered body image or to other mechanisms, in this example patient decision making is consistent with prospect theory. That is, individuals will gamble to avoid a sure loss, even when the uncertain alternative has a lower expected value.

An interesting phenomenon may occur when decision makers have differing perspectives on whether a potential outcome is a loss or a gain. The surgeon may consider transplantation of the

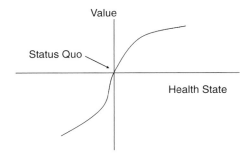

Fig. 5. This S-shaped value function shows that for gains people will be risk averse and for losses they may be risk seeking. More value is perceived for small gains or losses close to the status quo. The curve is steeper for losses than for gains.

hand as a gain for the patient and be risk averse, whereas the patient may consider the decision not to transplant as a sure loss and be willing to attempt the risky alternative [21].

It is important to consider prospect theory when undertaking decision analysis. The standard gamble, the advocated method of measuring utilities, and the use of decision modeling methods for medical decision analysis are based on expected value decision making. The impact of this apparent discrepancy between the theoretic problems suggested by prospect theory and our basic methods in decision analysis is still uncertain.

Regret theory

In expected value decision making, the value of each possible outcome is weighted by the probability that alternative will occur. The alternative with the highest expected value is chosen. In prospect theory, the weighted value and the direction of the alternative as a loss or gain are important. Each of these two methods assigns values to each possible outcome independent of other possible outcomes. In regret theory, the value of an outcome depends not only on the strength of the decision maker's preference for that outcome but also on which other outcomes are possible and how desirable they are [22]. The outcomes are compared, and each is assigned a regret factor or rejoicing factor depending on its relationship to other outcomes. A patient might be satisfied with a stiff finger if the alternative is amputation but will not be satisfied with the same degree of stiffness if the alternative is a normal finger. To achieve this comparison, the expected value of an alternative is weighted by a regret factor. Revisiting the decision tree for UCL injury, we see that a patient who has splinting with resulting ligamentous laxity might regret not having had surgery. The regret-weighted expected value of the splint branch could then be lower than the surgery branch. In the replantation tree, the regret-weighted expected value could be lower for amputation if the patient regrets not trying to have the digits replanted. If the regret balances across branches, the decision defaults to expected value decision making. Interestingly, the regret-weighted expected values change the expected values in a similar manner to prospect theory.

Summary

Understanding the way patients actually make decisions may improve the quality of the practice of medicine. Using the principles described here to understand how decisions are made creates an avenue for further study and holds the promise of improving patient satisfaction and health-related quality of life.

References

[1] Kahneman D, Slovic P, Tversky A. Judgement under uncertainty: heuristics and biases. New York: Cambridge University Press; 1982.

[2] Torrance GW. Utility approach to measuring health-related quality of life. J Chron Dis 1987; 40(6):593–600.

[3] Guyatt GH. A taxonomy of health status instruments. J Rheumatol 1995;22:1188–90.

[4] Torrance GW, Furlong W, Feeny DH, et al. Multi-attribute preference functions: Health Utilities Index. Pharmacoeconomics 1995;7:503–20.

[5] Gold MR, Siegel JE, Russell LB, et al. Cost-effectiveness in health and medicine. New York: Oxford University Press; 1996.

[6] Drummond MF, O'Brien B, Stoddart GL, et al. Methods for the economic evaluation of health care programmes. 2nd edition. New York: Oxford University Press; 2003.

[7] Hunink M, Glasziou P. Decision making in health and medicine. Cambridge (UK): Cambridge University Press; 2001.

[8] Keeney RL, Raiffa H. Decisions with multiple objectives: preferences and value tradeoffs. New York: Cambridge University Press; 1993.

[9] Ness RM, Holmes AM, Klein R, et al. Utility valuations for outcome states of colorectal cancer. Am J Gastroenterol 1999;94(6):1650–7.

[10] Tengs TO, Lin TH. A meta-analysis of utility estimates for HIV/AIDS. Med Decis Making 2002; 22:475–81.

[11] Torrance GW, Feeny DH, Furlong W, et al. Multi-attribute utility function for a comprehensive health status classification system. Health Utilities Index mark 2. Med Care 1996;34:702–22.

[12] Chapman GB, Elstein AS, Kuzel TM. A multi-attribute model of prostate cancer patients' preferences for health states. Qual Life Res 1999;8:171–80.

[13] Bellamy CA, Brickley MR, McAndrew R. Measurement of patient-derived utility values for periodontal health using a multi-attribute scale. J Clin Periodont 1996;23:805–9.

[14] MacPherson DW, McQueen R. Cryptoporidiosis: multiattribute evaluation of six diagnostic methods. J Clin Microbiol 1993;31(2):198–202.

[15] McCabe S, Rodocker G, Julliard K, et al. Using decision analysis to aid in the introduction of upper-extremity transplantation. Transplant Proc 1998;30(6):2783–6.

[16] Chung KC, Walters MR, Greenfield ML, et al. Endoscopic versus open carpal tunnel release: a cost-effectiveness analysis. Plast Reconstr Surg 1998;102(4):1089–99.

[17] Miller RJ. Dislocations and fracture dislocations of the metacarpophalangeal joint of the thumb. Hand Clin 1988;4(1):45–65.

[18] Kahneman D, Tversky A. Choices, values,

and frames. New York: Cambridge University Press; 2000.

[19] Kahneman D, Tversky A. Prospect theory: an analysis of decision under risk. Econometrica 1979;47(2):263–91.

[20] Treadwell JR, Lenert LA. Health values and prospect theory. Med Decis Making 1999;19: 344–52.

[21] Edgell SE, McCabe SJ, Breidenbach WC, et al. Different reference frames can lead to different hand transplantation decisions by patients and physicians. J Hand Surg 2001;26A(2):196–200.

[22] Loomes G, Sugden R. Regret theory: an alternative theory of rational choice under certainty. The Economic Journal 1982;92:805–24.

ELSEVIER
SAUNDERS

CLINICS IN
PLASTIC
SURGERY

Clin Plastic Surg 32 (2005) 463–470

Perspectives on Hand Transplantation

W.P. Andrew Lee, MD*, Vu T. Nguyen, MD

- Early clinical experience with composite tissue transplantation
- The modern era of hand transplantation
- Clinical assessment and functional outcomes
- Chronic rejection
- Tolerance induction
- Summary
- References

The hand, more than any other organ, embodies the human figure and acts as an extension of the human mind. Through its intricate mechanisms, our interaction with other individuals and the world around us is made possible. The loss of such a unique instrument is often viewed as catastrophic and is considered by many as second only to the loss of life itself. Therefore, the replacement of a lost limb or hand not only achieves a functional role but also acts to complete an individual.

Until recently, amputation of the upper extremity was addressed by replantation of the severed limb in the best of situations. However, such procedures are often impossible owing to a multitude of factors. Patients are then relegated to the use of prosthetics, which tend to be lacking in form or function and violate Sir Harold Gillies' reconstructive dictum of replacing "like with like." To address these issues, surgeons have long sought to "borrow" or transplant functioning organs, typically harvested from cadaveric sources. As early as the fourth century AD, the sainted brothers Cosmos and Damian were reported to have replaced the ailing limb of a parishioner with that of a recently deceased Moor [1]. Other attempts were undoubtedly made through the ages, apocryphal or not, including that of Gaspare Tagliacozzi, who in the

sixteenth century transplanted a flap of tissue from the forearm of a slave to reconstruct the nose of a nobleman, in exchange for the slave's freedom [2]. These and other attempts were likely doomed to failure without refined surgical techniques and modern immunosuppression regimens.

Early clinical experience with composite tissue transplantation

The first documented hand transplant was performed in Guayaquil, Ecuador in 1963, just before the modern era of calcineurin inhibitor-based therapy [3,4]. With immunosuppression consisting of azathioprine and corticosteroids, the hand only survived for 3 weeks. The subsequent discovery and introduction of cyclosporine A in the early 1980s ushered in a new era in both solid organ and composite tissue transplantation. In contrast to the homogeneity of the former, composite tissue allografts (CTAs) consist of any combination of a number of diverse tissues, such as bone, muscle/tendon, nerve, vessels, subcutaneous tissues, and skin.

Transplantation of a vascularized digital flexor tendon system was performed in two individuals in 1988 and 1989 by a French team led by Guimberteau [5]. Immunosuppression consisted of

Division of Plastic Surgery, University of Pittsburgh School of Medicine, 3550 Terrace Street, Scaife Hall, Suite 690, Pittsburgh, PA 15261, USA
* Corresponding author.
E-mail address: zimmerjm@upmc.edu (W.P.A. Lee).

doi:10.1016/j.cps.2005.05.005

6 months of cyclosporine, after which the authors documented improved function with a lack of rejection at 1 year. Subsequent CTAs, beginning in 1994, included three femoral diaphyses and five entire knee joint allografts by Hofmann and Kirschner [6] in Germany and culminated in the transplantation of a major histocompatibility complex–matched vascularized larynx allograft in 1998 by Strome [7]. Despite aggressive immunosuppression, consisting of cyclosporine, azathioprine, antithymocyte globulin, and methylprednisolone, all but two of the femur and knee allografts were lost at 2 years [8,9]. The laryngeal transplant, however, fared differently. The donor allograft, including five tracheal rings along with the thyroid and parathyroid glands, was anastomosed via bilateral superior thyroid arteries with multiple venous outflows. Both the superior laryngeal and the right recurrent nerve were connected to their respective recipient nerves. Induction therapy with a combination of anti-CD3 monoclonal antibodies (OKT3), cyclosporine, methylprednisolone, and mycophenolate mofetil (MMF) preceded maintenance immunosuppression with tacrolimus, MMF, and tapering doses of prednisone. Postoperatively, a rejection episode occurred at 15 months that was amenable to steroid therapy. Additional complications included transient hypertension, periodic tracheobronchitis, and *Pneumocystis carinii* pneumonia. A 40-month follow-up revealed the patient to have normal voice characteristics, active deglutition without evidence of aspiration, and a functional thyroid gland [10]. The patient, unemployed before the transplant, now functions as a motivational speaker. Although the case was complicated, the functional achievement of this individual gave credence to the notion that CTAs had become a clinical reality.

The modern era of hand transplantation

These clinical events, combined with data accumulated from various preclinical animal experiments, set the stage for the first hand transplant of the modern era. On September 23, 1998, an international group of surgeons in Lyon, France transplanted the right hand of a 41-year-old cadaveric donor onto that of a 48-year-old man [11]. This was followed by the first United States hand transplant, performed in Louisville, Kentucky in January of 1999 [12]. From 1998 to 2003, a total of 24 hand transplants in 18 patients (including six bilateral transplants) have been performed [Table 1]. The most recent transplant was a bilateral hand transplant performed in April 2003 in Lyon. The experience has been worldwide, with countries in Asia (China, Malaysia), Europe (France, Italy, Austria, Belgium), and North America (United States) taking part [Fig. 1].

The impetus for these events rested initially in the surgeons' confidence that limb transplantation

Table 1: Hand transplants performed			
Date	**Surgical team**		**Follow-up**
1998			
September	Lyon (France)	Unilateral	Removed at 28 mo
1999			
January	Louisville (USA)	Unilateral	
September	Guangzhou (China)	Unilateral	Removed at 20 mo
September	Guangzhou (China)	Unilateral	
2000			
January	Lyon (France)	Bilateral	
January	Guangxi (China)	Unilateral	
January	Guangxi (China)	Unilateral	
March	Innsbruck (Austria)	Bilateral	
May	Kuala-Lumpur (Malaysia)	Unilateral	
September	Guangzhou (China)	Bilateral	
October	Monza (Italy)	Unilateral	
2001			
January	Harbin (China)	Bilateral	
February	Louisville (USA)	Unilateral	
October	Monza (Italy)	Unilateral	
2002			
June	Brussels (Belgium)	Unilateral	
November	Milan (Italy)	Unilateral	
2003			
February	Innsbruck (Austria)	Bilateral	
April	Lyon (France)	Bilateral	

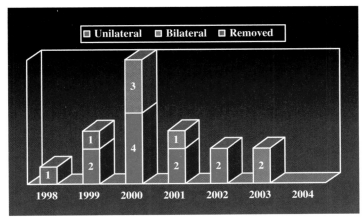

Fig. 1. The number of hand transplants performed per year since the first case in 1998. As of this writing, no hand transplants have been performed since the spring of 2003 to the author's knowledge.

could technically be performed. The replantation of digits and hands has occurred successfully since the replantations of an amputated arm by Malt in 1962 and of a distal radius/wrist amputation by Meredith in 1965 [13]. However, what was uncertain at the time and remains controversial today is whether we *should* be involved in the large-scale practice of human hand transplantation [14].

In the case of the first United States transplant, the Louisville group proceeded with human trials following their swine experiment with limb transplantation [15]. Of the nine recipients of a limb allograft, four died early of complications directly related to the immunosuppressive protocol. The remaining five animals achieved a rejection-free period of only 90 days, at the cost of complications that included pneumonia, septic arthritis, foot abscesses, diarrhea, and weight loss. An international symposium on composite tissue allotransplantation was convened in Louisville in 1997 [14]. Although some participants suggested caution in future hand transplants, proponents believed that "the time [was] ripe to proceed with the first human cadaveric hand transplantation" [14,16,17]. One argument for proceeding was that all tissue elements of a hand had been previously transplanted in humans, with each component exhibiting survival for several years [5,18–21]. Additionally, functional data comparing hand replantation versus prostheses favored the use of the former [22]. Some surmised that the function following allotransplantation would be of a similar caliber and therefore superior to prostheses.

Clinical assessment and functional outcomes

The immunosuppressive protocol for many of these patients consists of a synergistic regimen of drugs based on data extrapolated from preclinical CTAs and human solid organ transplants, particularly cadaveric renal transplants. Most of the human hand recipients have been treated with a combination of tacrolimus (FK506), MMF, and prednisolone, with several protocols adding various poly- and monoclonal antibodies during the induction phase [23]. Additional measures to combat rejection have included the use of donor irradiation, human leukocyte antigen (HLA) matching, and the removal of donor bone marrow [24].

Preliminary results have shown maintenance of allograft survival in the majority of patients. Of the 24 transplanted hands, two have undergone removal. The initial failure was the first hand transplant in Lyon, in which the patient underwent multiple episodes of acute rejection, treated each time with increased doses of both systemic and topical immunosuppression [24]. The patient was subsequently noncompliant with his postsurgical rehabilitation and immunosuppressive regimen, resulting in overall graft failure and amputation at 28 months. The second allograft removal occurred in a unilateral hand transplant performed in 1999 in Guangzhou, China. Circumstances surrounding the event are unpublished. However, in the author's interviews, the graft loss was attributed to subcutaneous injections of corticosteroids for irreversible hand erythema, which led to apparent arterial thrombosis and severe ischemic pain. Amputation of the limb was performed at 20 months. Overall, although 22 of 24 transplanted hands remain viable, the most recently published reports show that almost all patients have undergone one or more episodes of acute rejection following transplantation.

The combined French and Italian experience, consisting of eight transplants (four unilateral and two bilateral) in six patients, shows that skin rejection occurred at a mean period of 40 days postoperatively (range 25 to 76 days) [23]. Additional complications have included transient hyperglycemia and hypertension, cytomegalovirus (CMV) replication, *Clostridium* infection, anemia, and intermittent creatinine elevations. Excluding the two most recent patients, who were in the early postoperative period, all patients exhibited protective sensation in all fingers, with improved discriminative sensation beginning at approximately 18 months. Motor recovery was labeled "good" as assessed by activities of daily living (ADL). Excluding the latest two transplants, all patients have returned to work, including one patient who was previously unemployed.

Individual case reports of the bilateral transplant recipients in Lyon and Innsbruck showed similar results [25,26]. Both have undergone one or more episodes of acute rejection, again treated by bolus of increased immunosuppression. Postoperative complications included serum sickness and transient hyperglycemia in the French patient and CMV replication in the Austrian. However, the Austrian procedure was associated with surgical complications, including allograft skin necrosis and multiple arteriovenous fistulas necessitating surgical ligation. Functional results indicate protective sensation in all digits of both recipients, with electromyographic evidence of innervation of intrinsic musculature in both hands. Motor recovery in the French recipient indicates a mean total active range of motion (ROM) of fingers of 163° on the right and 158° on the left hand (out of a possible 265°); similar results were seen in the Austrian patient, who documented an average active ROM of 60.1% in both hands. This ROM reportedly translates into the ability to perform several ADLs, including holding small objects, such as a pen, eating with common utensils, drinking from a cup, and routine self-hygiene. Furthermore, both bilateral recipients have returned to work, and the Austrian recipient has resumed his hobby of motorbiking.

Similar to their European counterparts, the United States hand transplant recipients have experienced repeated episodes of acute rejection, treated with local and systemic increases in immunosuppression [27]. Additional complications included CMV infection, requiring long-term ganciclovir therapy, and recurrent *Tinea* fungal infections [12]. At 1 year, both recipients reported pain, temperature, and pressure sensation. Semmes-Weinstein monofilament testing exhibited scores ranging from 3.22 in the thumb to 3.61 in the index, middle, and ring fingers (diminished light touch) and 3.84 in the small finger (diminished protective sensation) in the first Louisville patient at 3 years. Car-

roll testing performed in these patients helps us to assess objectively the overall functional outcome following transplantation [22]. The maximum score, derived from objective ratings of 33 different tasks integrating mobility, motor function, and sensation, is 99, with "excellent" being greater than 84, "good" 74 to 84, "fair" between 51 and 74, and "poor" less than 51. Results have been published for the two Louisville recipients, in addition to early reports of the first two Guangzhou patients [27]. At 3 years, the first Louisville patient scored 65; the second Louisville recipient scored only 50 at 1 year. At only 7 months, the two Chinese recipients exhibited scores of 65 and 75, respectively. These scores are in comparison to published values of 51 for prosthetic limbs and 70 for distal replants.

More recent data from the Chinese have been lacking. Early reports indicated an improved outcome, with no reports of acute rejection during the first 8 months and improved Carroll testing early on [24]. Suggested reasons for this improvement include the use of higher doses of prednisone during the induction period and for maintenance therapy, the removal of bone marrow from the cavities of the donor radius and ulna, irradiation of one of the grafts, and, most importantly, the use of HLA-matching. Both of the initial transplants performed in Guangzhou were matched for three out of six HLA. As described earlier, one of these two recipients has required removal of the allograft.

Of additional clinical interest is the finding of cortical reintegration in the brain following transplantation. Following any sensory deprivation, cortical reorganization occurs. In the case of upper extremity amputation, cortical activation lateralizes toward the face locus, which is consistent with the finding that face stimulation induces symptoms of phantom hand in amputees. Six months following transplantation, functional magnetic resonance imaging scans exhibited progressive sensorimotor activation occupying the medial hand homunculus, indicating the reversible nature of cortical reorganization [28].

The senior author was given the opportunity by the American Society for Surgery of the Hand to independently assess the majority of hand transplant patients. From February to September 2003, 11 hand transplant recipients were evaluated at six transplant centers in Louisville, Guangzhou, Brussels, Lyon, Milan, and Innsbruck. The patients and transplant surgeons were interviewed, and the transplanted hands were evaluated in a standardized fashion. Mean active ROM was found to be +40/33° at the wrist and 174° in total finger flexion, with 35° of extension lag. Pulp to distal palmar crease distance ranged from 1.0 to 7.0 cm and averaged 3.7 cm. Intrinsic muscle recovery was generally poor, with only two patients exhibiting thumb palmar abduction and opposition against gravity. All but one patient reported protective sensation, and 6 out of 10 patients were able accurately to localize digits on touch. However, two-point discrimination was 12 to 15 mm in two patients and greater than 15 mm in all others. Nine of ten patients with transplants for more than 1 year have returned to work. Recent complications have included osteomyelitis of ulna requiring removal of the fixation plate before bony union, development of sustained diabetes requiring insulin treatment, and bilateral avascular necrosis of the hips. Most unilateral recipients cited enhanced self-image and hand function as the benefits of hand transplants, whereas the bilateral recipients cited self-reliance and ability to "feel" their world again [**Figs. 2 and 3**].

Chronic rejection

Although it has not yet been encountered clinically, a potentially critical complication of hand transplants is chronic allograft rejection. The pathogenesis of this phenomenon is not clearly known but appears to reflect a multifactoral causation. Chronic rejection is evidenced by the onset of vascular lesions showing intimal thickening and smooth muscle cell proliferation, culminating in the replacement of functional tissues with interstitial fibrosis, extracellular matrix deposition, and vascular neointimal hyperplasia [29]. Current hypotheses include the induction of B cells to produce alloantibodies and the activation of endothelial and smooth muscle cells by T-helper cell 2 (Th2) cytokines and growth factors. It should be noted that several of the current immunosuppressants, namely the calcineurin inhibitors, facilitate a Th2 type response. Others, including MMF, are capable of down-regulating the clonal expansion of B cells and the production of antibodies [30]. What is known is the impact chronic rejection has on current solid organ transplants, representing the most common cause of allograft loss among surviving patients. Greater than 50% of renal allografts succumb to chronic rejection 7 to 8 years following transplantation [31]. Additionally, the risks of chronic rejection appear to be directly related to acute rejection episodes, with increasing risk associated with increasing number of acute episodes and episodes occurring later (ie, more than 8 weeks after transplantation) [32]. Most reports indicate multiple episodes of acute rejection in the hand transplant recipients, in combination with late rejection episodes. Additionally, while solid organ transplants are known to harbor a substantial functional reserve, so that a significant amount of tissue may be compromised before loss of organ function, CTAs, and particularly that of the hand with its specialized neuromuscular interactions, may not be as resilient to tissue loss. With the longest surviving hand transplant just

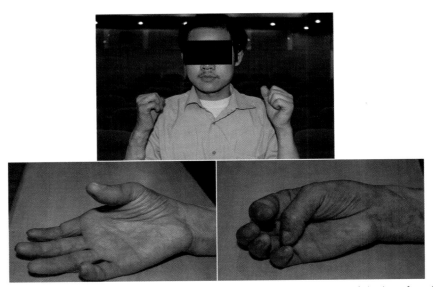

Fig. 2. One of the Chinese hand transplant patients, at 30 years of age, has had one of the best functional returns with convincing recovery of intrinsic muscle function. He uses his transplanted right hand to hold chopsticks and play mah-jong. He is able to unbutton, but not able to button his shirts. (Photographs taken by the authors in 2003).

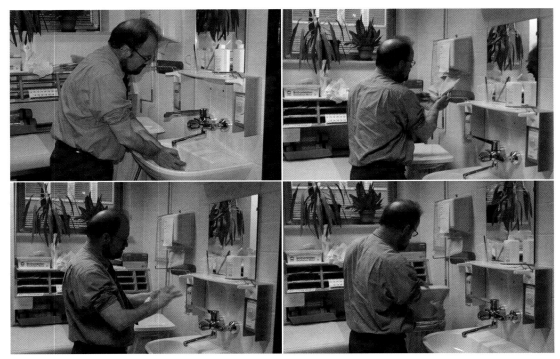

Fig. 3. One of the Austrian bilateral hand transplant patients, at 49 years of age, experienced profound work capacity improvement as a police dispatch person after the transplants. He is able to write, dress, and attend to personal hygiene. He has many hobbies, including riding a motorcycle on long-distance trips. (Photographs taken by the authors in 2003).

passing its sixth anniversary, the issue of chronic rejection deserves close monitoring.

Tolerance induction

As in all fields of transplantation, the attempt to reduce the inherent risk of the procedure has led many to focus on the concept of tolerance. Simply stated, tolerance is the ability to perceive what was originally deemed foreign (ie, an allograft) instead as part of oneself. Ideally, this would be "donor-specific" tolerance, in which an immune system could be directed to achieve tolerance toward a specific donor but maintain immunologic competency toward the spectrum of other foreign antigens.

Although examples exist of tolerance induction within the clinical arena, methods of achieving tolerance remain primarily experimental [33,34]. These methods include both central or thymic routes of deletion and peripheral routes. Centrally, complete elimination of all T-cell clones capable of alloantigen recognition is termed clonal deletion and focuses on the elimination of developing T cells within the thymus by means of the induction of full or mixed chimerism. Past methods have included toxic whole-body and lymphoid irradiation, in combination with hematopoietic stem cell

transfer, in an attempt to achieve full chimerism. More recent techniques have used reduced myelo-ablative conditioning to achieve a state of mixed chimerism, in essence a mutual sharing of the hematopoietic space between donor and recipient [35]. In rat and swine models of limb transplantation, for example, the authors' laboratory has achieved allograft survival without long-term immunosuppression by donor marrow infusion into prenatal or adult recipients, creating "chimeras" that possess both cell types [36–38].

Peripheral mechanisms for tolerance induction focus on the removal or modification of effector lymphocytes by means of veto cells and activation-induced cell death or on the induction of various regulatory cells and the use of costimulatory blockade. It has long been recognized that a particular subset of T cell inherently contains suppressive functions within the immune system [39]. Additionally, the character of the T-cell interaction via the T-cell receptor has been shown to cause deviation of the subsequent immune response, with blockade of key costimulatory signals inducing a state of suppression or anergy.

Regardless of the method used for tolerance induction, a key element is the capability to pretreat the recipient for immune modification yet to occur. In future hand transplants, the time constraints on using cadaveric sources of tissue may prohibit extensive preconditioning. Nevertheless, the induction of tolerance offers the best potential for obviating systemic immunosuppression with its concomitant adverse effects, while minimizing the likelihood of chronic rejection for future hand transplants.

Summary

The early experience of hand transplantation has yielded a mixture of successes and failures. No life-threatening adverse effects have been encountered from immunosuppression, yet additional medications were required in some cases with unknown long-term efficacy or side effects. Limited functional returns have been observed, but any effect of chronic rejection is too early to determine. Although the experience has confirmed the benefits of hand transplantation to patients and their families, the future of hand transplantation on a wide scale is dependent on further research to alter its risk-benefit balance.

References

[1] Kahan BD. Cosmos and Damian revisited. Transplant Proc 1983;15:2211–6.

[2] Gnudi M. The life and times of Gaspare Tagliacozzi. Los Angeles (CA): Zeitlin and Ver Brugge; 1976.

[3] Gilbert R. Transplant is successful with a cadaver forearm. Med Trib Med News 1964;5:20.

[4] Gilbert R. Hand transplanted from cadaver is reamputated. Med Trib Med News 1964;5:23.

[5] Guimberteau JC, Baudet J, Panconi B, et al. Human allotransplant of a digital flexor system vascularized on the ulnar pedicle: a preliminary report and 1-year follow-up of two cases. Plast Reconstr Surg 1992;89:1135–47.

[6] Hofmann GO, Kirschner MH, Wagner FD, et al. Allogeneic vascularized grafting of a human knee joint with postoperative immunosuppression. Arch Orthop Trauma Surg 1997;116:125–8.

[7] Strome M. Human laryngeal transplantation: considerations and implications. Microsurgery 2000;20:372–4.

[8] Kirschner MH, Brauns L, Gonschorek O, et al. Vascularized knee joint transplantation in man: the first two years' experience. Eur J Surg 2000; 166(4):320–7.

[9] Hofmann GO, Kirschner MH. Clinical experience in allogeneic vascularized bone and joint allografting. Microsurgery 2000;20:375–83.

[10] Strome M, Stein J, Esclamado R, et al. Laryngeal transplantation and 40-month follow-up. N Engl J Med 2001;344(22):1676–9.

[11] Dubernard JM, Owen E, Herzberg G, et al. Human hand allograft: report on first 6 months. Lancet 1999;353(9161):1315–20.

[12] Jones JW, Gruber SA, Barker JH, et al. Successful hand transplantation. One-year follow-up. Louisville Hand Transplant Team. N Engl J Med 2000;343(7):468–73.

[13] Meredith JH, Koman LA. Replantation of completely amputated distal forearm—1965. J South Orthop Assoc 1999;8(3):214–7.

[14] Siegler M. Ethical issues in innovative surgery: should we attempt a cadaveric hand transplantation in a human subject? Transplant Proc 1998; 30(6):2779–82.

[15] Jones Jr JW, Ustuner ET, Zdichavsky M, et al. Long-term survival of an extremity composite tissue allograft with FK506-mycophenolate mofetil therapy. Surgery 1999;126(2):384–8.

[16] Llull R. An open proposal for clinical composite tissue allotransplantation. Transplant Proc 1998; 30(6):2692–6. [discussion: 2697–703].

[17] Hewitt CW. Update and outline of the experimental problems facing clinical composite tissue transplantation. Transplant Proc 1998;30(6): 2704–7.

[18] Wendt JR, Ulich TR, Ruzics EP, et al. Indefinite survival of human skin allografts in patients with long-term immunosuppression. Ann Plast Surg 1994;32:411–7.

[19] Jones TR, Humphrey PA, Brennan DC. Transplantation of vascularized allogeneic skeletal muscle for scalp reconstruction in a renal transplant patient. Transplant Proc 1998;30:2746–53.

[20] Bain JR. Peripheral nerve and neuromuscular allotransplantation: current status. Microsurgery 2000;20:384–8.

[21] Hofmann GO, Kirschner MH, Wagner FD, et al. Allogeneic vascularized transplantation of human femoral diaphyses and total knee joints—first clinical experiences. Transplant Proc 1998; 30:2754–61.

[22] Graham B, Adkins P, Tsai TM, et al. Major replantation versus revision amputation and prosthetic fitting in the upper extremity: a late functional outcomes study. J Hand Surg [Am] 1998;23A:783–91.

[23] Lanzetta M, Petruzzo P, Vitale G, et al. Human hand transplantation: what have we learned? Transplant Proc 2004;36(3):664–8.

[24] Francois CG, Breidenbach WC, Maldonado C, et al. Hand transplantation: comparisons and observations of the first four clinical cases. Microsurgery 2000;20(8):360–71.

[25] Dubernard JM, Petruzzo P, Lanzetta M, et al. Functional results of the first human double-hand transplantation. Ann Surg 2003;238(1):128–36.

[26] Margreiter R, Brandacher G, Ninkovic M, et al. A double-hand transplant can be worth the effort! Transplantation 2002;74(1):85–90.

[27] Breidenbach III WC, Tobin II GR, Gorantla VS, et al. A position statement in support of hand transplantation. J Hand Surg [Am] 2002;27(5): 760–70.

[28] Shirwan H. Chronic allograft rejection. Do the Th2 cells preferentially induced by direct alloantigen recognition play a dominant role? Transplantation 1999;68:715–26.

[29] Giraux P, Sirigu A, Schneider F, et al. Cortical reorganization in motor cortex after graft of both hands. Nat Neurosci 2001;4(7):691–2.

[30] Meier-Kriesche H, Ojo AO, Arndorfer JA, et al. Mycophenolate mofetil decreases the risk of chronic renal allograft failure. Transplant Proc 2001;33:1005–6.

[31] Brenner MJ, Tung TH, Jensen JN, et al. The spectrum of complications of immunosuppression: is the time right for hand transplantation? J Bone Joint Surg Am 2002;84A(10):1861–70.

[32] Tejani A, Sullivan EK. The impact of acute rejection on chronic rejection: a report of the North American Pediatric Renal Transplant Cooperative Study. Pediatr Transplant 2000;4:107–11.

[33] Mazariegos GV, Reyes J, Marino IR, et al. Weaning of immunosuppression in liver transplant recipients. Transplantation 1997;63(2):243–9.

[34] Spitzer TR, Delmonico F, Tolkoff-Rubin N, et al. Combined histocompatibility leukocyte antigen-matched donor bone marrow and renal transplantation for multiple myeloma with end stage renal disease: the induction of allograft tolerance through mixed lymphohematopoietic chimerism. Transplantation 1999;68(4):480–4.

[35] Sachs DH. Mixed chimerism as an approach to transplantation tolerance. Clin Immunol 2000; 95:S63.

[36] Lee WPA, Butler PEM, Randolph MA, et al. Donor modification leads to prolonged survival of limb allografts. Plast Reconstr Surg 2001;108: 1235–41.

[37] Mathes DW, Randolph MA, Butler PEM, et al. Intravascular in utero injection of adult bone marrow leads to acceptance of fully mismatched composite tissue allografts. Surg Forum 2001; LII:529–31.

[38] Hettiaratchy S, Melendy E, Randolph MA, et al. Tolerance to composite tissue allografts across a major histocompatibility barrier in miniature swine. Transplantation 2004;77:514–21.

[39] Gershon RK, Kondo K. Cell interactions in the induction of tolerance. Immunology 1970;18: 723–37.

ELSEVIER
SAUNDERS

CLINICS IN
PLASTIC
SURGERY

Clin Plastic Surg 32 (2005) 471–483

Functional Evaluation in Children with Congenital Upper Extremity Malformations

Emily S. Ho, MEd, OT[a],
Howard M. Clarke, MD, PhD, FRCS(C), FACS, FAAP[b],*

- ■ Evaluation of existing outcome studies
  Level of evidence
  Literature review
- ■ Definition of hand function
- ■ Level of evidence
- ■ Measurement of function
  Essential components of functional hand assessment
  Measuring hand function

- ■ Developmental considerations
- ■ Future directions
- ■ References

Achieving optimal upper limb function is a priority in the management of children with congenital hand malformations [1–3]. Professionals need to be well equipped to help families understand the best surgical and rehabilitative options available for their child. Many parents come to the clinic with hopes that interventions will be provided to normalize the appearance of the hand. However, in some cases the best recommendation may be to abstain from any surgical intervention. One of the challenges, then, is to balance the family's need for cosmesis with concerns about jeopardizing optimal function. Lister [3] accurately summarizes this challenge when he identifies the need for professionals to assist families in viewing function as beauty, regardless of the limb differences that cannot be changed. Our ability as professionals clearly to define and evaluate the child's

optimal function will assist in achieving this balance. Objective outcome measures are essential to evidence-based practice. This article examines the existing literature to evaluate critically functional outcome studies of children with congenital upper extremity malformations and to address the challenges of defining and measuring functional outcome in this patient population.

Evaluation of existing outcome studies

Thumb hypoplasia and radial dysplasia are the most frequently seen congenital hand conditions requiring functional evaluations at the Hospital for Sick Children in Toronto, Canada. Functional evaluations provide valuable information to assist the plastic surgeon and occupational therapist in making recommendations for reconstructive sur-

[a] Department of Rehabilitation Services, The Hospital for Sick Children, University of Toronto, 555 University Avenue, Toronto, Ontario M5G 1X8, Canada
[b] Department of Surgery, The Hospital for Sick Children, University of Toronto, 555 University Avenue, Toronto, Ontario M5G 1X8, Canada
* Corresponding author. Division of Plastic Surgery, The Hospital for Sick Children, 555 University Avenue, 1524, Toronto, Ontario, Canada M5G 1X8.
E-mail address: howard.clarke@utoronto.ca (H.M. Clarke).

doi:10.1016/j.cps.2005.05.006

gery or therapy. Therefore, these two conditions were chosen as a comparative sample in evaluating functional outcome of children with congenital upper extremity malformations.

Level of evidence

Evidence-based practice demands that clinicians move beyond clinical experience and physiologic principles to evaluate the consequences of their clinical actions in a rigorous manner [4]. Critical evaluation of existing outcome studies of pollicization and centralization surgery in children with congenital thumb hypoplasia and radial aplasia is required to determine the effectiveness of this intervention. A systematic review of the literature was conducted using MEDLINE (1966–June 2003), CINAHL (1982–June 2003), and reference lists from secondary resources [5]. All literature pertaining to the functional outcome of patients with congenital malformations who had either pollicization or centralization surgery was eligible. Seven studies of children with index–thumb pollicization and three studies of children with centralization surgery were reviewed. The studies in this review were analyzed according to the levels of evidence for primary research introduced in the *Journal of Bone and Joint Surgery* [Box 1] [6].

Literature review

The review of the literature indicated inadequate rigor in research design and measurement of functional outcome. All 10 studies were conducted retrospectively, and the collection of preoperative data was lacking or varied in standardization. Of the 10 studies reviewed, only one study used a control group, thereby achieving a level 3 ranking. The remainder of the studies were ranked at level 4. Some of the studies in the latter group compared the performance of subgroups within the sample. Four of the ten studies reviewed had preoperative data available for comparison [7–10]. Three studies compared the outcomes of patients who had pollicization surgery with isolated thumb hypoplasia with those of patients who had associated conditions, such as radial dysplasia [11–13]. Two studies evaluated the impact of age at surgery on functional outcome [7,8]. Normative data, such as age-matched grip and pinch strength and sensation, were used by three studies [9,11,13]. Two studies compared the performance of patients on standardized upper extremity assessments (eg, Jebsen Taylor) with that of their peers [9,13].

The parameter and tools used to define function varied among the studies reviewed. The common measures of hand function used across studies were range of motion (ROM), prehension, pinch strength, and grip strength. Sensibility was included in six of the studies [7,8,11,12,14,15]. Semmes Weinstein monofilaments (Sammons Preston Roylan, Bolingbrook, Illinois and Connecticut Bioinstruments Inc., Danbury, Connecticut) and two-point discrimination were a common method used to assess sensation. Evaluation of cosmesis was reported in 6 of the 10 studies [7–11,14]. Most studies relied on parental report of satisfaction with the postoperative appearance of the child's limb. Goldfarb and colleagues [9] rated cosmesis and pain more objectively with a visual analogue scale. Activities of daily living (ADL) and performance of the hand during a task were measured in six of the studies [9–13,16]. Goldfarb and colleagues [9] was the only study that used a standardized assessment to evaluate this area. The evaluation of activity in the other studies was based on simple observational tasks or parental report.

Box 1: Levels of evidence for primary research questions

Therapeutic studies—investigating the results of treatment

Level 1

> Randomized controlled trial
> Systematic review[1] of Level 1 randomized controlled trials

Level 2

> Prospective cohort study
> Poor-quality randomized controlled trial (eg, <80% follow-up)
> Systematic review[1] of Level 2 studies or nonhomogeneous Level 1 studies

Level 3

> Case-control study[2]
> Retrospective cohort study[3]
> Systematic review

Level 4

> Case series (no or historical control group)

Level 5

> Expert opinion

[1] A study of results from two or more previous studies
[2] Patients with a particular outcome were compared with those who did not have the outcome.
[3] The study was initiated after treatment was performed.
From Wright JG, Swiontkowski MF, Heckman JD. Introducing levels of evidence to the journal. J Bone Joint Surg Am 2003;85A(1):2; with permission.

The review of the literature demonstrates (1) paucity of studies, (2) lack of consensus on the definition of function, (3) inadequate level of evidence in the present literature, and (4) inadequate tools to measure functional outcome in children with congenital hand malformations. Validation of surgical and therapeutic interventions in this population demands rigor in our research and clinical practice. Achieving these standards in our practice first requires a redefinition of functional outcome. Clinicians and researchers working with this population of children need to be unified with a clear and comprehensive definition of hand function. Moreover, professionals need to be intentional in evaluating their surgical and therapeutic interventions with rigorous research.

Definition of hand function

The term functional assessment has been used widely in literature pertaining to hand surgery and rehabilitation, but there is no consensus on what this term means [17]. The challenge of evaluating function in the child with upper extremity malformation is that the assessment needs to be specific enough to capture detailed individual differences in anatomy, movement, and prehension but also broad enough to capture the patient's day-to-day use of his or her hand.

The International Classification of Functioning, Disability, and Health (ICF) [18] provides useful terminology to define function. The ICF adopts a biopsychosocial model to capture the complexity of disability that involves appreciation of both the medical and social aspects of the individual and society [18]. The ICF model in **Fig. 1** synthesizes the idea of disability as interplay between features of the person and society. According to this model, functioning is classified as all body functions, activities, and participation. The formal definitions of these components of ICF are as follows: *Body functions* are physiologic functions of body systems, including psychologic function. *Activity* is the execution of a task or action by an individual. *Participation* is involvement in a life situation [**Fig. 2**] [18]. Disability is classified in these three domains as impairment, activity limitation, and participation restriction, respectively. Children with congenital hand malformations can experience disability at one or more of these levels. Impairments include alterations in musculoskeletal composition, joint ROM, muscle strength, and sensation. The presence of such impairment may lead to activity limitations. For example, a child with poor grasp may have difficulty with handwriting or manipulation of fasteners on clothing. Participation restrictions are more likely to occur when policy and infrastructure at the community or societal level pose barriers to the individual. A child with an upper limb malformation may require special instruction to learn to swim. When facilities or teachers are not available, a participation restriction results. The ICF model also recognizes that disability is defined within the parameters of personal factors (eg, gender, age, coping styles, social background) and environmental factors (eg, social attitudes, legal and social structures, climate, geography) [18].

The literature indicates that clinicians commonly use body functions, such as grip and pinch strength, ROM, sensation, cosmesis, and prehension, as the parameters to measure function. Measures of body functions are recognized as reliable baseline measures for clinical and research purposes to evaluate and monitor hand function

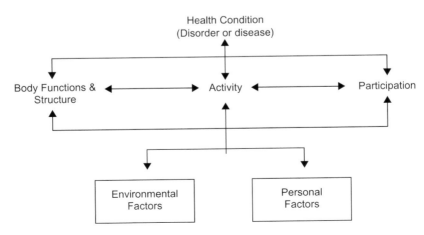

Fig. 1. ICF biopsychosocial model of disability. (*From* World Health Organization. International classification of functioning, disability, and health. Geneva [Switzerland]: World Health Organization; 2001; with permission.)

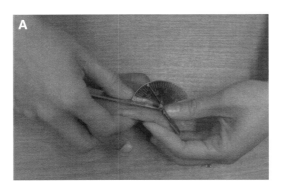
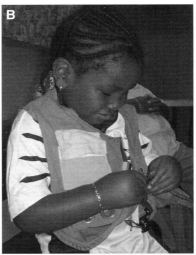
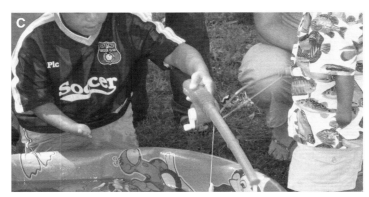

Fig. 2. Examples of measures of body functions, activity, and participation. (*A*) Body functions: evaluation of joint ROM, measured with goniometer. (*B*) Activity: evaluation of ADL skills, such as dressing. (*C*) Participation: evaluation of child performing an activity, such as playing fishing, with consideration of performance in the child's environment (ie, summer camp) with available resources.

[9,10]. For example, it is essential for therapists to document passive ROM of wrist deviation in a child with radial ray anomaly to evaluate stretching and splinting programs employed in preparation for centralization surgery. The benefits of this type of baseline measurement are obvious. The value of activity and participation measures is less apparent. Measures of activity and participation evaluate how the child uses his or her hand during a task. This information can assist the surgeon and therapist in identifying the need for surgery or for remediative and adaptive intervention. For example, an evaluation of body functions in a school-age child with a Blauth classification type 2 unilateral hypoplastic thumb may indicate a decreased ROM in first web space, below age-average pinch and grip strength, and decreased quality of pincer grasp. Pad-to-pad superior pincer grasp is not achieved, but an inferior pincer is attained. The evaluation of body function alone may suggest indications for surgical reconstruction to improve stability in the joint and deepening of the first web space to improve ROM and strength. However, an evaluation of activity and participation may reveal that this child has adequate strength and mobility in his or her thumb to perform daily activities. The child's first web space is sufficient to hold a cup and plastic containers of varying diameters. The child and family also report no difficulties in functioning, such as manipulating fasteners, printing, cutting, and participating in leisure activities. This information may change one's recommendations for surgery and could not be determined without an evaluation of activity and participation.

Measures of activity and participation are a necessary component of assessments of hand function. An assessment that only incorporates measures of body functions, such as ROM, strength, sensation, and prehension, is not a true reflection of the child's function in daily activities. Goldfarb and colleagues [9] allude to this dilemma in their discussion of the lack of correlation between measures of activity (ie, Jebsen-Taylor and Disabilities of the Arm, Shoulder, and Hand [DASH]) and those of body function (ie, forearm length, angulation of wrist, grip and pinch strength) in their study. Were the DASH and Jebsen-Taylor not sensitive enough to detect functional differences? Or were the body functions evaluated not a good measure of functioning? Limitations in body functions, whether physical or psychologic, do not define an individual's ability to function or describe his or her hand function repertoire [17].

A comprehensive definition of hand function requires an approach that evaluates body functions, activity, and participation. This approach recognizes the many facets of functioning. It recognizes that two children with the same congenital upper extremity malformation may present with differing hand function because of potential individual differences at the physiologic and psychologic levels, as well as differences in family or community environment. Uniform use of this definition of upper extremity function will improve the validity of clinical and research outcome measures of function in this population.

Level of evidence

Randomized control trials (RCT) represent the highest level of evidence in research [6]. However, there are many challenges in conducting RCT in a surgical population. McLeod and colleagues [19] report conditions and difficulties that limit the feasibility of RCT, including time, expense, ethical considerations, generalizability, rarity, and course of disease. Despite these challenges, researchers plan to examine alternatives that may be less rigorous than RCT but more rigorous than uncontrolled case series [19]. Ideally, postoperative functional outcome of children with congenital upper extremity malformations should be compared with a control group. This method raises the level of evidence and, more specifically, enhances the internal validity of the study [20]. However, the ethical implications of withholding potentially beneficial surgical procedures from patients are obvious. Parents are most likely to opt for reconstructive procedures if the option is presented [9]. Therefore, the next option is to strengthen research methods in design and measurement within each level of evidence. This option would improve the reliability and validity of the results reported. Comparison between subgroups in the sample, such as a contrast between the performance of children with isolated thumb hypoplasia and those with asso-

ciated conditions, should be used if a control group is unavailable. This method does not raise the level of evidence but increases the clinical usefulness of the research. Another method of comparison is the use of normative data available in literature or standardized assessments.

The rigor of functional outcome studies can also be improved with a prospective approach to research. All 10 studies reviewed were characterized by the evaluation of the group of patients after the surgery was performed. A retrospective approach can be attractive to clinicians because of the availability of data. However, interpretation and application of information from such studies must be viewed within the constraints of the data [20]. The researcher cannot control operational definitions of variables or the reliability of the data collected [20]. Furthermore, preoperative data are seldom available. Pre- and postoperative comparison increases the validity of the reported outcomes of the study [20].

Measurement of function

The validity and reliability of the tools used in both research and clinical settings are vital to the quality of outcomes reported [20]. Validity is the extent to which a tool measures what it is intended to measure [20]. Tools used to measure upper extremity function should reflect the children's ability to use their upper extremities in daily activities in their own environment. This assessment should encompass all the parameters of upper extremity function, including measures of body function, activity, and participation. Reliability is the degree to which a tool will yield similar results on repeated administration [20]. Professionals using these tools need to be confident that the change that is measured is indicative of true change in the child and not of inconsistency in the administration or development of the tool.

Essential components of functional hand assessment

Determining the essential components of an upper extremity functional evaluation is important to establish validity. The components used in the literature to measure upper extremity function are classified by the ICF model in the second column of Table 1. With the exception of pain, timed activity, and ADL, these items have also been identified by Skerik and colleagues [21] as necessary elements of a functional hand assessment in this population. In this review, hand size was also identified as essential. However, it was not used by any

Table 1: Essential components of hand function

ICF classification	Components used in literature	Essential components
Body function	Grip and pinch strength ROM Sensation Cosmesis Pain Static prehension: fine and gross grasp	Grip and pinch strength ROM Sensation Cosmesis Static prehension: fine and gross grasp
Activity	Dynamic prehension Bimanual activity Hand function during timed activity ADL	Dynamic prehension Bimanual activity ADL School Leisure
Participation	ADL	ADL School Leisure

of the 10 studies evaluated in the review. Next, the essential components of upper extremity function were determined by the frequency of use in the literature. The breadth of components of upper extremity function was determined by the defining framework of the ICF model. Column three of Table 1 is a list of essential components of upper extremity function. Evaluation of pain and timed activity were excluded from the essential list. Evaluation of pain was only used in one study with adults post–centralization surgery [9]. It is not a common issue in this population of children and was thus excluded. A timed-activity test was used in two studies to provide information regarding the performance of children postpollicization [9,13]. Timed-activity tests can be useful in determining qualitative hand performance during a task in comparison with a normative population. Although this information is valuable, it is not essential to determining whether a child requires further surgical or therapeutic intervention. For example, a poor score on the Jebsen Taylor timed-activity test may not translate to a child's requiring more time to manipulate buttons. A specific evaluation of ADL would be more important in identifying this qualitative difference in hand function. Furthermore, performance on timed activities in children is influenced by age and other developmental factors and must be normed on a general population for comparison.

Measuring hand function

Determining a consistent and reproducible means of measuring the components of function is essential for establishing reliability. The purpose of measurement is to attain a mechanism for achieving a degree of precision in describing a physical or behavioral characteristic according to its quantity, degree, capacity, or quality [20]. This process involves assigning a numerical value to variables to represent quantities of characteristics according to a certain rule [20].

Grip and pinch strength

Measures of grip and pinch strength are essential to documenting baseline strength for pre- and postoperative comparison, as well as for routine evaluations to investigate whether underlying muscle weakness is affecting optimal performance of daily activities. Grip and pinch strength should be quantified with standardized, commercially available equipment. Normative values are available for the hydraulic hand dynamometer and the Jamar Dynamometer (Sammons Preston Roylan, Bolingbrook, Illinois) to compare the children's performance to their peers [22,23]. Evaluations of pad-to-pad pincer and lateral pinch are necessary to evaluate the strength of thumb opposition [Fig. 3]. Depending on the child's hand anomaly, a tripod pinch may be included in the evaluation. Normative values for children aged 6 to 19 years are available [24].

Range of motion

Precise numerical documentation of active and passive ROM of involved joints in the upper extremity is essential. At the time of initial assessment, a detailed documentation of active and passive ROM is important regardless of whether surgical or therapeutic interventions will be initiated. Changes in ROM may also result from growth and development or injury. Routine ROM measurements are essential to evaluating the effectiveness of stretching, splinting, and therapy programs, as well as postoperative changes.

Sensation

Sensation was evaluated in 6 of the 10 studies reviewed and hence was included in the list

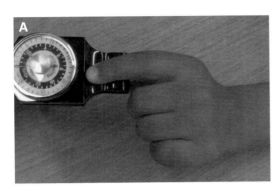
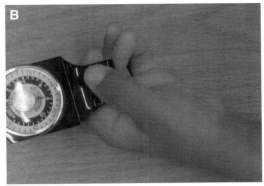
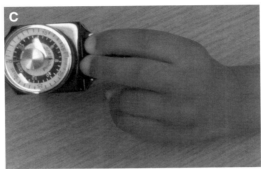

Fig. 3. Pinch strength. (*A*) Pad-to-pad pincer, (*B*) lateral pinch, (*C*) tripod pinch.

of essential components. The Semmes Weinstein monofilaments and two-point discrimination were used to test tactile sensation. However, it is generally recognized that children with congenital upper limb malformation have normal sensation [1]. Sensory evaluations are not necessary for routine assessments but may be used for pre- and postoperative baselines. Two-point discrimination is a reliable test for children older than 6 years [25].

Cosmesis

Psychosocial adjustment is an important aspect of function. Children with more attractive perceived physical appearance have lower depressive and anxious symptoms and higher general self-esteem [26]. Rubenfeld and colleagues [27] also found that a child's social support domains (ie, parent, teacher, close friend, and classmate) were significant predictors of self-esteem, whereas demographic variables and degree of limb loss were not. Attempts should be made to quantify evaluations of cosmesis routinely as well as pre- and postoperatively. Anecdotal evaluations may provide interesting information but are useless for evaluative purposes. It is important to measure both the parent's and child's view of the limb, because discrepancies may occur. Goldfarb and colleagues [9] used a visual analogue scale with adults to measure cosmesis. A similar approach can be successfully used with children, using graphics as visual indicators of their satisfaction with cosmesis.

Prehension

Prehension is the most important component of an upper extremity functional evaluation. It is the pattern of use of the hand during grasp. Routine observations of the child's prehension pattern are essential to determining the potential for reconstructive surgery and fine motor development. Prehension may be classified into two categories: static and dynamic prehension. Static prehension is defined as the basic acquisition of fine and gross grasp prehension patterns. Dynamic prehension is defined as the pattern of use during fine motor activity. Measurement in the first category focuses on how the quality of the child's prehension compares with developmentally appropriate prehension. Weiss and Flatt [28] made evaluations of static prehension, including hook grip, power grip, lateral pinch, tip pinch, and palmar pinch. Each task is objectively measured on a two-point Likehart scale: 0 = patient cannot grasp object; 1 = patient completes grasp in manner of his own adaptation; 2 = patient completes grasp in prescribed manner. This scale is helpful to compare the child's performance with the normal repertoire of grasps available to the general population.

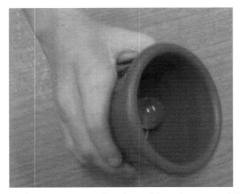

Fig. 4. Gross grasp: evaluation of hand span and first web space.

Is this a fair comparison? Children with congenital upper extremity malformations have altered musculoskeletal composition and may never attain normal prehension patterns. What is essential in an evaluation of static prehension are two basic components: gross and fine grasp. Gross grasp is defined as the maximum diameter of an object that a child can carry [**Fig. 4**]. Essentially, this measures a child's hand span and may be an indicator for reconstructive surgery, such as increasing the first web space. Fine grasp is an evaluation of the child's prehension that requires precision, such

as picking up a small peg or penny. The quality of fine grasp should be classified as pad-to-pad pincer grasp, lateral pinch, or interdigital grasp [**Fig. 5**]. The priority in reconstructing opposition between thumb and fingers is a pad-to-pad superior pincer grasp. If this is not attainable because of limitations on the thumb's mobility, a lateral pinch is a useful pinch to obtain [1]. A child who uses an interdigital grasp may benefit from reconstructive surgery to create opposition. Distinguishing between these three qualitative differences in a child's fine grasp will help determine potential reconstructive options. Descriptive evaluation of basic gross and fine grasp is sufficient in describing static prehension. Measures of dynamic prehension address whether the repertoire of the child's prehension is sufficient to perform daily activities.

Dynamic prehension

Observations of preferred patterns of hand use during a task are essential [28]. Standardized developmental tests that measure hand skills while engaged in a task have been developed. Examples of such tests are the Peabody Developmental Motor Scales–Fine Motor Scales and the Bruininks-Oseretsky Test of Motor Proficiency [29,30]. These tests look at a child's ability to engage in developmentally appropriate fine motor tasks, but they

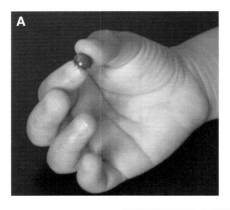

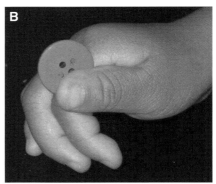

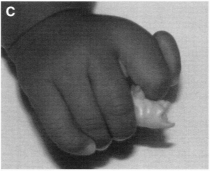

Fig. 5. Fine grasp. (*A*) Pad-to-pad superior pincer grasp, (*B*) inferior pincer grasp/lateral pinch, (*C*) interdigital pinch.

do not account well for children with differences in musculoskeletal composition of the hand. For example, a 4-year-old child with radial dysplasia may score poorly on the grasp subtest of the Peabody because of the inability to hold a pencil with a mature tripod grasp. This result is misleading, because this child may never attain a tripod grasp but still acquire a functional grasp for handwriting. The score of this test does not assist the clinician in making a conclusion regarding this child's grasp function. It may actually mislead the inexperienced clinician.

Dynamic prehension needs to be graded according to the quality of movement in reach, grasp, release, and manipulation of an object. Children should be evaluated by their ability to complete the task as well as the quality of positioning and movement of the limb. The ability to complete a task may be compared with age-expected performances. The movement pattern used to complete the task should not. The child in **Fig. 6** is demonstrating dynamic prehension. She is able to complete the task of reaching for an object, placing it in the container, and closing the lid. The pattern of use is a radial approach in reaching and grasp-

ing, with opposition of thumb against fingers. Precise voluntary release of the object into the container is observed. Manipulation skills are not demonstrated here.

Bimanual prehension

Observation of bimanual prehension is essential to evaluations of children with unilateral congenital upper extremity malformations. Bimanual tasks require the child to use his or her affected hand for activity to determine whether reconstructive surgery or adaptive strategies can be used to enhance function in the assisting hand. Bimanual evaluation is also useful in children with unilateral impairments, such as a forearm level transverse arrest, to evaluate the need for adaptive devices and techniques to enhance function. Bimanual prehension should be evaluated routinely, as well as pre- and postoperatively.

Activities of daily life, school, and leisure

All the activities that children perform in their daily living can be classified as self care, school, and leisure [31]. ADL include self-care tasks such as dressing, feeding, grooming, bathing, and toilet-

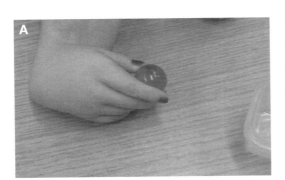
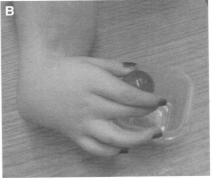
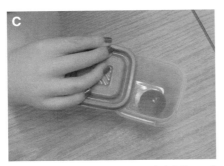
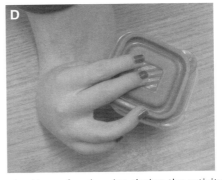

Fig. 6. Dynamic prehension observation of child's preferred pattern of prehension during the activity of placing an object into a container and closing the lid. (*A*) Radial approach to grasp with opposition of thumb and radial digits. (*B*) Active voluntary release with precision into a container. (*C*) Radial approach to grasp lid with opposition of thumb and digits. (*D*) Completion of task with adequate precision and strength.

ing. School activities include handwriting, scissor skills, and computer skills. Leisure activities include sports, music, and other pastimes. Measures of ADL and school and leisure activities outside the context of the child's social and personal environment are classified as activity measures. Participation measures consider the child's performance in these areas in context. Several studies use their own questionnaires or observation tools to capture activity and participation after reconstructive surgery [10,11,16]. Goldfarb and colleagues [9] used the DASH to evaluate function of adults who had centralization surgery for radial dysplasia as children. No studies have used a standardized assessment of global function for children with congenital hand malformations. Lack of awareness of the existence of appropriate scales or inadequacy of

existing scales may be reasons for the infrequency of use [32].

The essential components of an evaluation of ADL, school, and leisure are measures that provide both quantitative and qualitative assessment. First, a structured questionnaire that measures the child's level of difficulty of performance in ADL, school, and leisure activities is required to determine the child's activity limitation. Responses on the questionnaire should be quantified using an ordinal scale as a method of documenting change in level of difficulty. Collaboration between the professional, parent, and child is essential to completing such a questionnaire. Haley and colleagues [33] emphasize the need to rely on parental report of the child's function to gain an accurate assessment. Parents can provide information about

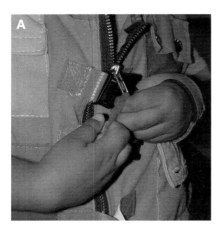
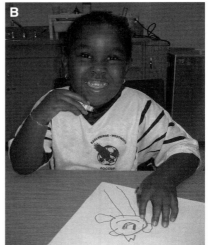
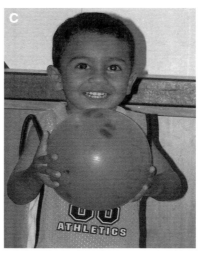

Fig. 7. Examples of ADL, school, and leisure skills that can be directly observed in clinic setting. (*A*) Zippering, (*B*) handwriting, (*C*) ball skills.

how the child functions in a variety of social and physical contexts, thereby increasing the reliability of the assessment. This assistance is helpful because it is often difficult to get a child to report on or perform ADL in a clinical setting [9]. However, it is important to recognize that parental report of function can be inadvertently skewed by underlying emotional involvement. Clinicians need to be discerning in interpreting reported information. Therefore, direct observation of the child engaged in key activities, such as manipulation of fasteners, printing, cutting, and catching a ball, is important to validate the responses obtained from the questionnaire [Fig. 7].

The measurement of ADL, school, and leisure also requires a qualitative approach to evaluation. It is difficult for a questionnaire to determine what is most important to a particular family and child. For example, the family of a child with Blauth type 4 hypoplastic thumb may not opt for pollicization surgery, even though the child demonstrates activity limitations due to loss of gross grasp and dexterity in his or her hand. Social, cultural, and religious factors may influence a family's decision. Identification of specific goals in leisure activities is another instance where a structured assessment may fail to identify the priorities of a family. A child may be interested in exploring numerous activities. A semistructured interview is necessary to identify the child's and family's specific needs and provide appropriate education, therapeutic remediation, or adaptive aids. The individual differences in this population of children warrant a qualitative component to evaluation of function.

Developmental considerations

All components of function should be evaluated within age-appropriate expectations. Professionals working with children with congenital upper extremity malformations should have an understanding of development. More specifically, expert knowledge of fine motor development is critical to evaluating prehension. Standardized assessments of grasp, release, manipulation, and visual motor integration, such as the Erhardt Developmental Prehension assessment, are useful references for normal development from birth to school age [34].

Future directions

Musculoskeletal evaluation of ROM, strength, and static prehension compose the traditional approach to functional evaluation of children with upper extremity malformations. In that approach, surgical and therapeutic decisions are made solely on the basis of the child's performance on measures of body functions. Clinicians find reassurance in using these measures because they are reliable and numerically based. After all, they are concrete measures of musculoskeletal change. However, this approach to evaluation fails to capture the full essence of function. A comprehensive functional evaluation should reflect the child's ability to perform day-to-day tasks at home, at school, and in the playground. Measures of activity and participation capture these qualitative components of function that measures of body function lack. A model for functional evaluation is illustrated in Fig. 8. Evaluation of function must incorporate the elements of body function, activity, and participation. Step 1 involves determining the child's deficits in the three components of function. If a deficit in body function, activity, or participation is found, step 2 involves determining appropriate surgical or therapeutic options to improve function. This step also includes consideration of the appropriateness of the child's developmental age for surgery. If timing for surgery is optimal and an appropriate intervention is found, step 3 involves the implementation of surgical and therapeutic recommendations.

Before taking this step, it is critically important to consider that implementation generally occurs when the child has demonstrated a deficit in activity or participation, as evaluated in step 1. If the child does not have deficits in either of these areas, surgical and therapeutic interventions are generally not recommended. However, there are occasional exceptions to this rule. These exceptions are represented graphically by the thin dotted arrows leading to step 3. For example, the family of a child with a unilateral symbrachydactyly may not opt for a toe-hand transfer, although the child is a surgical candidate. In this situation, the child has an activity limitation, such as bimanual activity. However, parents may still choose whether they wish to pursue this option, because this child will become efficient at using the unaffected limb and compensatory strategies to function at par with his or her peers. The other exception to this rule occurs when a child has no deficits in activity or participation and surgical intervention is pursued. For example, the family of a child with mild simple incomplete syndactyly of the long and ring fingers may opt for surgical release, although the child's use of the hand is not impaired. The family chooses to pursue treatment to improve cosmesis. Functional evaluation of children with congenital hand malformations is a balance of art and science. This model provides a generalized means of systematic evaluation in this population of children.

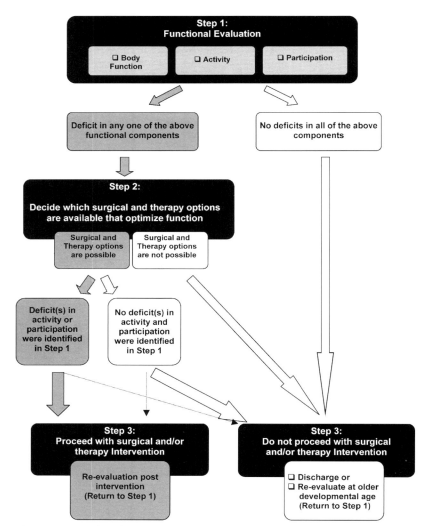

Fig. 8. Functional evaluation decision tree.

However, the uniqueness of each family and child may create exceptions.

Activity and participation play a key role in this approach to functional evaluation, which follows the principle that surgery and therapy are not required if a child does not demonstrate a barrier to his or her ability to engage in daily activities. Clinically, situations may arise where a surgical procedure is available potentially to enhance the child's musculoskeletal presentation. For example, an ilizarov procedure may give greater limb length, or a wedge osteotomy may help straighten the ulna of a child with radial aplasia. If this child demonstrates no difficulties in engaging in age-appropriate ADL and school and leisure activities, what does this child gain? This point is not made to disregard the value of such procedures. However, there are times when such interventions do not

truly offer the child a greater repertoire of functional ability. This approach to evaluation encourages clinicians to remember that an intervention is not always necessary or beneficial. This model of practice requires a paradigm shift toward comprehensive functional evaluations that fully capture the beauty of the child's function in everyday life.

References

[1] Watson S. The principles of management of congenital anomalies of the upper limb. Arch Dis Child 2000;83:10–7.
[2] Gallant GG, Bora FWJ. Congenital deformities of the upper extremity. J Am Acad Orthop Surg 1996;4(3):162–71.
[3] Lister G. Upper extremity. In: Mustarde JC, Jackson IT, editors. Plastic surgery in infancy and

childhood. London: Churchill Livingstone; 1988. p. 581–622.

[4] Oxman AD, Sackett DL, Guyatt GH. User's guide to the medical literature: 1. How to get started. JAMA 1993;270(17):2093–5.

[5] Ho ES, Clarke HM. Upper extremity function in children with congenital hand anomalies. J Hand Ther, in press.

[6] Wright JG, Swiontkowski MF, Heckman JD. Introducing levels of evidence to the journal. J Bone Joint Surg Am 2003;85A(1):1–3.

[7] Sykes PJ, Chandraprakasam T, Percival NJ. Pollicisation of the index finger in congenital anomalies. A retrospective analysis. J Hand Surg [Br] 1991;16(2):144–7.

[8] Manske PR, McCarroll HRJ. Index finger pollicization for a congenitally absent or nonfunctioning thumb. J Hand Surg [Am] 1985;10(5):606–13.

[9] Goldfarb CA, Klepps SJ, Dailey LA, et al. Functional outcome after centralization for radius dysplasia. J Hand Surg [Am] 2002;27(1):118–24.

[10] Lamb DW. Radial club hand. A continuing study of sixty-eight patients with one hundred and seventeen club hands. J Bone Joint Surg Am 1977;59(1):1–13.

[11] Clark DI, Chell J, Davis TR. Pollicisation of the index finger. A 27-year follow-up study. J Bone Joint Surg Br 1998;80(4):631–5.

[12] Kozin SH, Weiss AA, Webber JB, et al. Index finger pollicization for congenital aplasia or hypoplasia of the thumb. J Hand Surg [Am] 1992;17A:880–4.

[13] Manske PR, Rotman MB, Dailey LA. Long-term functional results after pollicization for the congenitally deficient thumb. J Hand Surg [Am] 1992;17(6):1064–72.

[14] Roper BA, Turnbull TJ. Functional assessment after pollicisation. J Hand Surg [Br] 1986;11(3):399–403.

[15] Buck-Gramcko D. Pollicization of the index finger. J Bone Joint Surg Am 1971;53A(8):1605–17.

[16] Bora FWJ, Osterman AL, Kaneda RR, et al. Radial club hand deformity. J Bone Joint Surg Am 1981;63A(5):741–5.

[17] Kimmerle M, Mainwaring L, Borenstein M. The functional repertoire of the hand and its application to assessment. Am J Occup Ther 2003;57(5):489–98.

[18] World Health Organization. International classification of functioning, disability, and health. Geneva (Switzerland): World Health Organization; 2001.

[19] McLeod RS, Wright JG, Solomon MJ, et al. Randomized controlled trials in surgery: issues and problems. Surgery 1996;119(5):483–6.

[20] Portney LG, Watkins MP. Foundations of clinical research: applications to practice. Upper Saddle River (NJ): Prentice-Hall; 2000.

[21] Skerik SK, Weiss MW, Flatt AE. Functional evaluation of congenital hand anomalies. Am J Occup Ther 1971;25(2):98–104.

[22] McCarron LT. McCarron assessment of neuromuscular development, revised edition. Dallas (TX): Common Market Press; 1982.

[23] De Smet L, Vercammen A. Grip strength in children. J Pediatr Orthop 2001;10(4):352–4.

[24] Mathiowetz V, Weimer DM, Federman SM. Grip pinch strength: norms for 6 to 19-year-olds. Am J Occup Ther 1986;40(10):705–11.

[25] Cope EB, Antony JH. Normal values for the two-point discrimination test. Pediatr Neurol 1992;8(4):251–4.

[26] Varni JW, Setoguchi Y. Correlates of perceived physical appearance in children with congenital/acquired limb deficiencies. J Dev Behav Pediatr 1991;12(3):171–6.

[27] Rubenfeld LA, Varni JW, Talbot D, et al. Variables influencing self-esteem in children with congenital or acquired limb deficiences. Journal of the Association of Children's Prosthetic-Orthotic Clinics 1988;23(4):85.

[28] Weiss MW, Flatt AE. Functional evaluation of the congenitally anomalous hand. I. Am J Occup Ther 1971;25(3):139–43.

[29] Folio MR, Fewell RR. Peabody developmental motor scales. Texas: Pro-Ed; 2000.

[30] Bruininks RH. Bruininks-Oseretsky test of motor proficiency. Minnesota: American Guidance Service; 1978.

[31] Canadian Association of Occupational Therapists. Enabling occupation: an occupational therapy perspective. Ottawa (Ontario): CAOT; 1997.

[32] Young NL, Wright JG. Measuring pediatric physical function. J Pediatr Orthop 1995;15(2):244–53.

[33] Haley DP, Coster WJ, Ludlow LH, et al. Pediatric evaluation of disability inventory. Boston: New England Medical Center Hospitals; 1992.

[34] Erhardt RP. Developmental hand dysfunction: theory, assessment and treatment. Tucson (Arizona): Therapy Skill Builders; 1994.

CLINICS IN
PLASTIC
SURGERY

Clin Plastic Surg 32 (2005) 485–493

ELSEVIER
SAUNDERS

Work-related Hand Injuries in Ontario: An Historical Perspective

Michel M.E. Schofield, MD, MSc[a,b,*]

- Development of the hand program at the Downsview Rehabilitation Centre
- Development of the specialty hand and upper extremity clinics
- Profiling work-related hand injuries in Ontario

- Postscript
- Acknowledgments
- References

When Albert Jenkins[1] came to Canada in September 1925, he had already completed several years of university in Leeds, England. He planned a career in the textile industry and began working in a woolen mill in Brantford, Ontario with the idea that he would gain practical experience of the trade from the ground up. But on November 16, 1925, Albert's left hand became caught in a picker cylinder machine, and he faced a setback he could hardly have imagined. His hand and wrist were held to the rest of his limb only by a tendon and muscle bridge and were crushed beyond repair. Twenty-year-old Albert ended up with a transradial amputation. Later, he was treated at the Department of Soldiers' Civil Re-establishment, where he received a prosthesis described as a "hook and rawhide hand."

The Workman's Compensation Board paid Albert Jenkins an initial sum of $75.00 and a small monthly life pension thereafter. Although it may be difficult for us to imagine today, if Albert had had his injury only 11 years earlier, he would not have received workers' compensation and would have had to bring a civil suit against his employer to have any hope of receiving damages for his injuries. Even an apparently straightforward case such as Albert Jenkins' would likely not have been litigated successfully. Before the enactment of worker's compensation legislation in Ontario in 1915, those injured at work were forced, for the most part, to rely on their own savings or handouts from family and friends to cover their lost wages when they were unable to work or to pay their medical bills. Before 1915 in Ontario, employers had only limited liability for providing payments to workers injured on the job, under the 1897 *Workmen's Compensation for Injuries Act*. Workers at this time still had the right to sue an employer after a workplace injury, but, in practice, three precedents in British law made it virtually impossible for an injured worker to succeed in a lawsuit against his or her employer. These three precedents, often referred to as the "Unholy Trinity," were as follows. First, in the instance of "contributory negligence," case law required that injured workers prove that they were not to some degree responsible for the injury. Second, the "fellow servant/common employment" doctrine was based on a legal precedent that effectively made it necessary for a worker

Michel Schofield is an employee of the Workplace Safety and Insurance Board of Ontario and worked at the Downsview Rehabilitation Centre from 1994 to 1998. The opinions are those of the author and not necessarily those of the Workplace Safety and Insurance Board of Ontario.

[a] Workplace Safety and Insurance Board of Ontario, Toronto, Ontario, Canada
[b] University of Toronto Hand Program, University Health Network, Toronto, Ontario, Canada
* Toronto Western Hospital, Fell Pavilion 4-178, 399 Bathurst Street, Toronto, Ontario, Canada M5T 2S8.
E-mail address: michel_schofield@wsib.on.ca
[1] Mr. Jenkins' name has been changed.

to prove that a co-worker was in no way responsible for the injury—and, by extension, the employer had to be proved directly culpable for the accident. Finally, the "assumption of risk" held that workers undertaking work known to be dangerous, such as mining or policing, should have made the appropriate financial arrangements beforehand, anticipating possible injury or death [1].

Throughout most of North America and Western Europe, there was considerable public sympathy for the plight of injured workers. Some countries had already implemented worker's compensation schemes, with Imperial Germany being the first in the 1880s [1]. The province of Ontario also felt these social pressures, and in 1910 the provincial government appointed Sir William Ralph Meredith (1840–1923) to review the matter and provide the government with recommendations. Meredith had served as leader of the Ontario Conservative Party from 1878 to 1894, had been Chancellor of the University of Toronto, and would later become Chief Justice of Ontario. Given his connections, surely none of Ontario's citizens were surprised by Meredith's appointment. Meredith surveyed models of worker's compensation law in other jurisdictions and received input from many employer and worker groups. Employers, not unexpectedly, pushed for a system that was not solely employer funded but had government or worker contributions as well; a system that had limits on the duration of compensation and one whose decisions could be appealed to the courts. Worker groups, again unsurprisingly, recommended an approach that was essentially the opposite.

If Ontario's citizens were not surprised by Meredith's appointment, surely many were taken aback by his Final Report, submitted in 1913. This document provided a forward-thinking set of recommendations that was to become the model for most of the worker's compensation statutes in Canada. Under Meredith's proposal, later termed the "Meredith Principles" [2], workers gave up their right to sue employers in exchange for almost everything else they had desired: a no-fault system that was entirely employer funded and provided wage replacement for as long as their disability lasted. Under a no-fault scheme, workers and employers would no longer have to argue over who was responsible for an injury. Meredith's system was to be administered by an independent body called the Workmen's Compensation Board (WCB) with an internal appeal structure. This structure denied employers the recourse of appealing the WCB's rulings to the courts, potentially using their greater financial resources to delay or deny benefits. Under Meredith's plan, most employers had the advantage of a collective liability for compensation that allowed them to share the financial responsibility for benefits to injured workers. Employers were to fund the system by levies on their payrolls, with the amount per worker determined by the risk of injury in that industry [1–4]. The Workmen's Compensation Act, encompassing Meredith's recommendations effectively intact, was passed by the Ontario provincial parliament in 1914 and became law in January of 1915. Meredith's legislation has survived, with only minor changes, to the present day. In Ontario, approximately 70% of the workforce is covered by the Act, which became the Workplace Safety and Insurance Act by an amendment passed in 1997.

One of the earliest changes to the Act was the inclusion of coverage for costs of medical care, medical benefits not being covered under the original Act. This oversight was corrected 2 and a half years after the original legislation came into force [5].

We take many of the medical advances made in the first half of the twentieth century for granted, forgetting how, at that time, infection after minor injuries could lead to disfigurement or death. The 1922 Annual Report of the Ontario WCB tells us that "The figures respecting blood poisoning cases are startling. From six to nine per cent of all compensation cases have infection at some stage, and the cost of such cases is at least one-eighth of the total accident cost amounting probably to three-quarters of a million dollars a year…. By far the worst record was that of the packing house class, in which the percentage of 1920 was 24.86" [6]. The toll of blood poisoning, as well as the number of ankylosed joints, amputations, and deaths attributable to sepsis, was accounted yearly in a separate table in the Annual Report of the WCB until 1937. Surviving records do not indicate how many of these infections were secondary to hand injuries or how many of the amputations and ankylosed joints involved the upper extremities.

Development of the hand program at the Downsview Rehabilitation Centre

Early commentaries in the Annual Reports also describe the importance of expert medical attention. "Whether a broken bone, a severed tendon…is to result in loss or impairment of function depends in many cases upon the skill and care of the surgeon who is looking after the case. This, as we all known [sic], varies very greatly, and it is good business and a great benefit to the workman to make sure that none but the most capable and painstaking surgeons are called to deal with accident cases" [6]. Although the role of medical and surgical expertise was recognized early on, medical rehabilitation following an injury was a practice that was still in its infancy. In 1932, the WCB created a small physiotherapy unit to treat injured workers who did not have access to such services in their own communities. Three years later, occupational therapy services were added to evaluate and improve a worker's vocational and physical status. These services continued to expand, and by 1940 over 100 patients attended a daily outpatient program of therapy in midtown Toronto [7].

In 1947, the Ontario WCB established its own rehabilitation center in Malton, just northwest of Toronto, to provide injured workers with an expanded space and provision of care from well-trained physicians, surgeons, and therapists. The earliest specialized service provided here was the Amputee Clinic. In 1958, the treatment center was relocated to a 62.5-acre property purchased by the WCB in northwest Toronto. Here the WCB established the Downsview Rehabilitation Centre.

In 1974, Dr. James Murray, one of Canada's first hand surgeons, established a Hand Clinic for injured workers at the Downsview Rehabilitation Centre. Dr. Murray's skills as a hand surgeon have been recognized internationally, but his work in developing the multidisciplinary Hand Clinic at Downsview is less well known. Dr. Murray and his surgical colleagues assessed workers with hand injuries, and therapists provided rehabilitation that focused on activities of daily living, recreational pursuits, and vocational activities. In Dr. Murray's zeal to ensure that workers with hand injuries had the best possible care, it was not uncommon for him, in the midst of a busy Hand Clinic, to call one of his former residents and "give them hell" when he believed that the treatment that had been provided was not up to his standards (Sandy Griffiths, former Clinical Coordinator, Hand and Amputee Program, Downsview Rehabilitation Centre, personal communication, 1994).

Several other hand programs operated in the province at this time, but these programs tended to treat patients with acutely injured and postsurgical hands, rather than the longer-term problems that appeared to face many WCB claimants. Specialized services to benefit workers with severe hand injuries included the provision of aesthetic prostheses and custom gloves, as well as tool adaptations to assist a worker in returning to the workplace.

As the Hand Clinic program grew, further services were provided to help workers with hand injuries return to productive lives. A dominance transfer program was developed to help workers with a serious injury to their dominant hand strengthen their previously subdominant hand and use it in a more coordinated manner for both gross and fine motor activities. The significant psychologic impact of many hand injuries was recognized by the clinicians in the Hand Clinic at Downsview, and the services of psychologists and social workers formed an important part of the team approach.

As new work-related hand problems emerged, Hand Clinic staff strove to meet these needs. An example is the development of keyboard assessments and training when computer use became ubiquitous in the 1990s. Workers with severe hand injuries often could not easily navigate a traditional keyboard, and at Downsview they were provided with special keyboards and trained in their use. With increased computer use, Canada, like other jurisdictions, saw an increase in claims from workers who developed computer-related upper extremity injuries [8]. These workers were also assessed and provided with devices or treatment that would help them return to keyboarding.

Both general and specialized services were provided at Downsview Rehabilitation Centre over the years; in addition to the Amputee Clinic, specialized services for workers with acquired brain injuries, chronic pain, and posttraumatic stress disorder were developed. The Centre was a model of the provision of care to injured workers, and visitors from many other countries came to learn from the Downsview experience. The clinicians performed considerable research that appeared in peer-reviewed journals. Residents in orthopedic surgery and rehabilitation medicine at the University of Toronto rotated through the programs. The Centre was associated with the University of Toronto Department of Rehabilitation Medicine in the training of physiotherapists. Beginning in the early 1970s, the Downsview Centre cosponsored an annual course in "Hand Injuries" with the University of Western Ontario.

But the work being done at the Downsview Rehabilitation Centre was not universally admired. In 1986, a representative of the Canadian Auto

Table 1: **Number of lost-time hand injuries in Ontario Workplace Safety and Insurance Board claimants by year and sex**

Year of injury	1996	1997	1998	1999	2000	2001	2002	2003
Total both sexes	23,083	23,009	22,309	23,481	24,365	22,257	21,570	19,810
Women	6885	6935	6760	7404	7947	7304	7210	6644
Men	16,181	16,067	15,547	16,075	16,415	14,952	14,360	13,166

Table 2: **Number of lost-time claims by part of body and number of total Workplace Safety and Insurance Board lost-time claims by all body parts affected (1996–2002)**

Part of body affected	Year of injury or illness						
	1996	*1997*	*1998*	*1999*	*2000*	*2001*	*2002*
	Number of injuries						
Upper extremities							
Fingers, fingernails	10,550	10,510	10,270	10,585	10,799	9706	9340
Arms	5030	4926	4482	4753	5013	4822	4556
Hands, except fingers	4405	4638	4430	4831	5063	4661	4545
Wrists	3947	3812	3714	4184	4286	4046	4063
Upper extremities, unspecified, NEC	861	793	766	746	809	722	714
Subtotal	24,793	24,679	23,662	25,099	25,970	23,957	23,218
Total All injuries	103,080	101,806	97,190	100,726	104,154	98,359	95,568

This table shows the number of allowed lost-time claims by part of body injured or affected for each year as of March 31 of the following year. 2003 data were not available at the time of this writing.
Abbreviation: NEC, not elsewhere classified.
Data from Statistical supplement to the Annual Report of the Workplace Safety and Insurance Board 2002. Available at: www.wsib.on.ca/wsib/wsibsite.nsf/LookupFiles/DownloadableFile2002StatisticalSupplement/$File/SS2002.pdf.

Workers Union reported allegations of improprieties from injured workers who had been treated at Downsview, including reports of drug abuse among patients, sexual harassment of patients by staff, and inappropriate questioning by psychologists [9,10]. The allegations were followed by a flurry of external and internal reviews of activities at the Downsview Centre, as well as a police investigation [9–13]. Former patients and Downsview staff were interviewed, and procedures were analyzed in depth. The reports were finally submitted, with some critics charging that the reviews were a "whitewash" [9] and others believing that their criticism was vindicated, pointing to one report's descriptions of Downsview as lacking "focus and direction" [14]. Although none of the specific accusations had been supported by the evidence, and no charges were ever laid, the reputation of the Downsview Centre never fully recovered from this episode.

Unsurprisingly, there were calls at this time to have the Downsview Centre shut down [15], and the WCB began seriously to consider closing the Centre. Partially in response to this scandal, the WCB developed a new medical rehabilitation strategy in the late 1980s that focused on the provision of therapy services closer to injured workers' homes, rather than centralized in one location. One important difference was that the health care professionals staffing these facilities were not WCB employees, perhaps reducing the perception of biased opinions and care.[2] Senior management at the WCB reasoned that, if workers could be seen at medical facilities throughout the province, there would be no need for services at Downsview. Indeed, Regional Evaluation Centers were established in many larger cities in Ontario, and workers were sent to these facilities by their own physicians or the WCB for assessment by specialists. Community clinics were also set up across the province as part of this strategy, and these programs provided an early and active approach to workplace injuries.

The WCB recognized, however, that there were some injured workers whose care could not be readily obtained in many smaller communities. Limited numbers of health care providers in the province had the skills to treat workers with these more complex injuries, including the difficult hand injuries seen in the Hand Clinic at Downsview. The WCB pondered various options for locating the specialized clinics from 1990 until the Downsview clinical programs were finally closed at the end of 1997. Conflicting forces led to delays and reversals in decision making. Concerns existed about the cost of relocating the specialized programs or renovating the Downsview site versus the expense of having programs provided by either private or hospital-based clinicians. In addition, falling real estate prices during the early 1990s reduced the value of the Downsview property, making its sale less desirable for the WCB. In the meantime, the clinical work at Downsview went on; during this period of uncertainty, the Centre received a 3-year accreditation from the Canadian Council on Health Facilities Accreditation, the highest level then awarded.

Development of the specialty hand and upper extremity clinics

Ultimately, the concerns that the services at Downsview were too expensive and could be provided

---

[2] The consulting hand surgeons at the Downsview Hand Clinic were not employees of the WCB.

Table 3: Percentage of lost-time Workplace Safety and Insurance Board claims by part of body affected for hand and wrist injuries

Part of body affected	Year of injury or illness						
	1996	*1997*	*1998*	*1999*	*2000*	*2001*	*2002*
	% of total of all injuries						
Upper extremities							
Fingers, fingernails	10.2	10.3	10.6	10.5	10.4	9.9	9.8
Arms	4.9	4.8	4.6	4.7	4.8	4.9	4.8
Hands, except fingers	4.3	4.6	4.6	4.8	4.9	4.7	4.8
Wrists	3.8	3.7	3.8	4.2	4.1	4.1	4.3
Upper extremities, unspecified, NEC	0.8	0.8	0.8	0.7	0.8	0.7	0.7
Subtotal	24.1	24.2	24.3	24.9	24.9	24.4	24.3

This table shows the number of allowed lost-time claims by part of body injured or affected for each year as of March 31 of the following year. 2003 data were not available at the time of this writing.
Abbreviation: NEC, not elsewhere classified.
Data from Statistical supplement to the Annual Report of the Workplace Safety and Insurance Board 2002. Available at: www.wsib.on.ca/wsib/wsibsite.nsf/LookupFiles/DownloadableFile2002StatisticalSupplement/$File/SS2002.pdf.

with less controversy by non-WCB staff persisted, and the clinical programs were closed at the end of 1997. The Workplace Safety and Insurance Board (WSIB) decided to move the services from Downsview into academic centers of excellence, and proposals to provide specialized services for injured workers were obtained from a number of teaching hospitals in Toronto. The WSIB Hand Program at the Toronto Western Hospital was one of the first

specialty clinics to operate outside Downsview, opening its doors to injured workers in January 1998. This program, staffed by some of the former Downsview Hand Clinic therapists, continues to provide high quality patient care. The model established by Dr. Murray also endures, with consulting hand surgeons from several hospitals travelling to one site where the surgeon will assess workers and workers can receive hand therapy. The WSIB

Table 4: Canadian labor force and participation rates by sex and age group

	1999	2000	2001	2002	2003
			Thousands		
Labor force	15,721.2	15,999.2	16,246.3	16,689.4	17,046.8
Men	8534.0	8649.2	8769.2	8989.8	9135.9
Women	7187.2	7350.0	7477.1	7699.6	7910.9
Participation rates			%		
15 years and older	65.6	65.9	66.0	66.9	67.5
Men	72.5	72.5	72.5	73.3	73.6
Women	58.9	59.5	59.7	60.7	61.6
15–24 years	63.5	64.4	64.7	66.3	67.0
Men	65.3	65.9	66.1	67.7	68.0
Women	61.7	62.9	63.3	64.9	66.0
25–44 years	85.8	86.0	86.3	86.8	87.1
Men	92.1	92.1	92.1	92.4	92.5
Women	79.6	80.0	80.4	81.2	81.6
45 years and older	47.8	48.5	48.9	50.3	51.7
Men	56.6	56.9	57.1	58.6	59.6
Women	39.9	40.9	41.5	42.8	44.6
65 years and older	6.2	6.0	6.0	6.7	7.3
Men	9.8	9.5	9.4	10.5	11.5
Women	3.4	3.3	3.4	3.7	4.1

Statistics Canada information is used with the permission of Statistics Canada. Users are forbidden to copy the data and redisseminate them, in an original or modified form, for commercial purposes, without the expressed permission of Statistics Canada. Information on the availability of the wide range of data from Statistics Canada can be obtained from Statistics Canada's Regional Offices, its World Wide Web site, and its toll-free access number 1-800-263-1136.
Data from Statistics Canada, CANSIM, table.282–0002. Available at: http://www.statcan.ca/english/Pgdb/labor05.htm. Accessed November 13, 2004.

Table 5: Number of lost-time hand injuries for both sexes in Ontario Workplace Safety and Insurance Board claimants by year and age at time of injury

Both sexes	1996	1997	1998	1999	2000	2001	2002	2003
All ages	23,083	23,009	22,309	23,481	24,365	22,257	21,570	19,810
Under 20 years	1371	1,586	1836	2078	2,357	2092	2038	1787
20–29 years	6677	6,479	6228	6355	6441	5718	5308	5041
30–39 years	7093	6,893	6522	6588	6637	5968	5531	4749
40–49 years	4832	4,849	4679	5166	5339	5066	5213	4834
50–59 years	2557	2,613	2526	2726	2978	2833	2873	2743
60 years and over	544	553	516	568	613	579	607	655
Average age at time of injury	35.4	35.4	35.1	35.3	35.6	35.7	36.1	36.4

Hand Program, under the direction of Dr. Brent Graham, is also involved in training of surgical residents and occupational therapy and physiotherapy students and carries out research, studying outcomes of interventions in the hand-injured worker population.

Recognizing the expertise available at other academic teaching centers in Ontario, the WSIB has partnered with the Hand and Upper Limb Center in London at the University of Western Ontario, under the leadership of Dr. James Roth, and at Hotel Dieu Hospital in Kingston at Queen's University with Dr. David Pichora to provide assessment and treatment for workers with upper extremity injuries. The developing network of hand and upper limb WSIB specialty programs has allowed workers outside of the greater Toronto area to stay closer to home when they seek specialized care.

The WSIB and its specialty program partners developed a validated patient satisfaction survey to help monitor the quality of care from an injured worker's perspective. The results have consistently shown high levels of patient approval, with 98% of workers surveyed rating the overall quality of the care and services received in the specialty programs as "good to excellent" (Brenda Perkins-Meingast, manager of the Specialty Programs Liaison Office in the Health Services Division of the Workplace Safety and Insurance Board of Ontario, personal communication, 2005).

Profiling work-related hand injuries in Ontario

Work-related injuries are coded by the WSIB using the National Work Injuries Statistics Program, a coding system used by most of the WCB of Canada. The system describes a claimant's injury using four primary factors: (1) the nature of the injury or disease (eg, amputation, sprain, neoplasm, or infection), (2) the body part, namely the anatomic region or regions involved by the injury or disease, (3) the source of injury (eg, machinery, container, bodily motion of the worker), and (4) the event (eg, fall, overexertion, exposure to a harmful substance). For example, de Quervain's tenosynovitis in a meatpacker could be coded as a tenosynovitis (nature of injury) in the wrist (body part) as a result of repetitive motion of the worker (source of injury) related to repetitive grasping of moving objects (event code).

Statistical coding of WSIB claims is only done for injuries that result in wage replacement benefits paid for time lost from work; in 2003 there were approximately two no-lost-time claims for every lost-time claim [16]. Coverage for health care expenses may ensue from a worker's no-lost-time claim. This coding system, adopted by the Ontario WCB in 1996,

Table 6: Number of lost-time hand injuries for female Workplace Safety and Insurance Board claimants by year and age at time of injury

Women	1996	1997	1998	1999	2000	2001	2002	2003
All ages	6885	6935	6760	7404	7947	7304	7210	6644
Under 20 years	430	508	550	619	764	662	668	576
20–29 years	1606	1567	1531	1645	1646	1475	1398	1348
30–39 years	1956	1908	1831	2048	2099	1975	1757	1452
40–49 years	1693	1760	1656	1861	2037	1876	2015	1843
50–59 years	1019	1011	1021	1067	1211	1146	1177	1186
60 years and over	176	169	170	164	190	169	195	238
Average age at time of injury	37.1	37.0	36.8	36.8	36.9	37.2	37.7	38.2

Table 7: Number of lost-time hand injuries for male Workplace Safety and Insurance Board claimants by year and age at time of injury

Men	1996	1997	1998	1999	2000	2001	2002	2003
All ages	16,181	16,067	15,547	16,075	16,415	14,952	14,360	13,166
Under 20 years	939	1078	1286	1459	1592	1430	1370	1211
20–29 years	5065	4910	4697	4710	4795	4243	3910	3693
30–39 years	5133	4983	4690	4539	4537	3993	3774	3297
40–49 years	3136	3088	3022	3305	3301	3189	3198	2991
50–59 years	1538	1600	1505	1658	1767	1687	1696	1557
60 years and over	367	384	346	404	423	410	412	417
Average age at time of injury	34.6	34.7	34.4	34.6	34.6	34.9	35.3	35.5

allows the WCBs that use it across Canada to compare data. Unfortunately, however, because different diagnostic coding systems are used by almost everyone else, it prevents the WSIB from comparing its data with those of other organizations.

The data on hand injuries presented here come from a subset of the WSIB database obtained from the Research and Evaluation Division at the WSIB in July 2004. The information includes diagnostic coding as well as demographic information, such as age at time of injury, occupational code, sex, and geographic location, for all WSIB hand, wrist, and forearm injury claims between January 1, 1996 and December 31, 2003.

As seen in Table 1, claims for work-related hand injuries in Ontario are declining. Data for all of 2003 may be incomplete and do not include claims that are still "pending" (ie, those that are awaiting an adjudicative decision). The decline in injuries is more evident in male workers than in females, whose numbers of work-related hand injuries appear to be in a holding pattern. Tables 2 and 3 show the breakdown of hand, finger, and wrist injuries by year and compare these figures with the total number of WSIB claims for all types of bodily injury.

Recent data from Statistics Canada indicate that the population is aging [17], and, as Table 4 from Statistics Canada shows, the labor force is getting older as well; rates of participation in the workforce are increasing for all age groups. These data suggest that not only is Canada's populace aging but, increasingly, Canadians are staying in the workforce longer and not retiring as early as they once may have. This trend is echoed in workers with hand injuries, as outlined in Tables 5, 6, and 7, which demonstrate rising numbers of workers aged 60 and older with hand injuries. Even in the setting of a decrease in WSIB claims of all types, including most hand injuries (see Table 2), the only group with a growth in work-related hand injuries in recent years is that of

workers aged 60 and older. Table 6 suggests that female hand-injured workers account for most of this increase.

A closer look at the group of female WSIB claimants who were older than 60 at the time of their hand injuries offers a view of types of hand pathologies we may be seeing more of in the future. In 2003, the most common industry sector in which hand injuries in women older than 60 occurred was the services industry, with 31.1% of all the claims in this group (24.6% of WSIB claims for all ages and injury or illness types were in this industry [16]), followed by health care with 18.9% (9.4% overall), Schedule II[3] with 18.5% (16.4% overall), and manufacturing with 17.2% (17.8% overall).

One worrisome finding about the over-60 female hand-injured group for 2003 is that the most common injury was not the degenerative or repetitive type of problem that might be expected in this age group (although there were 25 cases of carpal tunnel syndrome diagnosed, or 10.5% of the overall total). Rather, the most common injuries were fractures, with a total of 60 cases or 25.2% of all claims. For all ages, both sexes, and all body parts, fractures made up a total of 7.1% of all WSIB claims from 2003 [16], so fractures are disproportionately represented in this group of older women with hand injuries. By far the most common event code (ie, information on the mechanism of the injury) for the older-than-60 women with hand injuries group was a "fall to a floor, walkway or other surface." The energy involved in this type of impact is low compared with other types of fall that occur from a height or down stairs. The injured women older than 60 do not, therefore, appear to be experiencing an unexplained increase in high-impact injuries; it seems more likely that they are

---

[3] Schedule II employers are large and mostly public sector employers that are self-insured under the WSIB and therefore pay claimant's costs on a dollar-for-dollar basis.

Table 8: Average wage replacement benefit costs and health care costs per claim by year and sex for lost time Workplace Safety and Insurance Board hand injuries

Year of injury	1996	1997	1998	1999	2000	2001	2002	2003
Average wage replacement costs in $ per claim	2640	2538	3817	3843	3670	3105	2560	1486
Average health care costs in $ per claim	996	948	1063	1153	1113	1086	864	430
Average wage replacement benefit costs in $ per claim—women	2942	2676	4163	4196	3769	3162	2411	1346
Average health care costs in $ per claim—women	1057	909	1016	1144	1090	1066	881	427
Average wage replacement benefit costs in $ per claim—men	2515	2480	3667	3681	3622	3077	2635	1553
Average health care costs in $ per claim—men	973	963	1083	1157	1123	1095	856	432

sustaining more serious injuries from minor accidents. It is interesting to speculate that the increase in hand and wrist fractures in this group is, at least in part, due to their more fragile bones.

The reported prevalence of osteoporosis varies, with the National Osteoporosis Foundation in the United States estimating that 55% of those aged 50 and older have the diagnosis [18] and the Osteoporosis Society of Canada providing an estimate of one in four women over the age of 50 with probable osteoporosis [19]. In any case, osteoporosis is a common condition, and the aging of our labor force, along with the growing participation of those older than 50, may make it increasingly a workplace issue.

Table 8 shows the wage loss benefit costs and health care costs per claim from 1996 to 2003. This table suggests that the costs may have decreased in the last 2 years, after peaking in 2000. These data should be viewed with caution, however. The costs are real costs, not adjusted for inflation, and are cumulative, so that the costs indicated for 1996 claims reflect the charges to the claim from the period of 1996 to July 2004. More recent claims have not had the same time to accumulate potential longer-term charges. In addition, data related to claims that are less than 15 months old are considered "immature" and may have incomplete costs associated with them, because of delays in adjudication decisions that may occur when the information on file is incomplete. The health care costs are even less reliable than the wage replacement costs. Manktelow and colleagues' [20] study of WSIB carpal tunnel syndrome claims showed that Ontario health care providers frequently did not bill their services to the WSIB, leading to a gross underestimation of health care costs when using WSIB data.

Postscript

When Albert Jenkins lost his hand in 1925, there was no legal obligation for employers to re-employ an injured worker.[4] Fortunately, Albert's employer agreed to train him as a wool buyer when he returned to work early in 1926. His employer made it clear that they would not pay Albert's wages during this apprenticeship and expected the WCB to provide him with ongoing lost-wage benefits until the training was completed. He continued working as a wool buyer until 1930, when changes in the Canadian textile market made wool manufacture less profitable. Albert made the switch to fabric designer and obtained employment with another textile manufacturer when his original employer closed the plant in 1959. He married and never allowed his amputation to prevent him from achieving his goals. Albert's daughter recalls her father putting down hardwood flooring in her bedroom. He golfed (although apparently not very well), curled, and became a member of the Rotary Club after his retirement at age 80. For more than a decade, he has been living in a long-term care facility. Now 99 years old, Albert recalls having a total of four or five prostheses from the time of his injury at age 25. He is a widower but remains an active participant in the lives of his daughter, son-in-law, and two grandsons, as well as listening to his favorite classical music.

Acknowledgments

The author is grateful for the assistance of Carolyn Murphy, manager, and Irene Yu, research analyst, from the Research and Evaluation Branch of the Workplace Safety and Insurance Board of Ontario for obtaining the WSIB hand injury data for this project. Irene Yu also prepared Table 2, taken from the Statistical Supplement to the 2002 Annual Report of the Workplace Safety and Insurance

---

[4] Limited vocational rehabilitation services began to be offered to WCB claimants as of 1923, but the legal obligation to re-employ injured workers did not come until considerably later, as part of Bill 162, which came into effect in January 1990.

Board. The author also wishes to thank Linda Kacur, Medical Statistics Coder Analyst, for explaining many of the nuances of the National Work Injuries Statistics Program.

References

[1] A short history of workers' compensation. Butterworth's workers' compensation in Ontario service. Toronto: Butterworth; 1998.

[2] Saskatchewan Workers' Compensation Board. Available at: http://www.wcbsask.com/About_Us/Meredith_Principles.html. Accessed November 10, 2004.

[3] Workers' Compensation Board. Alberta. Available at: http://www.wcb.ab.ca/about/prince.asp. Accessed November 10, 2004.

[4] Workers' Compensation Board of Nova Scotia. Available at: http://www.wcb.ns.ca/annual report1997/meredith.html. Accessed November 10, 2004.

[5] Report for 1917 of the Workmen's Compensation Board. Ontario, Toronto: A.T. Wilgress; 1918.

[6] Report for 1922 of the Workmen's Compensation Board. Ontario, Toronto: C.W. James; 1923.

[7] Kaegi E. Staff discussion paper prepared for the Downsview review team: the future role of the Downsview Rehabilitation Centre. 1987.

[8] Ashbury FD. Occupational repetitive strain injuries and gender in Ontario, 1986 to 1991. J Occup Environ Med 1995;37(4):479–85.

[9] Ontario Hansard. November 6, 1986. Transcripts from the Ontario Provincial Legislature. Available at: http://www.ontla.on.ca/hansard/index.htm.

[10] Ontario Hansard. December 10, 1986. Transcripts from the Ontario Provincial Legislature. Available at: http://www.ontla.on.ca/hansard/index.htm.

[11] Kummel E, Wellman P, Hagan A. Downsview Rehabilitation Centre (DRC) inquiry report. Toronto: Worker's Compensation Board of Ontario; November 28, 1986.

[12] Minna M, Majesky W, chairs. Ontario Task Force on Vocational Rehabilitation Services of the Workers' Compensation Board of Ontario. An injury to one is an injury to all: Toward dignity and independence for the injured worker. Toronto: Government of Ontario; September 2, 1987.

[13] Stoughton V, Garber R, Persichilli A, et al. Downsview Review Team. Final Report of the Ontario Review Team. Toronto: commissioned by the Ontario government to provide an external review of the Downsview Rehabilitation Centre; 1987.

[14] Ontario Hansard. December 11, 1986. Transcripts from the Ontario Provincial Legislature. Available at: http://www.ontla.on.ca/hansard/index.htm.

[15] Ontario Hansard. April 29, 1987. Transcripts from the Ontario Provincial Legislature. Available at: http://www.ontla.on.ca/hansard/index.htm.

[16] Workplace Safety and Insurance Board of Ontario. Statistical Supplement to the 2003 Annual Report. 2004. Available at: http://www.wsib.on.ca/wsib/wsibsite.nsf/LookupFiles/DownloadableFile2003StatSupp/$File/StatSupp03.pdf.

[17] Statistics Canada. CANSIM. 2004. Population by sex and age group, by provinces and territories. Table 051-0001. Available at: http://www.statcan.ca/english/Pgdb/demo31g.htm. Accessed November 30, 2004.

[18] National Osteoporosis Foundation. About osteoporosis: fast facts. Available at: http://www.nof.org/osteoporosis/diseasefacts.htm. Accessed November 30, 2004.

[19] Osteoporosis Society of Canada. About osteoporosis. Available at: http://www.osteoporosis.ca/english/about%20osteoporosis/default.asp?s=1. Accessed November 30, 2004.

[20] Manktelow RT, Binhammer P, Tomat LR, et al. Carpal tunnel syndrome: cross-sectional and outcome study in Ontario workers. J Hand Surg [Am] 2004;29(2):307–17.

CLINICS IN PLASTIC SURGERY

Clin Plastic Surg 32 (2005) 495–502

ELSEVIER
SAUNDERS

Musculoskeletal Injury Associated with Fluoroquinolone Antibiotics

Yasmin Khaliq, PharmD[a,b], George G. Zhanel, PhD[c,d],*

- Scope of problem and risk factors
- Mechanism of musculoskeletal injury
  - *Clinical reports*
  - *Animal and in vitro studies*
- Clinical overview
  - *Clinical aspects of tendon injury and onset*
  - *Patient demographics*

- *Fluoroquinolones implicated and duration of treatment*
- *Type of tendon injury*
- Therapy overview
- Legal implications
- Summary
- References

The fluoroquinolone antimicrobials were first introduced in the 1980s and have since been used extensively in gram-negative bacterial infections [1]. With the introduction of the newer-generation agents, their use has expanded to include gram-positive and anaerobic infections [2]. Guidelines now recommend these newer-generation respiratory fluoroquinolones for use in community-acquired pneumonia and acute exacerbations of chronic bronchitis, in some cases as first-line therapy [3,4]. The use of these agents in patients with asthma or chronic obstructive pulmonary disease receiving corticosteroids is of concern, because concurrent use of these agents may increase the incidence of tendon injuries. In this article, the authors review the literature describing any association found between the use of fluoroquinolones and tendon injury, particularly that occurring in the hands.

Scope of problem and risk factors

The prevalence of fluoroquinolone-induced tendon injury is not well established in the literature, but reports suggest it is low, ranging from 0.14% to 0.4% [5–7] in an otherwise healthy population. A number of factors have been suggested to predispose a patient to fluoroquinolone-associated injury. In the renal transplant population, a prevalence of 12.2% to 15.6% is reported, as compared with 0.6% to 3.6% for transplant patients not receiving fluoroquinolones [8,9].

[a] Department of Pharmacy, Ottawa Hospital General Campus, 501 Smyth Road, Ottawa, Ontario K1H 8L6, Canada
[b] Faculty of Medicine, University of Ottawa, Ottawa, Ontario, Canada
[c] Department of Medical Microbiology, Faculty of Medicine, University of Manitoba, Winnipeg, Manitoba, Canada
[d] Departments of Medicine and Clinical Microbiology, Health Sciences Centre, 820 Sherbrook Street, Winnipeg, Manitoba R3A 1R9, Canada
* Corresponding author. Microbiology, Health Sciences Centre, MS673, 820 Sherbrook Street, Winnipeg, Manitoba R3A 1R9, Canada.
E-mail address: ggzhanel@pcs.mb.ca (G.G. Zhanel).

doi:10.1016/j.cps.2005.05.004

Other risk factors include age, renal failure or hemodialysis, diabetes mellitus, hyperparathyroidism, rheumatic disease, gout, and sports [9–14]. The concurrent use of corticosteroids has also been highly implicated in tendinopathy [14]. The addition of a fluoroquinolone to the regimen of a patient with any risk factor potentially creates additive or synergistic toxicity.

Mechanism of musculoskeletal injury

Clinical reports

The mechanism by which fluoroquinolones cause tendon injury is not established, although a number of suggestions have been made and are summarized in Table 1. An investigation by Jorgensen and colleagues [15] indicated that the pathology in a 68-year-old man who had received 3 months of pefloxacin demonstrated degenerative lesions, fissures, interstitial edema without cellular infiltration, necrosis, and neovascularization. Beuchard and colleagues [16] described, in a 54-year-old man who had received only 1 week of pefloxacin therapy, normal tendon tissue without degenerative lesions, thickening of the vasculature, hyaline deposits, and inflammatory infiltrate. It was suggested that an ischemic vascular process was the cause in these patients. Necrosis has also been noted in other patients who have received norfloxacin and ciprofloxacin [17,18]. LeHuec and colleagues [11] suggest that the mechanism may be related to direct toxicity to the collagen because of the rapid onset of tendon injury. In renal transplant patients, reduced clearance of the fluoroquinolone possibly results in elevated concentrations that might play a role in toxicity as the incidence increases in this population.

Animal and in vitro studies

The use of pefloxacin in a mouse model demonstrated a change in proteoglycan synthesis in the Achilles tendon [19]. Oxidative damage was also found, suggesting the involvement of a reactive oxygen species. The authors proposed that age, sports, and corticosteroid therapy play a role in preventing repair in the tendon. This damage could lead to irreversible matrix changes and rupture. Oxidative damage is supported by in vitro work, pointing to intrinsic or direct toxicity [20].

The toxic effects of various fluoroquinolones were evaluated in a juvenile rat model [21]. Edema and increased mononuclear cells were often found in the tendon sheath of the Achilles. Pefloxacin, fleroxacin, levofloxacin, and ofloxacin were found to induce the greatest number of lesions. Enoxacin, norfloxacin, and ciprofloxacin had little or no effect. The authors suggested that the substituent at the seventh position of the fluoroquinolone molecule might play a role: the agents with the highest toxicity all share a methylpiperadinyl moiety at this position, whereas the other three have a piperadinyl substituent. Table 2 summarizes the substituents found at the seventh position for each fluoroquinolone discussed [22]. Nitric oxide and 5-lipoxygenase were also found to play a role. Another animal study described alterations in the viability of rabbit tenocytes by quinolones that are fluorinated but not by those that are not fluorinated [23]. Further studies are required to elucidate whether a structure activity relationship exists.

Investigators have hypothesized that the chelating properties of fluoroquinolones with multivalent cations such as magnesium disturb the integrity of the tendons, suggesting that the pathophysiology of this process is similar to that of chondrotoxicity [24]. Correction of baseline magnesium deficiency has even been suggested to help prevent fluoroquinolone-associated tendon injury [25]. Irregular collagen alignment is also implicated, suggesting an adverse effect on fibroblast function in the tendon [26].

Table 1: Pathologic changes in tendons associated with fluoroquinolones [11,15–18]

Human findings	Animal findings
Degenerative lesions	Change in proteoglycan synthesis
Fissures	Oxidative damage
Interstitial edema without cellular infiltration	Edema
Necrosis	Increased mononuclear cells
Neovascularization	Alterations in the viability of tenocytes
Thickening of the vasculature	Irregular collagen alignment—adverse effect on fibroblast function
Hyaline deposits	Associations with nitric oxide and 5-lipoxygenase
Inflammatory infiltrate	

Clinical overview

The first case report regarding tendinopathy associated with fluoroquinolones was published in 1983 [12]. The general features of fluoroquinolone-associated tendinopathy appear to be similar across

Table 2: **Fluoroquinolones in Canada and the United States**

Fluoroquinolone	Current market status (# prescriptions dispensed)	Substituent in seventh position of quinolone ring[a]
Norfloxacin	Marketed	1-piperazinyl
Ofloxacin	Marketed	4-methyl-1-piperazinyl
Ciprofloxacin	Marketed (>700 million)	1-piperazinyl
Levofloxacin	Marketed (>500 million)	4-methyl-1-piperazinyl
Moxifloxacin	Marketed (>12 million)	(4aS,7aS)-octahydro-6H-pyrrolo[3,4-b]pyridin-6-yl
Gatifloxacin	Marketed (>5 million)	3-methyl-1-piperazinyl
Gemifloxacin	Marketed (<1 million)	3-(aminomethyl)-4-(methoxyimino)-1-pyrrolidinyl
Fleroxacin	Not marketed	4-methyl-1-piperazinyl
Pefloxacin	Not marketed	4-methyl-1-piperazinyl
Enoxacin	Not marketed	1-piperazinyl
Clinafloxacin	Withdrawn due to adverse effects	3-amino-1-pyrrolidinyl
Grepafloxacin	Withdrawn due to adverse effects	3-methyl-1-piperazinyl
Sparfloxacin	Withdrawn due to adverse effects	(3R,5S)-3,5-dimethyl-1-piperazinyl
Trovafloxacin	Use restricted due to adverse effects	(1α,5α,6α)-7-6-amino-3-azabicyclo[3.1.0]hex-3yl

[a] Methylpiperadinyl substituent postulated to be associated with increased incidence of toxicity.
Data from Kashida Y, Kato M. Characterization of fluoroquinolone-induced Achilles tendon toxicity in rats: comparison of toxicities of 10 fluoroquinolones and effects of anti-inflammatory compounds. Antimicrob Agents Chemother 1997;41(11):2389–93.

agents and locations of injury. Cases of injury to the hands are discussed in detail. Detailed aspects of cases found in other parts of the body can be found elsewhere [27].

Clinical aspects of tendon injury and onset

Tendon injury manifests most commonly with pain that is severe and of sudden onset [27]. Other frequent signs and symptoms include tenderness to palpation, edema, and difficulty with movement of the involved area. Painful nodules, thickened tendon sheaths, warmth, stiffness, and erythema are also reported. Diagnosis is made primarily by physical examination, although occasionally radiography, ultrasound, nuclear scanning, or magnetic resonance imaging has been used.

The mean onset of symptoms after the initiation of fluoroquinolone therapy is 9 to 18 days [27,28]. Tendon rupture is reported to occur in 40% of subjects with a mean onset of about 17 to 26 days (median 6 days) after the initiation of fluoroquinolone treatment. Tendon injury has been reported to occur from as early as 2 hours after the first dose of a fluoroquinolone (ciprofloxacin) [29] to as late as 6 months after treatment had been terminated [17].

Patient demographics

The mean age of patients experiencing fluoroquinolone-associated tendinopathy is about 60 years [27,28]. The ratio of males to females is as high as 2:1. About 33% of patients have received systemic or inhaled corticosteroids before and during fluoroquinolone administration; however, in most cases, treatment with steroids was long-term [27]. More than 50% of patients with tendon rupture have received corticosteroids.

Fluoroquinolones implicated and duration of treatment

Most fluoroquinolones have been implicated in causing tendinopathy. Pefloxacin and ciprofloxacin are the foci of most reports [5,6,8,27,28,30]; however, the newer levofloxacin has recently had a number of cases reported [30–33]. Most reports are European; underreporting in North America might bias the data. Injury associated with pefloxacin primarily occurred at doses of 800 mg daily, although one case reported the use of 400 mg daily [27]. The dose at which ciprofloxacin has caused injury ranges from 500 to 2000 mg. Levofloxacin doses were 500 mg once or twice daily [30–33]. Cases have also been reported with norfloxacin (800 mg/d), ofloxacin (400 mg/d), fleroxacin, enoxacin, and, most recently, moxifloxacin [27,34]. Injury occurred regardless of the use of normal therapeutic doses and with treatments that were

of standard, shorter than normal, and longer than normal duration.

Type of tendon injury

The Achilles tendon is the most common site of injury, cited in about 90% of patients; about 40% of cases are bilateral. **Figs. 1 and 2** show the histology and location of tendon injury. Cases that have occurred in the lower extremities also include the patellar (n=1) and quadriceps (n=1) [11,35]. Cases in the upper extremities include, in the hand, the flexor tendon sheath and the extensor tendons of the fingers (n=3) and the thumb, including the extensor pollicis longus (n=3), as well as the lateral epicondyle (n=2), supraspinatus tendon (n=1), subscapularis (n=1), and rotator cuff (n=1) [11–13,17,36–38]. The cases that occurred in the upper extremities were infrequent compared with those in the lower extremities. Those specific to the hand are summarized in Table 3 [12,13,36,38,39]. Five patients had tendons in the hands affected by fluoroquinolone therapy. One patient had involvement of both a finger and a thumb (de Quervain's tenosynovitis) [38]. The same patient also exhibited tendinopathy in several other tendons, including the supraspinatus and the Achilles, demonstrating that injury can occur in multiple sites simultaneously. As with fluoroquinolone-associated tendinopathy in other body parts, the average age of the patients whose hands were affected was 55.4 years. Patient demographics and risk factors were similar, as were the clinical manifestations of the injury. The small number of

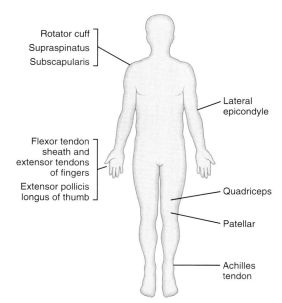

Fig. 1. Locations of fluoroquinolone-associated tendinopathies.

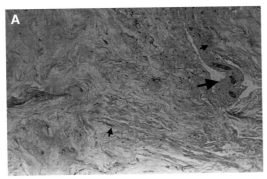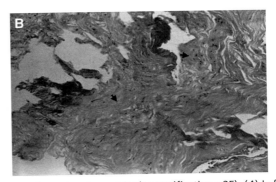

Fig. 2. Pathologic analyses of both Achilles tendons (hematoxylin and eosin, original magnification ×25). (*A*) Left side. (*B*) Right side. The fibers of both Achilles tendons were sparse and meandering, with edema and imbibition (*small arrows*). This degenerative change was marked on the right side (*B*). There was no marked stenosis of intratendinous blood vessels (*A, large arrow*) and no infiltration of inflammatory cells. (*From* Kowatari K, Nakashima K, Ono A, et al. Levofloxacin induced bilateral Achilles tendon rupture: a case report and review of the literature. J Orthop Sci 2004;9:188; with permission.)

cases in the hand makes it difficult to draw specific conclusions.

Therapy overview

Intervention is similar regardless of location of injury. Immediate discontinuation of the implicated fluoroquinolone is recommended. Nonsurgical interventions (analgesics, physical therapy, heel raise, cast or immobilization) have been instituted regularly, and, surgery has been used less frequently. In one case, symptoms were alleviated with a reduction in the dose of the fluoroquinolone (norfloxacin) from 400 mg twice daily to 200 mg daily [13]. Rechallenge at the higher dose resulted in recurrence; however, once the dose of 200 mg daily was reinstituted, treatment was successfully continued. In another case, treatment with ciprofloxacin for 7 days resulted in improvement when instituted 2 weeks after a course of pefloxacin that was associated with tendon injury [40]. Most authors, however, do not recommend rechallenge with any fluoroquinolone, because recurrence has occurred even when the agent is switched [34]. Recovery is described as occurring in a mean of 60 days (range 2–600). Sequelae have been reported in as many as 13% of patients, including pain on exertion as long as 1 year after the event [40].

Legal implications

Adverse drug reactions continue to cause injury and harm to patients regardless of careful patient evaluation, prescription, and drug administration. New drugs always represent unknown risks; sometimes infrequent but serious adverse reactions only

become apparent after prolonged postmarketing surveillance. Musculoskeletal injury with fluoroquinolones is a good example. Increasing numbers of cases are being reported in the literature, including events secondary to newer-generation agents [30,31,34]. Tendon disorders associated with the use of fluoroquinolones have even been described as one of the most frequent serious reactions to these agents [41]. Patients who are at risk are becoming easier to identify, although underreporting remains a problem [42]. Thus, incidences of these events and specific documented patient risk factors may not fully reflect the impact on those who have received the agents. It is the responsibility of the physician to be aware of the risks of fluoroquinolones when prescribing to patients [42]. The widespread prescribing of ciprofloxacin for anthrax prophylaxis after September 11th, 2001 is a good example of potential overuse, which could be paired with inadequate patient evaluation in a time of fear. Fluoroquinolone-associated musculoskeletal injury has been documented in the literature for more than 20 years, suggesting that there has been ample opportunity to learn of this infrequent complication.

A physician's best defense in cases of malpractice or negligence is to demonstrate that practice was within a reasonable standard of care and that any deviations from approved indications were documented at the time of care with literature support [42]. Action against the practitioner may also be minimized by ensuring adequate patient education or "informed consent." Fluoroquinolone-associated musculoskeletal injury should be described to the patient, particularly those at risk, and signs or symptoms should be described so that patients understand what should prompt them to revisit the physician. Informed consent assumes

Table 3: Fluoroquinolone-associated tendinopathy in the hand

Age	Gender	Drug	Dose	Duration (d)	Tendon	Tendonitis	Unilateral/Bilateral	Rupture
67	N	Norfloxacin	800 mg qd	N	Long extensor of thumb	N	N	Y
34	M	Norfloxacin	400 mg bid	31	Flexor tendon sheath (finger)	Y	B	N
53	F	Ofloxacin	N	8	Achilles, finger, thumb, supra-spinal muscle	Y	B	N
55	M	Ciprofloxacin	N	N	Extensor hallucis longus of thumb	Y	B	N
68	F	Pefloxacin	N	2	Extensor tendons of two fingers	Y	N	Y

Table 3: (continued)

Age	Steroids	Onset (d)	Diagnosis	Recovery (wk)	Risk factors	Intervention	Sequelae	Country	Reference
67	N	4	N	N	Age	Surgery	N	France	[30]
34	N	post	Clinical	<1	Renal transplant, chronic renal failure	Dc drug	N	NZ Med J	[31]
53	Y inhaled beclomethasone	14 d post	Clinical	8	N	Acetaminophen	N	France	[33]
55	Y prednisone 20 mg d	2	N	4	Renal transplant, chronic renal failure	Dc drug	N	Switzerland	[29]
68	N	2	Clinical, radiography	104	? Long-term history of FQ use	Splint, surgery, physiotherapy	Y	France	[38]

Abbreviations: B, bilateral; dc drug, drug discontinued; F, Female; FQ, Fluoroquinolone; M, male; N, no/information not available; post, after drug discontinued; U, unilateral; Y, yes.

adequate provision of information, such that a reasonable person can make a rational decision with an understanding of the intervention, its risks and benefits, and any alternative course of action [43]. The physician has a duty to warn the patient regarding side effects, including uncommon ones with serious complications, such as fluoroquinolone-associated tendinopathy. A breach of this duty that causes harm is the basis for negligence [42].

Finally, when a drug does cause harm to a patient, the responsibility of the physician is to discontinue the agent or to investigate the cause of the harm [42]. In most cases of fluoroquinolone-associated musculoskeletal injury, the practice has been discontinuation of the agent and institution of a range of treatments, depending on the severity of the injury. Of concern is the report in the literature of a patient whose quality of life was sufficiently diminished that the individual committed suicide [30]. Caution must be practiced with regard to adequate patient assessment and intervention. Psychologic support may also be necessary.

Legal action may be minimized with careful patient evaluation when prescribing with regard to this increasingly reported adverse effect of fluoroquinolones, adequate patient education with consent, and rapid intervention when a patient demonstrates signs or symptoms of tendon injury.

Summary

Fluoroquinolone antibiotics are now well documented to cause serious tendinopathy. Tendinopathy is usually reported in the Achilles tendon but is also known to occur in other tendons, including those of the hand. Several risk factors should be kept in mind, including, most importantly, age, prior tendon injury with previous fluoroquinolone use, and use of corticosteroids. Careful consideration must be given to prescribing these agents and to treating musculoskeletal injury secondary to fluoroquinolones.

References

[1] Zhanel GG, Walkty A, Vercaigne L, et al. Fluoroquinolones in Canada: a critical review. Can J Infect Dis 1999;10:207–38.

[2] Zhanel GG, Ennis K, Vercaigne L, et al. Critical review of fluoroquinolones: focus on respiratory infections. Drugs 2002;62(1):13–59.

[3] Mandell LA, Marrie TJ, Grossman RF, et al. Canadian guidelines for the initial management of community-acquired pneumonia: an evidence-based update by the Canadian Infectious Diseases Society and the Canadian Thoracic Society. Clin Infect Dis 2000;31:383–421.

[4] Bartlett JG, Dowell SF, Mandell LA, et al. Practice guidelines for the management of community-acquired pneumonia in adults. Clin Infect Dis 2000;31:347–82.

[5] Wilton LV, Pearce GL, Mann RD. A comparison of ciprofloxacin, norfloxacin, ofloxacin, azithromycin and cefixime examined by observational cohort studies. Br J Clin Pharmacol 1996;41: 277–84.

[6] van der Linden PD, van der Lei J, Nab HW, et al. Achilles tendonitis associated with fluoroquinolones. Br J Clin Pharmacol 1999;48:433–7.

[7] Lafon M. Tendinopathies et fluoroquinolones. Concours Med 1993;115:819–25.

[8] Donck JB, Segaert MF, Vanrenterghem YF. Fluoroquinolones and Achilles tendinopathy in renal transplant recipients. Transplantation 1994; 58(6):736–7.

[9] Leray H, Mourad G, Chong G, et al. Ruptures spontanées du tendon d'Achille après transplantation rénale: rôle des fluoroquinolones. Presse Med 1993;22(36):1834.

[10] Zabraniecki L, Negrier I, Vergne P, et al. Fluoroquinolone induced tendinopathy: report of 6 cases. J Rheumatol 1996;23:516–20.

[11] Le Huec JC, Schaeverbeke T, Chauveaux D, et al. Epicondylitis after treatment with fluoroquinolone antibiotics. J Bone Joint Surg [Br] 1995; 77B:293–5.

[12] Cattaneo F, Serna M, Stoller R. Fluoroquinolone associated tendon rupture and bilateral tendinitis in a hemodialysis patient and two renal transplant recipients. Kidney Int 1990;50:1429.

[13] Bailey RR, Kirk JA, Peddie BA. Norfloxacin-induced rheumatic disease. N Z Med J 1983; 93:590.

[14] van der Linden PD, Sturkenboom MCJM, Herings RMC, et al. Fluoroquinolones and risk of Achilles tendon disorders: case-control study. BMJ 2002;324:1306–7.

[15] Jorgensen C, Anaya JM, Didry C, et al. Arthropathies et tendinopathie achilénne induites par la péfloxacine. Rev Rhum 1991;58(9):623–5.

[16] Beuchard J, Rochcongar P, Saillant G, et al. Tendinopathie achilénne bilatérale chronique à la péfloxacine, sans rupture spontanée, traitée chirurgicalement. Presse Med 1996;25:1083.

[17] Casparian JM, Luchi M, Moffat RE, et al. Quinolones and tendon ruptures. South Med J 2000;93(5):488–526.

[18] Petersen W, Laprell H. Insidious rupture of the Achilles tendon after ciprofloxacin-induced tendinopathy. A case report [abstract]. Unfallchirurg 1998;101(9):731–4 [in German].

[19] Simonin MA, Gegout-Pottie P, Minn A, et al. Pefloxacin-induced Achilles tendon toxicity in rodents: biochemical changes in proteoglycan synthesis and oxidative damage to collagen. Antimicrob Agents Chemother 2000;44(4):867–72.

[20] Pouzard F, Bernard-Beaubois K, Thevenin M,

et al. In vitro discrimination of fluoroquinolone toxicity on tendon cells: involvement of oxidative stress. J Pharmacol Exp Ther 2004;308:394–402.

[21] Kashida Y, Kato M. Characterization of fluoroquinolone-induced Achilles tendon toxicity in rats: comparison of toxicities of 10 fluoroquinolones and effects of anti-inflammatory compounds. Antimicrob Agents Chemother 1997; 41(11):2389–93.

[22] O'Neil MJ, Smith A, Heckelman PE, editors. The Merck index. An encyclopedia of chemicals, drugs, and biologicals. 13th edition. Whitehouse Station (NJ): Merck; 2001.

[23] Kahn M-F, Hayem G. Tendons and fluoroquinolones: unresolved issues. Rev Rhum [Br] 1997; 64(7–9):437–9.

[24] Stahlmann R. Clinical toxicological aspects of fluoroquinolones. Toxicol Lett 2002;127:269–77.

[25] Deresinski S. Fluoroquinolones and tendinopathies [comment]. Available at: http://www. hospital-consult-pda.com/PDAima78.htm. Accessed November 18, 2004.

[26] Williams RJ, Attia E, Wickiewicz TL, et al. The effect of ciprofloxacin on tendon, paratendon, and capsular fibroblast metabolism. Am J Sports Med 2000;28(3):364–9.

[27] Khaliq Y, Zhanel GG. Fluoroquinolone-associated tendinopathy: a critical review of the literature. Clin Infect Dis 2003;36:1404–10.

[28] Pierfitte C, Royer RJ. Tendon disorders with fluoroquinolones. Therapie 1996;51:419–20.

[29] Jagose JT, McGregor DR, Nind GR, et al. Achilles tendon rupture due to ciprofloxacin. N Z Med J 1996;109(1035):471–2.

[30] Melhus A, Apelqvist J, Larsson J, et al. Levofloxacin-associated Achilles tendon rupture and tendinopathy. Scand J Infect Dis 2003;35(10): 768–70.

[31] Haddow LJ, Chandra Sekar M, Hajela V, et al. Spontaneous Achilles tendon rupture in patients treated with levofloxacin. J Antimicrob Chemother 2003;51:747–8.

[32] Gold L, Igra H. Levofloxacin-induced tendon rupture: a case report and review of the literature. J Am Board Fam Pract 2003;16(5):458–60.

[33] Kowatari K, Nakashima K, Ono A, et al. Levofloxacin-induced bilateral Achilles tendon rupture: a case report and review of the literature. J Orthop Sci 2004;9:186–90.

[34] Burkhardt O, Kohnlein T, Pap T, et al. Recurrent tendonitis after treatment with two different fluoroquinolones. Scand J Infect Dis 2004;36(4): 315–6.

[35] Fleisch F, Hartmann K, Kuhn M. Fluoroquinolone-induced tendinopathy: also occurring with levofloxacin. Infection 2000;28:256–7.

[36] Chaslerie A, Bannwarth B, Landreau JM, et al. Ruptures tendineuses et fluoro-quinolones: un effet indésirable de classe. Rev Rhum Mal Osteoartic 1992;59:297–8.

[37] Tonolli-Serabian I, Mattei JP, Poet JL, et al. Rupture de la coiffe des rotateurs au cours d'un traitement par quinolone. Collection de pathologie locomotrice 1993;26:147–50.

[38] Schwald N, Debray-Meignan S. Suspected role of ofloxacin in a case of arthralgia, myalgia, and multiple tendinopathy. Rev Rhum [Br] 1999;66(7–9):419–21.

[39] Levadoux M, Carli PH, Gadea JF, et al. Rupture iterative des tendons extenseurs de la main sous fluoroquinolones. Ann Chir Main 1997;16(2): 130–3.

[40] Meyboom RHB, Olsson S, Knol A, et al. Achilles tendonitis induced by pefloxacin and other fluoroquinolone derivatives. Pharmacoepidemiology and Drug Safety 1994;3:185–9.

[41] Leone R, Venegoni M, Motola D, et al. Adverse drug reactions related to the use of fluoroquinolone antimicrobials. Drug Saf 2003;26(2): 109–20.

[42] Kaufman MB, Stoukides CA, Campbell NA. Physicians' liability for adverse drug reactions. South Med J 1994;87(8):780–4.

[43] Fink S, Chaudry TK. Medical characteristics of 61 unwarranted malpractice claims. South Med J 1995;88(10):1011–9.

CLINICS IN PLASTIC SURGERY

Clin Plastic Surg 32 (2005) 503–514

ELSEVIER
SAUNDERS

The Management of Web Space Contractures

Loree K. Kalliainen, MD[a,b,*], Warren Schubert, MD[a,b]

- Anatomic features of the web space
- Prevention of web space contractures
- Effects of first web space contractures
- Surgical techniques
  Skin grafts
  Local flaps
  Regional and free flaps

- *Management of first web space contractures*
- *Tissue expansion in the hand*
- Digital amputation as an important consideration
- Summary
- References

Web space contractures result from a variety of hand deformities: burns, neuromuscular deficiencies, scleroderma and rheumatoid arthritis, congenital anomalies, and traumatic soft tissue loss. Preventive measures can frequently be taken to minimize the effect and degree of web space contractures, but it is difficult to reverse a long-standing contracture with nonsurgical means. The likelihood that therapy and splinting alone prevent or reverse web contracture depends on the time from injury and depth of tissue involvement. Contracture may initially result from skin loss, but lack of motion may contribute to the pathology by promoting joint stiffness and muscle wasting or fibrosis. More extensive reconstruction is needed in these situations. This article reviews the anatomy and functional deficits associated with web contracture and summarize currently accepted surgical practices.

Anatomic features of the web space

The normal distal-most extent of the web skin is approximately at the midpoint of the proximal phalanx [1]. This has been more recently calculated by Richterman and coworkers [2] using X-rays. They calculated normal web height as a ratio between the distance from the distal ossification center of the metacarpal to the distal end of the web and the distal ossification center to the fingertip. They found significant differences between the second through fourth webs and between children of different ages. Limitations of their study are the need for serial X-rays in a population that normally does not need them; lack of consideration of the first web (most likely because of the rarity of this event); and unclear applicability to populations other than simple syndactyly. In one of the author's experience (LKK), the arc of the second through the fourth webs is that of a circle. If the hand is placed on a piece of paper and the distal ends of the webs are marked with the fingers completely abducted, the amount the abnormal web needs to be shortened is the distance from the existing to the predicted normal point on the arc. This does not follow for the first web but is useful for the other digits. Assuming that some web creep occurs, the depth is overcorrected by a few milli-

a Department of Plastic and Hand Surgery, Regions Hospital, USA
b Division of Plastic and Reconstructive Surgery, The University of Minnesota, Mail Stop 11503 B, 640 Jackson Street, St. Paul, MN 55101–2505, USA
* Corresponding author. Division of Plastic and Reconstructive Surgery, The University of Minnesota, Mail Stop 11503 B, 640 Jackson Street, St. Paul, MN 55101–2505.
E-mail address: loree.k.kalliainen@healthpartners.com (L.K. Kalliainen).

doi:10.1016/j.cps.2005.06.002

meters to create more of a straight line between the distal web heights.

Web skin receives its blood supply from dorsal and volar branches. Dorsal digital arteries are fed from perforating branches from the volar aspect of the hand through the intermetacarpal spaces and the dorsal carpal arch formed by connections between the dorsal carpal branches of the radial and ulnar arteries [3–5]. This arch is less consistent than that found volarly.

Dorsal sensory innervation is by the dorsal radial sensory and ulnar sensory branches. Volar innervation of the webs is by branches from the common digital nerves, which are the terminations of the median and ulnar nerves. The first web space is mostly innervated by the median nerve but receives contributions from the dorsal radial sensory nerve [3,6].

The extensor expansion is the terminal extent of the extensor digitorum communis tendons, with contributions from the lumbrical and interosseous muscles. It extends to the middle and distal phalanges. On the volar aspect of the hand, the palmar aponeurosis contains longitudinally directed fibers, the fibers of Legueu and Juvara [3,7], which bifurcate at the proximal extent of the fingers, fusing with the tendon sheaths and tissues around the metacarpophalangeal joints volarly and dorsally. They are the terminations of the deep fibers of the pretendinous fascia. Finger abduction is limited by Bourgery's transverse subcutaneous band, a component of the natatory ligament. This forms the distal extent of the web, and its arciform fibers create the arches between the fingers. These fibers become the volar digital septum of Grayson and the dorsal digital septum of Cleland [3]. Dupuytren's contractures are created in part by the aforementioned fibers at the level of the web and proximal phalanx, but a review of Dupuytren's diathesis is beyond the scope of this article. In the first web, discrete fibers travel in an anteroposterior direction and connect the volar and dorsal skin. These are superficial to the muscle fascia. The reader is directed to Zancolli and Cozzi's [3] atlas for deeper understanding of the anatomy of this region.

Prevention of web space contractures

Early postburn reconstructive surgery minimizes hypertrophic scar formation and muscle and joint disturbance, allowing faster healing. Decreasing the time the tissues spend in the inflammatory phase of healing potentially optimizes ultimate functional recovery. In patients with nerve injury or congenital neuromuscular problems, appropriate early splinting and passive range of motion exercises preserve muscle and joint compliance. Contracture prevention focusing on the first web has recently been reviewed by del Piñal and coworkers [8]. They stress techniques to reduce edema and optimize thumb positioning, and recommend splinting, timely wound debridement, and closure with stable tissues.

Multiple forms of splinting have been described: internal stabilization with K-wires, external static and dynamic splints, and pressure gloves. K-wire fixation may be useful for first web defects or where deeper tissue release was performed in addition to skin release. It is generally desirable to mobilize the tissues relatively quickly following contracture release, but for children or noncompliant adults, up to 2 weeks of K-wire fixation may be useful. By 2 weeks postoperatively, the skin grafts should be well adherent and vigorous active motion and dynamic splinting can be initiated [9,10]. Inexpensive dynamic splints for the first web have been described by Bhattacharya and coworkers (the clothespin) [10] and Kalisman and coworkers (Joint Jack) [11]. Both act as external spacers and allow for active motion. Adequate longitudinal pressure in the webs is difficult to achieve with compression gloves because of mobility of the glove with hand motion. Both Alexander and coworkers [12] and Cheng and coworkers [13] have used interdigital straps to optimize pressure within the web. Elastic bands are passed dorsovolarly and secured to a wristband. The longitudinal bands are tightened to maintain pressure in the web. Alexander and coworkers [12] believe that it is most important to focus forces on the dorsal aspect of the web. It may also be beneficial to insert silicone pads into the depth of the webs if there is difficulty in maintaining the glove's fit into the web. Splints and compression should be used until scars are supple.

In elective surgery involving the web it is important to make optimal incisions. Incisions should be at 45- to 90-degree angles to the web [14]. Incisions should not be made along the border of the web because this results in contracture and hooding.

Effects of first web space contractures

Jensen and coworkers [15] studied 125 normal hands to define the mean first web angle. They found that the angle decreased with age from 105 to 95 degrees ($P < .0001$), but there were no differences with respect to gender or handedness. They simulated joint space contractures with splints and had volunteers do multiple repetitions of the Jebsen-Taylor test. They discovered that greater degrees of functional impairment were related to increasing web space contractures. Interestingly, there was some evidence that subjects were able to adapt to the contractures and improve their scores on certain subtests with practice. It follows that scores might worsen if multiple tissues were involved and if there were neuromuscular deficiencies or joint contractures. Alexander and coworkers [12] reviewed 190 web contracture releases performed by multiple surgeons. They compared the reconstructive techniques with outcome based on anatomic extent and cosmesis and were most satisfied with the V-M plasty. Unfortunately, functional outcome was not measured, and no mention was made on whether or not deep tissues were released.

Surgical techniques

It is generally advisable to create the surgical defect before harvesting skin grafts or distant flaps because the amount of tissue needed is often underestimated (especially by surgeons who do not perform these procedures frequently). As is true with other hand operations, tourniquet control is advisable. The tourniquet should be released before applying the skin graft so as to ensure hemostasis in the graft bed. Coverage may be achieved solely with Z-plasties or other local flaps, but the consideration should be made preoperatively and during skin preparation to the potential need for skin graft or flap harvest.

Skin grafts

Split-thickness skin grafts are not ideal as the sole reconstructive choice for web space contractures because of their propensity to contract during healing. Full-thickness skin grafts contract less and are generally more useful. Jang and coworkers [9] found that primary reconstruction with full-thickness skin grafts required fewer delayed reconstructive procedures than did primary split-thickness grafts. Full-thickness skin grafts are

useful in syndactyly and interdigital releases in combination with local flaps [**Fig. 1**].

Split-thickness skin grafts are harvested using standard techniques with a Padgett or Zimmer dermatome. Harvesting split-thickness skin grafts with a knife is an alternative when a dermatome is not available. Commonly used knives are the Blair-Brown, the Watson, the Cobbett, and Silver's Miniature. The split-thickness skin graft may be more useful as coverage for the donor site of a local transposition flap rather than as the primary coverage of a wound.

Multiple donor site dressings have been described and are left in place for 10 to 14 days until re-epithelialization occurs. Semiocclusive dressings, such as OpSite or Tegaderm, limit pain. Xeroform is relatively inexpensive but can be uncomfortable as it dries. One surgeon (WS) uses a combination of Xeroform covered by OpSite or Tegaderm and is pleased with how comfortable this is for patients. The authors recommend preparing the skin surrounding the donor site with benzoin to promote adherence of the OpSite or Tegaderm. Benzoin can cause skin irritation, and its use should be avoided in patients with known sensitivity to it and similar allergens [16]. Biobrane is a more expensive dressing but is reasonably comfortable and allows early motion.

Full-thickness skin grafts are widely used in syndactyly release to resurface adjacent sides of digits. Attempts should be made to match the recipient site skin in color and thickness with that of the donor if the luxury of choice is available. The ulnar and thenar eminences are good sources of small skin grafts as is the ulnar border of the distal forearm. The medial upper arm is also a reasonable site. If a male child has not yet been circumcised when evaluated by the hand surgeon but circumcision is planned, the foreskin is a very reasonable source of donor skin [17]. The foreskin can provide up to 25 cm² of tissue [18]. If groin skin is to be used as

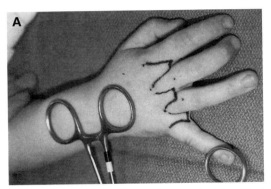
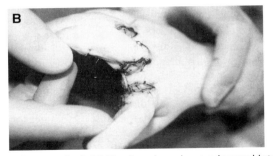

Fig. 1. (*A*) An example of incomplete syndactyly with dorsal flaps marked. (*B*) The flaps have been advanced into the webs with small full-thickness skin grafts at the bases of the fingers.

the source of a full-thickness skin graft for web reconstruction in the prepubertal child, the surgeon should try to stay lateral in the groin crease to avoid eventual inclusion of pubic hair. If large amounts of skin are needed, the lower abdomen is a good source. Inject the donor site with local anesthesia containing epinephrine to control local blood loss and provide for postoperative pain control. Hydrodissection with local anesthesia also makes graft elevation easier. One of the authors (LKK) has found it expedient to elevate the full-thickness skin graft in the lower level of the dermis, leaving a minimal layer of dermis down. Not elevating fat with the graft precludes the need to dissect fat off of it. The remaining dermis then can be incised around the borders of the donor site and the wound closed with the surgeon's preferred technique. There have been no problems with inclusion cysts or scar cosmesis using this technique. If fat is left on the deep surface of the graft, it can be easily be debrided by snapping fine hemostats onto the graft tips, hanging the graft over the surgeon's nondominant index finger, and using the curved surface of small, curved tissue scissors to defat the graft.

A recently described technique incorporates the use of Integra as a primary or secondary reconstructive template on which is placed a thin split-thickness skin graft [19,20]. The authors of that article believe that the use of Integra below a skin graft inhibits contracture and promotes improved range of motion. The limitations were lack of comparison with standard techniques. A learning curve is involved in the use of Integra, and it may be better to attempt this technique on less irregular parts of the hand or body than the digital web until facility is gained.

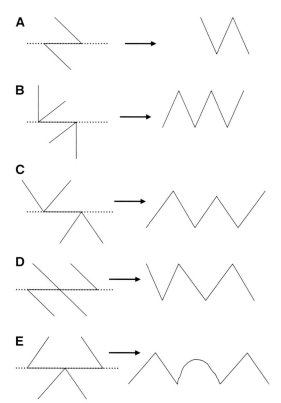

Fig. 2. Variants of Z-plasties. (*A*) The classic 60-degree angle Z-plasty. (*B*) The 90-90 degree four-flap Z-plasty. (*C*) The 120-120 degree four-flap Z-plasty. (*D*) The Z-plasty in series. (*E*) Double-opposing Z-plasties (butterfly flap). The dotted line refers to the axis of contracture. The figures on the right reflect the appearance after flap rotation.

Local flaps

Local random or pedicled flaps more closely match native web space tissue but may be in short supply, especially in burn or trauma situations. Local flaps are classically described as transposition, rotation, and advancement flaps. Transposition flaps are defined as flaps that require closure of their donor site and may "jump" over an area of uninvolved tissue. They can either be random, in which a named vessel is not included, or axial, containing a known vessel. Examples of the random transposition flap include the rhomboid (Limberg or Dufourmentel); the Z-plasty and its variants [**Fig.** 2]; and the bilobed flap [21–23]. Multiple axial transposition flaps have been described; the most useful ones for web space reconstruction include the first and second dorsal metacarpal artery flaps [4]. These flaps are based on the first and second dorsal metacarpal arteries. These run along the radial and ulnar as-

pects of the second metacarpal and overlie the first and second dorsal interossei, respectively. The flaps can be designed with a distal skin island on the proximal pedicle or as a larger cutaneous flap, which does not have the pedicle skeletonized proximally. Distally based dorsal island flaps have also been described for coverage of the web [4,5,24].

Rotation flaps are random and rely on the subcutaneous vascular plexus instead of a single vessel. They are dissected below dorsal veins and superficial to cutaneous nerves. Local tissue pliability is required. Back-cuts with excision of a small Burrow's triangle can increase their effective length, but care must be taken not to compromise the base width. Rotation flaps need to be larger than their recipient site, and pure rotation flaps are not generally useful for the reconstruction of web space defects.

Advancement flaps use local tissue to close the wound, but the tissue does not pivot. Advancement flaps are random or axial and are commonly used in hand reconstruction. They include the V-Y [Fig. 3], the V-M [Fig. 4], and the Moberg flaps. The Moberg flap is best used for reconstruction of thumb tip defects and is minimally applicable in the setting of web space contractures.

The local flaps that have been discussed extensively in the literature for the reconstruction of web contractures are primarily Z-plasties and combinations of Z-plasties with advancement flaps. Mustardé [25] described the jumping man flap, which has been modified into the five-flap by Hirshowitz and coworkers [26] [Fig. 5]. V-M flaps have been described by Alexander and coworkers [12], Lewis and coworkers [27], and Onishi and coworkers [28]. Three-flap web-plasties have been described by Ostrowski and coworkers [29] and Housinger and coworkers [30] [Fig. 6]. Housinger's "goalpost" flap is effectively an advancement of a rectangular tissue flap with rotation of small flaps from its distal end along its sides. The flap can either be advanced dorsal to volar or the reverse. The apex of the rectangular flap is marked at the edge of the web, and a linear extension is made to the point of desired advancement of the flap. A "T" extension is then made at the far end of the extension parallel to the line of the web. The rectangular flap is advanced and secured in place, and the flaps created by the "T" are rotated into the web alongside the advancement flap. V-Y advancements have been used for syndactyly correction by Savaci and coworkers [31] and Sherif [32]. Savaci and coworkers

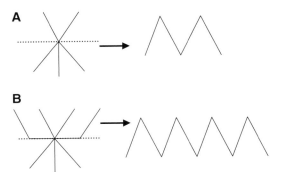

Fig. 4. V-M advancement flaps. (*A*) Standard V-M flap. (*B*) Seven-flap V-M variant described by Suliman [38]. The dotted line refers to the axis of contracture. The figures on the right reflect the appearance after flap advancement.

[31] described dorsal and volar V-Y flaps to meet in the center of the web [see Fig. 3A]. Sherif described an island flap advanced in a V-Y fashion to resurface the web [see Fig. 3B].

Local flaps are elevated in the relatively avascular plane deep to the dermis and superior to paratenon. Vascular arborization occurs in the subdermis, so a small amount of fat should be left on the flap to avoid turning the flap into a full-thickness skin graft. Dissection can be performed sharply with a knife or by blunt spreading with scissors. Littler scissors are useful because of their combination of delicate slightly blunted tips and sturdiness. When dissecting with scissors, insert them into the subdermal plane closed and then open them. Beware of closing the scissors while their tips are encased within the tissue for fear of damage to neurovascular structures. Elevate the tissue in a plane parallel with the edge of the flap so as not to dig oneself into a hole. The use of electrocautery dissection is common, but if the tissue is delicate or has been injured previously, the heat cone may cause further microscopic injury. Dissection in the proper plane loses minimal blood. Tissue that has been burned but has healed and is mature can be used for Z-plasties and local flaps as long as undermining is minimal. Care must be taken to use a minimal-touch technique when handling this tissue.

Regional and free flaps

Regional or free fasciocutaneous flaps may have greater bulk than is desirable. One of the more commonly used regional flaps is the groin flap [Fig. 7]. This is especially useful if a soft tissue envelope is required and if there is a later need for tendon transfers or free functioning muscle transfers. The groin flap and the random abdominal or chest wall flap have the benefits of supple

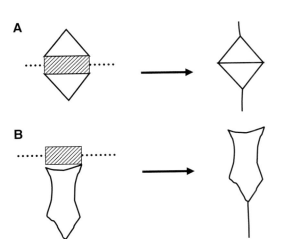

Fig. 3. V-Y advancement flaps. (*A*) Opposing V-Y islands as described by Savaci and coworkers [31]. (*B*) V-Y island advancement as described by Sherif [32]. The dotted line refers to the axis of contracture. The shaded area represents excised scar tissue. The figures on the right reflect the appearance after flap advancement.

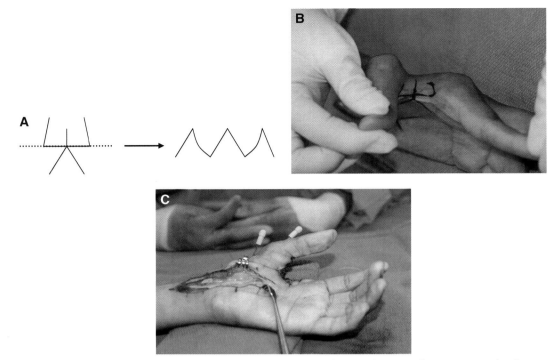

Fig. 5. The five-flap "jumping man" flap. (*A*) The dotted line refers to the axis of contracture. The figure on the right reflects the appearance after flap rotation. (*B*) Preoperative end-on markings. (*C*) Immediate postoperative result.

tissue, minimal donor defect, and large size, but their downsides include soft tissue bulk and discomfort during the 2- to 3-week time in which the extremity is secured to the body wall. Both normal and mature burned tissue can be used for these flaps. If done in children, the authors have found it feasible to apply an external fixator between the

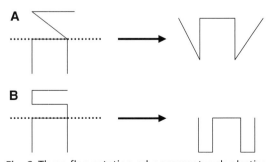

Fig. 6. Three-flap rotation-advancement web-plasties. (*A*) Triangular flaps of tissue are rotated around the advanced rectangular flap. (*B*) Rectangular flaps of tissue are rotated around the rectangular flap. The flaps in (*B*) may be more tenuous and care should be taken in elevating these flaps in tissue that has previously been injured. The dotted line refers to the axis of contracture. The figures on the right reflect the appearance after flap rotation.

forearm and iliac crest. The cross-arm flap is also a reconstructive option for first web defects. It may be more comfortable than the groin and abdominal flaps. The injured arm is crossed to the contralateral upper arm. A flap in the shape of the defect is drawn on the upper arm, and the inferior half is elevated and sutured to the dorsal aspect of the web defect. After a 2- to 3-week period, the flap is divided and the superior aspect rotated into the volar web defect. In the aforementioned cases, the flap may need to be debulked of soft tissue to optimize digital motion and appearance. This may need to be done in several stages to avoid devascularizing the tissue.

If distant tissue is sought because local tissue is unavailable, efforts should be made to use the thinnest flaps possible for web reconstruction. The web most amenable to reconstruction with free tissue transfer or regional flap is the thumb-index. The other interdigital spaces are too narrow to have large amounts of tissue interposed and yet retain function. The best options for first web reconstruction are the reverse radial forearm flap, posterior interosseous artery flap, dorsalis pedis free flap, or temporalis free flap [33,34]. If added tissue bulk is desired for concomitant bone or tendon exposure, the lateral arm flap, scapular or parascapular flap, and various muscle free flaps are

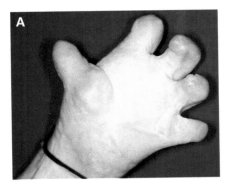
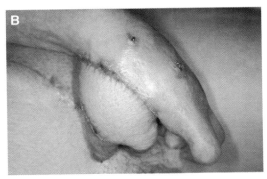
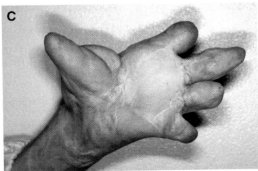

Fig. 7. (*A*) Preoperative view of young woman with severely burned hand and first web contracture. (*B*) After elevation and inset of groin flap. Notice that the groin skin had been burned and grafted but was mature. (*C*) Improved first web width after flap detachment.

reasonable options. In situations where there is extensive digital bony comminution and soft tissue loss, covering the injured tissues with a "mitten" of soft tissue and later creating webs with local tissue rearrangement or full-thickness skin grafts is a reasonable option. Even mature burn tissue can be used for such a purpose [35,36]. Partial release of the intermetacarpal ligaments may be considered to increase hand span in cases of amputation at the level of the metacarpal heads [Fig. 8].

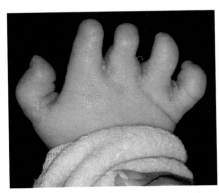

Fig. 8. Web deepening using local flaps and grafts in child with congenital brachydactyly caused by amniotic bands.

Management of first web space contractures

First web contracture can create functional deficits in the use of the hand [15]. The degree and impact of functional impairment has not been published for web contracture of the fingers, but it seems logical that the deficiency is less for an incomplete syndactyly than for a tightly adducted thumb. For minor contractures only involving skin, the Z-plasty and tissue advancement variants are useful techniques [Fig. 9]. Fraulin and Thomson [37] measured the gain achieved by four-flap and five-flap Z-plasties and concluded that the 120-degree four-flap Z-plasty doubled the deepening compared with the five-flap. The seven-flap plasty is a type of V-M advancement flap that has recently been described by Suliman [38] for use across large joints. Whereas there is not enough room between the fingers for this flap, it could be useful in the first web [see Fig. 4B].

If the contracture is significant with poor quality of the soft tissue envelope, resurfacing the defect requires a larger quantity of higher-quality tissue (ie, more normal in consistency). Pedicled flaps used for resurfacing the first web have been described rotating ulnarly from the dorsal aspect of the thumb [39] or radially from the dorsal aspect of the index finger and proximal phalanx and

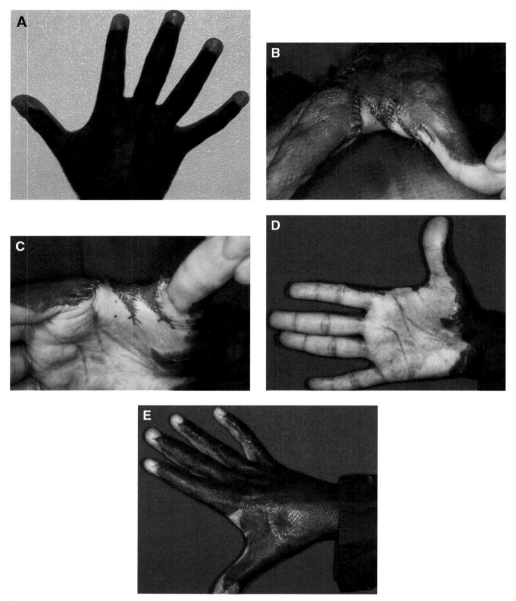

Fig. 9. (*A*) Preoperative view of thumb-index web contracture. (*B*) Immediate view after web deepening with five-flap plasty, dorsal view. (*C*) Volar perspective. (*D*) Postoperative view of resolved thumb-index web contracture, volar view. (*E*) Note hypopigmentation on dorsal view of (*D*).

metacarpal [40]. The web defect is created by incising the web at a 90-degree angle to the line of contracture. Soft tissues are released as needed. A full description of the technique of muscle and joint contracture release is beyond the scope of this article. The length of the flap needed is estimated using a template of gauze held in place at the pivot point, the base of the metacarpal. Both flaps have wide bases extending from the base of the thumb to the base of the middle finger metacarpal. Elevation is at a level superior to the exten-

sor paratenon. Care is taken to maintain the veins within the flap to promote drainage. The donor site is generally covered with a split- or full-thickness skin graft. One group advocated the use of undermining the dorsal skin of the hand to close the donor site [41]. The tourniquet should be deflated before complete closure because the collection of a hematoma beneath the flap can cause tissue necrosis. One author recommends the use of a K-wire to maintain full palmar abduction of the thumb for 3 weeks [40]. The pseudokite flap is a variant of the rhomboid flap, which can be used to resurface the first web space [42]. It is an axial flap based on the first dorsal interosseous artery on the dorsoradial shaft of the second metacarpal. The key technical point of this flap is to maintain the vascular supply by staying deep to the aponeurosis of the first dorsal interosseous muscle. A more ulnar flap is then elevated to close the donor defect, and this site is closed primarily. This flap is a variant of the bilobed flap, also a reconstructive option for this location [Fig. 10]. It is important to create the defect first, and then estimate flap length with a gauze sponge. It may be necessary to carry the flap up to or beyond the index metacarpal joint to obtain adequate length.

Cosmetic restoration has been described for patients with atrophy of the first web space resulting from ulnar nerve deficits caused by war injuries and leprosy [43,44]. Ghobadi and coworkers [43] used free fat grafts with initial overcorrection. Although perfect symmetry was not achieved and the final volume on the operated side was less than that of the normal side, patients were satisfied, volume maintenance was achieved at a mean follow-up of 5 years, and complications were minimal.

Duerksen and Virmond [44] described the insertion of carved solid silicone implants in 15 hands with atrophy caused by leprosy. They saw one complication caused by an oversized implant. Neither technique improves hand function.

Tissue expansion in the hand

Tissue expansion has wide application in the trunk and scalp but is used less frequently in the extremities because of the perception of increased risk of complications. Depending on the size of the area undergoing expansion, either small off-the-shelf expanders or custom-made expanders may be used. Complications of tissue expansion include pain, seroma, hematoma, infection, and exposure [45].

Several case series examining the use of tissue expanders in the hand and upper extremity have been reported. No complications were noted by four authors who had small series of patients in whom expanders were used to treat first web deformities and recurrent syndactyly [46–49]. Basic principles followed include subcutaneous placement of the expander on the dorsum of the hand with a buried port proximal to the expander; delay

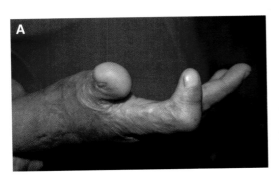
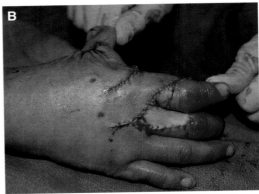
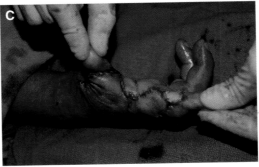

Fig. 10. (A) Thumb-index contracture with index flexion contracture in young adult burned 15 years prior. The index finger was malrotated, but the proximal interphalangeal joint had remodeled to allow anteroposterior flexion; there was no scissoring. (B) Bilobed flap elevated from the index and middle fingers. Full-thickness skin grafts were used to cover the donor defects on the index and middle fingers. (C) A full-thickness graft was used to cover the volar proximal interphalangeal joint of the index finger.

of initiation of expansion for 2 weeks; injection of small volumes of saline once or twice a week (5–10 mL aliquots per expansion); and removal of saline if there was evidence of excess pressure on the skin. One author (Borenstein) used a K-wire temporarily to maintain the web space following reconstructive surgery. Rates of complications in larger series range from 6% to 31% [50,51].

External tissue expanders have been described [52,53]. They have been promoted to be easy to use, well-tolerated by patients, and inexpensive but all indications have yet to be prospectively analyzed.

Digital amputation as an important consideration

The ultimate way to address a web space contracture, especially in a hand with severe burns, is to perform a digital amputation. It is often easy to become seduced into consideration of various modalities of web space reconstruction before seriously considering whether the patient may be better off with the amputation of a digit. This is particularly true when considering the serious burn and scar contracture of the index and small fingers. A ray amputation may improve both function and aesthetics.

In the case of a significant first web space contracture, where the function of the index finger is also significantly compromised, a ray amputation may result in a significant increase in space of the first web space. Skin from the index finger may also be used as a filet flap in the release of dorsal or volar hand contractures.

In the case of a significant burn scar with a stiff small finger, it is unlikely that the patient will achieve good function, regardless of the patient's motivation and the extent of postoperative hand therapy. The therapy is painful and the strength of the muscles too weak to gain meaningful active range of motion. In one of the author's 14 years of experience with burn hand reconstruction (WS), he has never had a patient who regretted secondary ray amputation of the contracted index or small digit.

Although there may be some benefit to giving the patient a trial period of hand therapy, early introduction of the concept of amputation as an alternative treatment may lead to an earlier and better acceptance of amputation as a treatment option. In many cases, early amputation may obviate unnecessary therapy and pain on a digit that has little chance for improvement, and allow faster rehabilitation, with a concentration of therapy on salvageable structures. Use of the skin from the fifth digit as a filet flap may be an important consideration for the release of other hand contractures [Fig. 11].

Summary

Whether congenital or acquired, basic principles must be followed in the management of web space contractures. Nonoperative methods are often effective in preventing or limiting the degree of web contractures if initiated early after the traumatic event. Nonoperative methods include early splinting and passive and active range of motion exercises. If operative intervention is required for established contractures or for conditions where contractures are likely to form, the options that allow for durable coverage and minimal postoperative contracture formation are the most desirable. Many variations and combinations of Z-plasties, V-Y, and V-M advancements have been described. The surgeon should follow principles of reconstruction and be versed in several options to optimize the outcome. The first web space has the added challenge of the need for thumb motion in multiple planes. Local rotation-advancement flaps are useful for minor skin contractures, but greater degrees of adduction require larger amounts of

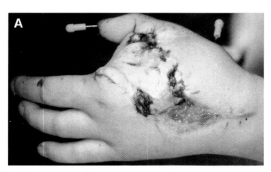
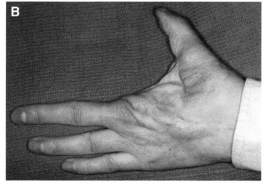

Fig. 11. The index finger was not salvageable and there was a complex dorsal wound. (*A*) Acute wound with filet flap. (*B*) Well-healed filet flap several years after the original procedure.

high-quality tissue, such as that of a regional flap or free tissue transfer. These procedures should be done in the acute phase in trauma situations where it is obvious that tissue loss leads to first web contracture.

References

[1] Moss ALH, Foucher G. Syndactyly: can web space creep be avoided? J Hand Surg [Br] 1990; 15:193–200.

[2] Richterman IE, DuPree J, Thoder J, et al. The radiographic analysis of web height. J Hand Surg [Am] 1998;23:1071–6.

[3] Zancolli EA, Cozzi EP. The retinaculum cutis of the hand. In: Zancolli EA, Cozzi EP, editors. Atlas of surgical anatomy of the hand. 1st edition. New York: Churchill Livingstone; 1992. p. 1–135.

[4] Dautel G, Merle M. Direct and reverse dorsal metacarpal flaps. Br J Plast Surg 1992;45:123–30.

[5] Chang LY, Yang JY, Wei FC. Reverse dorso-metacarpal flap in digits and web-space reconstruction. Ann Plast Surg 1994;33:281–9.

[6] Moore KL. The upper limb. In: Clinically oriented anatomy. Baltimore: Williams & Wilkins; 1980. p. 764–807.

[7] Bilderback KK, Rayan GM. The septa of Legueu and Juvara: an anatomic study. J Hand Surg [Am] 2004;29:494–9.

[8] del Piñal F, García-Bernal F, Delgado J. Is posttraumatic first web contracture avoidable? Prophylactic guidelines and treatment-oriented classification. Plast Reconstr Surg 2004;113: 1855–60.

[9] Jang YC, Kown OK, Lee JW, et al. The optimal management of pediatric steam burn from electric rice-cooker: STSG or FTSG? J Burn Care Rehabil 2001;22:15–20.

[10] Bhattacharya S, Bhatnagar SK, Pandey SD, et al. Management of burn contractures of the first web space of the hand. Burns 1992;18:54–7.

[11] Kalisman M, Chesher SP, Lister GD. Adjustable dynamic external splint for control of first web contracture. Plast Reconstr Surg 1983;71:266–7.

[12] Alexander JW, MacMillan BG, Martel L. Correction of postburn syndactyly: an analysis of children with introduction of VM-plasty and postoperative pressure inserts. Plast Reconstr Surg 1982;70:345–54.

[13] Cheng JC. Dynamic pressure therapy for scars in the finger web spaces. J Hand Surg [Am] 1991; 16:176–7.

[14] Yu HL, Chase RA, Strauch B. Skin incisions in hand surgery. In: Yu HL, Chase RA, Strauch B, editors. Atlas of hand anatomy and clinical implications. 1st edition. St. Louis: Mosby; 2004. p. 87.

[15] Jensen CB, Rayan GM, Davidson R. First web space contracture and hand function. J Hand Surg [Am] 1993;18:516–20.

[16] Scardamaglia L, Nixon R, Fewings J. Compound tincture of benzoin: a common contact allergen? Australas J Dermatol 2003;44:180–4.

[17] Oates SD, Gosain AK. Syndactyly repair performed simultaneously with circumcision: use of foreskin as a skin-graft donor site. J Pediatr Surg 1997;32:1482–4.

[18] Mak AS, Poon AM, Tung MK. Use of preputial skin for the release of burn contractures in children. Burns 1995;21:301–2.

[19] Dantzer E, Queruel P, Salinier L, et al. Dermal regeneration template for deep hand burns: clinical utility for both early grafting and reconstructive surgery. Br J Plast Surg 2003;56: 764–74.

[20] Frame JD, Still J, Lakhel-LeCoadou A, et al. Use of dermal regeneration template in contracture release procedures: a multicenter evaluation. Plast Reconstr Surg 2004;113:1330–8.

[21] Lister GD, Gibson T. Closure of rhomboid skin defects: the flaps of Limberg and Dufourmentel. Br J Plast Surg 1972;25:300–14.

[22] Furnas DW. Z-plasties and related procedures for the hand and upper limb. Hand Clin 1985;1: 649–65.

[23] Hudson DA. Some thoughts on choosing a Z-plasty: the Z made simple. Plast Reconstr Surg 2000;106:665–71.

[24] Quaba AA, Davison PM. The distally-based dorsal hand flap. Br J Plast Surg 1990;43:28–39.

[25] Mustardé JC. The treatment of ptosis and epicanthal folds. Br J Plast Surg 1959;12:252.

[26] Hirshowitz B, Karev A, Rousso M. Combined double Z-plasty and Y-V advancement for thumb web contractures. Hand 1975;7:291–3.

[27] Lewis RC, Nordyke MD, Duncan KH. Web space reconstruction with a M-V flap. J Hand Surg [Am] 1988;13:40–3.

[28] Onishi K, Maruyama Y, Chang CC. Further application of VM-plasty. Ann Plast Surg 1987; 18:480–7.

[29] Ostrowski DM, Feagin CA, Gould JS. A three-flap web-plasty for release of short congenital syndactyly and dorsal adduction contracture. J Hand Surg [Am] 1991;16:634–41.

[30] Housinger TA, Ivers G, Warden GD. Release of the first web space with the "goalpost" procedure in pediatric burns. J Burn Care Rehabil 1993;14: 353–5.

[31] Savaci N, Hosnuter M, Tosun Z. Use of reverse triangular V-Y flaps to create a web space in syndactyly. Ann Plast Surg 1999;42:540–4.

[32] Sherif MM. V-Y dorsal metacarpal flap: a new technique for the correction of syndactyly without skin graft. Plast Reconstr Surg 1998;101: 1861–6.

[33] Upton J, Havlik RJ, Coombs CJ. Use of forearm flaps for the severely contracted first web space in children with congenital malformations. J Hand Surg [Am] 1996;21:470–7.

[34] Woo SH, Seul JH. Optimizing the correction of severe postburn hand deformities by using ag-

gressive contracture releases and fasciocutaneous free-tissue transfers. Plast Reconstr Surg 2001; 107:1–8.

[35] Yongwei P, Jianing W, Junhui Z, et al. The abdominal flap using scarred skin in the treatment of postburn hand deformities of severe burn patients. J Hand Surg [Am] 2004;29:209–15.

[36] Pribaz JJ, Pelham FR. Use of previously burned skin in local fasciocutaneous flaps for upper extremity reconstruction. Ann Plast Surg 1994; 33:272–80.

[37] Fraulin FOG, Thomson HG. First webspace deepening: comparing the four-flap and five-flap Z-plasty. Which gives the most gain? Plast Reconstr Surg 1999;104:120–8.

[38] Suliman MT. Experience with the seven flap-plasty for the release of burns contractures. Burns 2004;30:374–9.

[39] Sandzén SC. Dorsal pedicle flap for resurfacing a moderate thumb-index web contracture release. J Hand Surg [Am] 1982;7:21–4.

[40] Friedman R, Wood VE. The dorsal transposition flap for congenital contractures of the first web space: a 20-year experience. J Hand Surg [Am] 1997;22:664–70.

[41] Marble K, Fudem G. First web space release with the dorsal hand rotation flap: closing the donor site. Ann Plast Surg 1995;35:83–5.

[42] Foucher G, Medina J, Navarro R, et al. Correction of first web space deficiency in congenital deformities of the hand with the pseudokite flap. Plast Reconstr Surg 2001;107:1458–63.

[43] Ghobadi F, Zangeneh M, Massoud BJ. Free fat autotransplantation for the cosmetic treatment of first web space atrophy. Ann Plast Surg 1995; 35:197–200.

[44] Duerksen F, Virmond M. Carvable silicone rubber prosthetic implant for atrophy of the first web in the hand. Lepr Rev 1991;62:436–7.

[45] Argenta LC. Tissue expansion. In: Georgiade GS, Riefkohl R, Levin LS, editors. Georgiade plastic, maxillofacial and reconstructive surgery. 3rd edition. Baltimore: Williams & Wilkins; 1997. p. 87–98.

[46] Morgan RF, Edgerton MT. Tissue expansion in reconstructive hand surgery: case report. J Hand Surg [Am] 1985;10:754–7.

[47] Fernandez-Villoria JM, Abad Morenilla JM. Tissue expansion for thumb and first web space reconstruction. J Hand Surg [Am] 1994;19:663–4.

[48] Coombs CJ, Mutimer KL. Tissue expansion for the treatment of complete syndactyly of the first web. J Hand Surg [Am] 1994;19:968–72.

[49] Borenstein A, Yaffe B, Seidman DS, et al. Tissue expansion in reconstruction of postburn contracture of the first web space of the hand. Ann Plast Surg 1991;26:463–5.

[50] Meland NB, Loessin SJ, Thimsen D, et al. Tissue expansion in the extremities using external reservoirs. Ann Plast Surg 1992;29:36–9.

[51] Zoltie N, Chapman P, Joss G. Tissue expansion: a unit review of non-scalp, non-breast expansion. Br J Plast Surg 1990;43:325–7.

[52] Brongo S, Pilegaard J, Blovqvist G. Clinical experiences with the external tissue extender. Scand J Plast Reconstr Surg Hand Surg 1997; 31:57–63.

[53] Ogawa Y, Kasai K, Doi H, et al. The preoperative use of extra-tissue expander for syndactyly. Ann Plast Surg 1989;23:552–9.

ELSEVIER
SAUNDERS

CLINICS IN
PLASTIC
SURGERY

Clin Plastic Surg 32 (2005) 515–527

The Burned Hand: Optimizing Long-term Outcomes with a Standardized Approach to Acute and Subacute Care

Robert Cartotto, MD, FRCS(C)[a,b,*]

A burn to the hand, whether it is in isolation or associated with a major systemic thermal injury, continues to pose one of the greatest challenges to the surgeon and the rehabilitation team. Burns to the hand are common and are excessively represented relative to other parts of the body. At the Ross Tilley Burn Centre, of 970 acute burn admissions between January 1, 1998 and December 31, 2003, burns to one or both hands were present in 57% of cases. Other burn centers report similar or higher incidences of hand burns, ranging from 54% to 90% of all burn admissions [1–3]. Furthermore, even though the total surface area of the hands is small, burns to the hand and their sequelae have an immense impact on subsequent func-

tional outcome, quality of life, and ability to return to work [4]. Finally, because the hand is a highly visible body part that cannot be hidden under clothing (much like the face), the aesthetic outcome and quality of scars on the hand are tremendously important to the patient and of much greater significance than burn scars on other parts of the body.

The purpose of this article is to promote the concept that good functional results can be reliably obtained for the burned hand when it is treated by an experienced team of burn surgeons, rehabilitation therapists, and nurses using a standardized protocol. This idea is by no means new [5–8], but it is worth repeating because the margin for error

a Ross Tilley Burn Centre, Sunnybrook and Women's College Health Sciences Centre, 2075 Bayview Avenue, Toronto, Ontario M4N 3M5, Canada
b University of Toronto, Toronto, Ontario, Canada
* Room D 710, Ross Tilley Burn Centre, Sunnybrook and Women's College Health Sciences Centre, 2075 Bayview Avenue, Toronto, Ontario, Canada M4N 3M5.
E-mail address: robert.cartotto@sw.ca

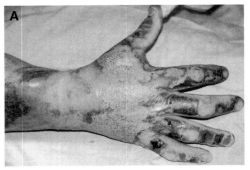 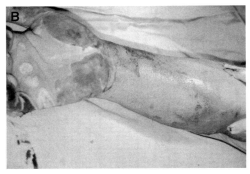

Fig. 1. Typical distribution of deep dermal and full-thickness burns to the hand, predominantly involving the dorsum (*A*), with slight palmar extension onto the thenar and hypothenar eminences and minor blistering of the palm (*B*).

in treating the burned hand is small, with substantial consequences for the patient who receives inadequate early treatment. For the purposes of this article, the author has reviewed late outcomes for patients on whom he operated and who were managed in a standardized fashion by the nurses and rehabilitation team between April 1, 1999 and April 1, 2004, where at least 1 year had elapsed since the patient's injury. This article focuses solely on the management and late outcomes of deep partial-thickness and full-thickness burns to the hand, which make up the bulk of hand burns that are seen day in and day out by the plastic surgeon. Sheridan and colleagues [6], in a study of 1047 hand burns, found that 48% of all hand burns fall into this category. Superficial burn injuries to the hand that heal within 2 weeks without the need for surgery (which composed 47% of all hand burns in Sheridan and colleagues' study) uniformly do well and are not included in this review. Similarly, severe fourth degree burn injuries that involve tendons, joint capsules, or bone are not included. These injuries are uncommon and make up only about 5% of hand burns [6]. Detailed reports on the management and outcomes of these severe injuries are available [1,6,7], and discussion of this subset of hand burns is beyond the limits of this article.

Injury patterns and anatomic considerations

The overwhelming majority of deep partial-thickness and full-thickness burns to the hand involve the dorsal aspects of the hand and digits; they occasionally creep onto the palmar surface of the hand along the hypothenar and thenar eminences [Fig. 1A]. Deep burns to the palmar surfaces are distinctly uncommon, first because the palm is relatively protected by the clenched-fist posture that is

often assumed at the time of the injury, and second by the thick palmar stratum corneum. Hence, palm burns, although they initially present with blisters and bullae [Fig. 1B], typically turn out to be superficial and heal spontaneously within 10 to 14 days. Normally, the dorsal skin is loose and mobile while the palmar and digital palmar skin is tightly attached to the underlying fascia. Hence, following a burn, edema tends to develop preferentially on the dorsal surfaces of the hand and fingers. The immediate consequence is that the skin's capacity to stretch over the flexed metacarpal-phalangeal (MCP) joint is compromised, and the digits assume an extended position at the MCP joints. Meanwhile, the relative strength of the wrist and digital flexors places the interphalangeal (IP) and wrist joints into gentle flexion. Finally, as the skin over the first dorsal web-space becomes tight, the thumb assumes an adducted position. The net result is a perilous hand posture, sometimes referred to as the "position of comfort," wherein the patient has a flexed wrist, extended MCPs, flexed IPs, and an adducted thumb [Fig. 2]. This position is a recipe for disaster, and active steps must be taken through

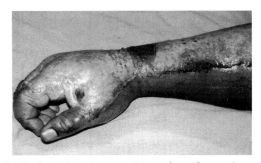

Fig. 2. The deleterious "position of comfort" adopted by the patient with a burned hand: slight wrist flexion, MCP extension, IP flexion, and adduction of the thumb.

all phases of acute and subacute treatment to combat the tendency for the hand to assume it.

Standardized approach to the management of the burned hand

Initial evaluation

Early clinical evaluation of the burned hand is secondary to careful attention to the primary and secondary survey of the burn patient as a whole. Immediate attention is always devoted to assessment of the airway, breathing, and circulation, followed by evaluation of the overall extent of the burn injury and the presence of associated trauma. Evaluation of the burned hand may then take place and should include careful observation of the depth and distribution of the burns on the hand. Identification of deep circumferential and near-circumferential burns is essential, because vascular compromise may develop from edema forming beneath the noncompliant eschar. Evaluation of both the *current* circulatory status of the hand and the *potential* for subsequent compromise of the hand circulation is the most important part of the physical examination. For example, near-circumferential deep dermal burns to the digits, when in isolation, may not pose much risk of impairing digital perfusion. However, in a patient with a major systemic injury where large volumes of resuscitation fluid may be administered, the same burn might warrant performance of prophylactic digital escharotomies. Hence, evaluation of the burned hand must always be within the context of the patient and the burn as a whole. The well-perfused burned hand is soft, warm, and pliable, with good nail-bed capillary refill, whereas a poorly perfused hand is cool, usually tense and swollen, and often held in a clawed position. Palpation of the radial pulse at the wrist should be complemented by Doppler examination of the ulnar, palmar arch, and digital pulses.

Inpatient versus outpatient care

Burns to the hands are considered an indication for referral to a burn center in the current practice guidelines of the American Burn Association [9]. The author's bias is to favor early inpatient burn unit care for all but the most minor hand burns. Prompt attention to splinting and elevation, pain control, and early range of motion (ROM) exercises, along with wound care and dressings by a skilled burn nurse, may avert early problems and a more prolonged recovery. Even if admission is only for 24 to 36 hours, the attention to early care may pay large dividends for patients by keeping them out of a vicious cycle of pain, swelling, and loss of hand mobility that may occur with inadequate early care. Outpatient care may be suitable in selected instances where the burn to the hand is limited and clearly superficial, where the patient is well motivated and compliant and has good support at home, and where pain is controlled with oral analgesics. Daily dressings are arranged through a home care nurse, and the patient is given careful instructions on hand mobilization exercises and the importance of hand elevation. Follow-up will initially be arranged roughly every 2 days but can be spread out if the patient is making good progress with healing and ROM at home.

Inpatient care: escharotomy

The decision to perform an escharotomy is based either on the presence of impaired hand or digital perfusion from circumferential or near-circumferential deep burns or on anticipated impairment of perfusion from these burns. The usual clinical signs of impaired perfusion in the burned hand include coolness, diminished or absent nail-bed capillary refill, a tense, nonpliable hand, often held in the claw position, and absence of wrist, palmar arch, or digital pulses by Doppler examination. Determining which hand or digits may have the potential for future development of circulatory compromise is more difficult and requires careful clinical judgment based on experience. Escharotomies performed for this indication are essentially prophylactic. The author generally will perform a prophylactic escharotomy when all the following conditions are met: (1) there are circumferential or near-circumferential burns that are clearly deep partial thickness (DPT) or full thickness (FT), (2) a large fluid volume resuscitation is expected based on the extent of the associated burn injury, and (3) serial reassessment of the hand may be difficult because of the patient's diminished level of consciousness, dressings, and the contributing effects of systemic hypothermia and hypotension.

The technique of forearm, hand, and digital escharotomy has been described in detail [2,6,10]. In an adult, the author does the procedure at the bedside after preparing with povidone-iodine and sterile draping. For digital escharotomies, the author prefers to use a number-15 scalpel or, if available, a needle point cautery. The standard cautery tip is not conducive to placing the incision in the exact plane deep to the eschar but superficial to the lateral edges of the digital extensor mechanisms. Standard cautery may be used on the hand and forearm. The digital incisions are placed on the radial side of the thumb and ulnar sides of the digits, mainly to avoid inadvertent injury to the digital nerve on the functionally more important pinch aspects of the fingers and thumb. The incision is made in a line dorsal to the neuro-vascular bundle but volar to the edge of the extensor mechanism. This line may be approximated by flexing the digit and marking the dorsal tip of each flexion crease, then connecting these points. Digital escharotomies may be extended onto the dorsum of the hand if necessary. Forearm escharotomies follow the standard midaxial lines, placing the ulnar incision just anterior to the medial humeral epicondyle to avoid injury to the ulnar nerve in the cubital tunnel. Some authors advocate placement of the forearm escharotomies first before proceeding to digital escharotomies, in the hope that adequate perfusion will be restored to the hand and digits by the proximal release alone, obviating a digital escharotomy [6,7]. Although this technique may work in certain instances, the author's experience is that full release to the distal extent of the burn is usually required. The escharotomy procedure is completed with meticulous hemostasis using cautery.

Inpatient care: standard nonoperative measures

The acute burn wound is debrided by removing any loose bits of tissue and by unroofing ruptured blisters and bullae. Intact blisters are left alone unless they are so large as to impair hand exercises and movement or make the hand dressing difficult. The hand is gently cleansed under tap water with chlorhexidine soap. Analgesia is usually provided by frequent administration of small doses (25 to 50 mcg every 5–10 minutes) of parenteral fentanyl as needed. If the burn is superficial, a tulle gauze layer (Jelonet, Smith, and Nephew, Hull, United Kingdom) is applied to the wound, followed by a single layer of saline-soaked gauze, then a layer of dry gauze. For deep partial-thickness and full-thickness burns, silver sulfadiazine is applied to the wound, again followed by the wet and dry gauze layers. The dressing is completed with a layer of kling bandages (Kendall: Tyco Healthcare, Mansfield, Massachusetts), and the digits are dressed individually with stretch net. Dressings are then changed twice a day. The importance of a good dressing is underemphasized. A dressing that is too bulky, where the hands are bunched together in a mitt, hampers hand therapy and early motion, whereas a dressing that is too tight can impair circulation, worsen edema, and limit hand mobility. The opportunity to have a good hand dressing [Fig. 3A] applied by a professional burn nurse is part of the author's rationale for favoring early admission (even if of short duration) for most hand burns.

Once dressed, the hand should be elevated at all times. Foam wedges or pillows work perfectly well [see Fig. 3A], but more elaborate devices that suspend the hand and forearm from overhead hooks [3] can be fabricated. Whatever the method, the most practical point is that the nurses caring for the patient be educated about the need to ensure that the patient's hand and forearm remain elevated at all times.

Within 12 hours of admission, the occupational therapist will make a thermoplastic resting splint to fit on the palmar surfaces of the dressed hand. The splint places the wrist in approximately 20° of extension, the MCPs in 70° to 90° of flexion, the IPs neutral, and the thumb abducted with the first web-space spread [see Fig. 3A]. The role of the

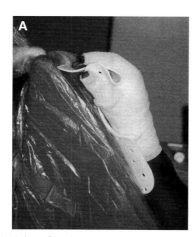
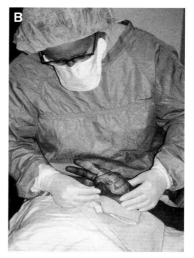

Fig. 3. Critical principles of early nonoperative management of the acutely burned hand, including a tidy dressing that does not impair mobility, hand elevation, and a "safe-position" resting splint (*A*), as well as regular stretching by an occupational therapist (*B*).

splint is to counteract the tendency of the hand to assume the deleterious position of comfort described earlier. As with hand elevation, it is essential that the bedside nurse understand the correct placement and application of the splint. Digital photographs [11] or drawings placed in the patient's room may help in this respect. The splint is only useful if it fits and is correctly applied to the hand.

At each dressing change, the occupational therapist takes the burned hand through active and gentle passive ROM exercises once the dressings are off [**Fig. 3B**]. The only contraindication to mobilization is the scenario of obviously deep burns to the dorsal fingers where there is suspicion of injury to the underlying extensor mechanism. IP flexion in this situation may promote rupture of the central slip and production of a boutonniere deformity and should therefore be avoided. Otherwise, mobilization of the hand and digits may proceed, and use of parenteral analgesics for the dressing change may allow the patient to participate in more effective hand therapy. Between hand dressing changes, patients who are able to cooperate are encouraged to remove their splints and do active ROM exercises throughout the day and early evening.

Inpatient care: surgical decisions

Within 24 to 48 hours of injury, the surgeon caring for the patient with burned hands needs to consider whether surgical intervention is necessary. Burns that are superficial and appear to be capable of healing within 2 weeks should be left alone and managed with the standardized conservative care principles described earlier. Following a short period of burn center admission, this care may continue on an inpatient basis or in an outpatient setting, depending on the individual case. As reported by Goodwin and colleagues [12], hypertrophic scarring after these burns is essentially nonexistent, and functional outcomes approach normal. At the other end of the spectrum, burns that are clearly full thickness and appear to have no possibility of healing within 2 weeks should be treated by excision and skin grafting at the earliest opportunity. The considerations in staging this procedure are discussed in the next section.

Disagreement and controversy continue to surround the management of burns to the hand that are neither clearly superficial nor obviously full thickness and where the ability to heal spontaneously by 2 weeks is uncertain. Most of these burns are deep dermal burns with a variety of possible clinical features, including pallor, hemorrhagic staining, sluggish but present capillary refill, and diminished sensation. The question is whether there are adequate viable dermal reserves to allow healing of the wound within 2 weeks, recognizing

that healing delayed beyond this point is associated with an increased risk for hypertrophic scars and contractures [13]. Two general approaches to these deep partial-thickness and "indeterminate" hand burns exist. The first and more aggressive approach is to excise and skin graft at an early stage, accepting that a proportion of these burns might have gone on to heal within 2 to 2.5 weeks without surgery. Proponents of this approach argue that early surgery results in less hypertrophic scarring and reduced need for secondary reconstruction [14,15]. An alternative and more conservative approach is to treat the hand expectantly and proceed with excision and grafting at 2 to 2.5 weeks if healing is not complete. Proponents of this approach suggest that, with an experienced rehabilitation team that can provide early vigorous physiotherapy, functional results with the conservative approach are as good as those with the early approach; moreover, frequency of late complications and need for secondary reconstructive surgery is no different [16–19].

The author uses an aggressive early surgical approach for practically all deep partial-thickness or "indeterminate" hand burns. In rare instances, where the hand burn is truly indeterminate but there is a reasonable suspicion that the burn may heal by 2 weeks, the hand is followed expectantly, continuing basic nonoperative care, to the 5-day point when it is reassessed. If the burn remains indeterminate or now appears deep, excision and grafting are performed between days 5 and 7. If, conversely, the wound has made progress and appears capable of healing by 2 weeks, dressings and physiotherapy continue.

The author favors the early surgical approach for deep partial-thickness and "indeterminate depth" hand burns for the following reasons: (1) early excision and closure of these burns will shorten the overall time to wound healing and result in fewer dressings, shorter hospitalization, and faster return to work and school [20]; (2) spontaneous healing of the deep partial-thickness and indeterminate depth burn is unpredictable, with nearly half of these burns remaining open at 3 weeks post–burn injury [20]; (3) wound closure at or beyond 2.5 to 3 weeks is associated with an unacceptably high risk of hypertrophic scar formation [13]; in two studies of conservative management, some patients did not spontaneously reepithelialize their wounds until 4 or 5 weeks postburn [16,18]; (4) some studies suggest that late complications and need for secondary reconstructive surgery are higher with the conservative approach [14,15], although it should be noted that two prospective randomized studies have suggested that early excision and grafting and the conservative approach produced comparable outcomes for this subset of hand burns [17,18]. In the prospective study by Salisbury and Wright [17], 12 of the 28 patients originally entered did not complete the study, leaving a comparison among only eight hands in the early excision group and 12 hands in the conservative group. Although total active motion (TAM), pinch strength, and grip strength were similar at 12-month follow-up in both groups, the findings should be interpreted with some degree of caution because of the high drop-out rate and small number of hands studied. In the prospective study by Edstrom and colleagues [18], which showed similar rates of late complications for conservatively versus aggressively managed deep dermal hand burns, the "early" excision group had surgery at approximately 14 days postburn, which is not a true measure of early excision. Also, although late complication rates in the groups were comparable, there were important qualitative differences in the nature of these complications [10,21]. Those in the conservative group mostly had diffuse hypertrophic scarring and unstable scars, which are, in the author's opinion, more difficult to treat than the complications seen in the early surgery group, such as web contractures and linear scar bands. Finally, and in contrast, several recent large series have shown that an aggressive approach to early surgical excision and closure of the deep partial-thickness burn wound of the hand is a reliable strategy with predictable results and good functional outcomes when undertaken by an experienced team of surgeons, nurses, and rehabilitation therapists using a standardized protocol [6–8].

In summary, the author's position is that the risk of operating unnecessarily on an "indeterminate" or deep dermal hand burn that might have healed on its own within 2 to 2.5 weeks is outweighed by the risks of waiting 2 weeks or longer for wound closure. The single most important goal is to have the wound healed and closed by 2 weeks postburn. In all cases, these concepts must be explained and discussed in an understandable manner with patients or their proxies, as part of obtaining informed consent for the procedure.

Surgery: sequence, timing, and priorities

Once the decision to operate has been made, consideration needs to be given to the staging and timing of surgery for the hand burns, as this will be influenced by the presence of associated burns and the medical status of the patient. If only the hands are burned, surgery should be done at the earliest opportunity. Each hand will require 2 to 2.5 hours of operating time, from harvest of the skin graft to completion of the dressing. Therefore, a bilateral procedure may be a lengthy operation unless two surgical teams can work simultaneously. When there are associated deep partial- or full-thickness burns on the forearm or upper arm, the author's preference is to excise and graft these burns simultaneously with the hand. The reason is that, when the arm and hand are done in separate stages, at the second stage a tourniquet may have to be placed over fresh grafts on the arm. Conversely, when the hand is done first, the freshly grafted hand is subjected to relatively aggressive manipulation and dependent positioning during the excision and grafting of the arm. Simultaneous grafting of the arm and hand is considerably more laborious than repairing the hand alone and is best performed as two procedures when it is bilateral, unless two operating teams are available.

When the patient has more extensive and potentially life-threatening burns, excision and closure of the large surface areas, such as the trunk and legs, always takes priority over surgery for the hands. In this situation, it is essential to plan the graft donor sites with care preoperatively. The author always uses unmeshed sheet grafts for the hand and reserves adequate donor sites for this purpose. When the patient's burn is so extensive as not to allow preservation of future donor sites for the hand, excision and grafting of the hand burns may need to wait until a donor site is healed and can be recropped. Alternatively, the hand burns could be excised early and temporarily covered with allograft or closed with a dermal regeneration template such as Integra (Integra Life Sciences Corp., Gainsborough, New Jersey) [22] until skin autograft sites become available. In certain situations, a critically ill and unstable patient may require debridement of hand and upper extremity burns. Here, the priority is rapid excision of the burns, deferring the time-consuming meticulous hemostasis and careful graft application that are mandatory for sheet autografting of the hand. Instead, the excised wounds may be rapidly and temporarily closed with a biosynthetic skin substitute

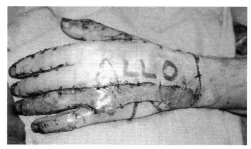

Fig. 4. Temporary coverage of an excised burn wound of the hand with cadaveric allograft.

such as Biobrane (Bertek Pharmaceuticals, Morgantown, West Virginia) or alternatively with cadaveric allograft [Fig. 4]. Later, when the patient has stabilized, definitive autografting may be performed.

Operative technique

After subcutaneous infiltration of the planned donor site with 1:500,000 epinephrine solution [23], skin grafts are harvested first. Obtaining a high-quality and adequately thick split-thickness graft of sufficient length and width is crucial to a successful outcome. Graft thickness is usually set between 0.014 and 0.016 of an inch. A randomized prospective study has found that harvesting very thick grafts (eg, 0.025 of an inch) conferred no advantages but was associated with significant donor-site healing problems [24]. The author has traditionally used the 4-in wide guard for the dermatome (Zimmer Instruments, Dover, Ohio), which will provide a sheet capable of covering approximately one half to two thirds of the hand dorsum and two or three adjacent digits. Recently, however, the author has switched to the 6-in wide dermatome (Padgett Instruments, Kansas City, Missouri) [Fig. 5A], which provides a sheet large enough to cover the entire dorsal hand and index, long, ring, and small digits simultaneously without a seam.

Next, debridement of the hand and digits begins. The areas to be excised are marked with Bonney's Blue. Then a tourniquet above the elbow is inflated to 250 mm Hg. In the author's experience, use of the tourniquet has significantly reduced operative blood loss during limb burn excision [23]. The wound margins marked with ink are now lightly scored with a scalpel [Fig. 5B], and tangential, layer-by-layer excision is performed using the Goulian blade, as originally described by Janzekovic [25] [Fig. 5C], the only variation being that tissue viability is based on gross appearance rather than on the bleeding pattern, as was originally described.

This technique is not as difficult as some might believe. Healthy dermis has a pristine, pearly-white appearance, with no evidence of hemorrhagic staining. Healthy fat should have a pale yellow, moist appearance, whereas injured fat is typically golden-brown, dry, and sometimes hemorrhagically stained. Finally, subdermal vessels should be demonstrated to be patent and not thrombosed. The author's team's skin-graft take rate for excisions done under tourniquet or with epinephrine tumescence, where they do not assess viability based on bleeding, is 96% [23], indicating that adequacy of excision can be reliably assessed without using the bleeding pattern. For most hand burns, the tangential technique works well and creates a fresh surgical wound, usually at the level of the deep dermis

or the upper fat, with preservation of the subcutaneous dorsal venous plexus of the hand [Fig. 5D]. Less often, generally when the burn is deep and involves the fat, with clear evidence of thrombosis of the subcutaneous veins, a plane of dissection must be obtained deep to the subcutaneous veins of the dorsal hand and digits but superficial to the paratenon over the extensor tendons. This procedure is most easily performed by sharp scalpel dissection with a number-15 blade. Attempting the tangential technique in this plane usually results in exposure of or injury to the extensor tendons. Sometimes it is necessary to interchange the tangential and sharp techniques, when different-depth burns are encountered as the excision proceeds. For the portions of the dorsal hand burn that creep in a palmar direction onto the hypothenar or thenar eminences, tangential excision may be continued. However, when there are more extensive full-thickness burns on the palm, sharp scalpel dissection of the eschar off the palmar fascia is the preferred technique.

If there are burns on the forearm, these are next excised, also tangentially while the tourniquet is still inflated, but now switching to the Braithwaite blade. Depending on the extent and distribution over the forearm, the author may elect to place a temporary Steinman pin through the distal radius and ulna and attach this pin to a horseshoe bracket that may then be suspended from an overhead hook, thus facilitating elevation of the limb [Fig. 5E]. This method of elevation may be used for excision of burns on the proximal arm as well, if necessary.

When excision is complete, the wounds are wrapped with Telfa pads (Kendall: Tyco Healthcare, Mansfield, Massachusetts) soaked in epinephrine/saline solution and secured with a circumferential wrapping of kerlex, while the tourniquet remains inflated. After 5 minutes, the tourniquet is deflated, and the laborious process of obtaining hemostasis begins. This process involves sequential application of epinephrine-soaked Telfa pads to the excised wounds, alternating with light use of cautery. The author relies heavily on time, epinephrine, and elevation of the hand and less on cautery in obtaining hemostasis. This part of the procedure is the most time consuming and requires patience and persistence.

When hemostasis is complete, the unmeshed sheet grafts are applied to the wound in longitudinal strips. With grafts from the 4-in dermatome, one sheet may be wrapped around the ulnar border of the hand and then stretched radially to cover about two thirds of the dorsal hand and the small through long digits. A second sheet is used to cover the index finger, thumb, first web-space, and remaining dorsal hand, wrapping the sheet around

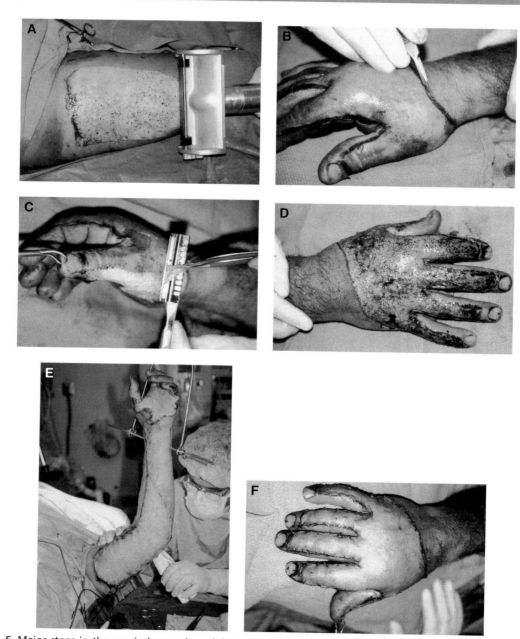

Fig. 5. Major steps in the surgical procedure. (*A*) Donor site following skin harvest with 6-in wide dermatome. (*B*) Scoring the marked margins of the burn wound to be excised. (*C*) Tangential debridement of the burn wound under tourniquet control. (*D*) Completed excision, following hemostasis, with patchy preservation of deep dermis. (*E*) Steinman pin and bracket elevation of the upper limb to allow excision and grafting of the remainder of the arm. (*F*) Sheet graft (6-in wide) sutured to wound. Note the absence of seams.

the thenar border of the hand if needed. If a 6-in wide graft is harvested, the sheet will cover the entire dorsal hand and index through small digits, with a small piece required to cover the thumb separately. In a smaller hand, the 6-in piece may cover the entire hand and all five digits, and only a small dog-ear fold needs to be trimmed along the proximal edge of the graft [**Fig. 5F**]. The thickest

parts of the harvested grafts should be used on the palmar surfaces if possible. When the palmar wound is large, the author applies a full-thickness graft here, using a split-thickness graft to close the full-thickness donor site.

Checking the length–tension relationships of the sheets is essential before making the final cuts to the graft for it to fit the defect. The wrist, MCPs,

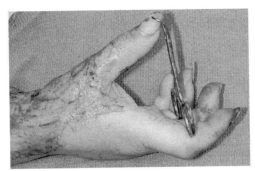

Fig. 6. Demonstration of principle of placing first web-space in maximum spread before cutting graft to fit excised burn wound, ensuring adequate length and tension of graft across the web-space.

and IPs are flexed, with the sheet loosely applied to make sure the graft is long enough over the dorsum of the hand and digits to allow composite flexion without undue tightness of the graft dorsally. Similarly, the first web is placed in maximal spread when applying the graft here [**Fig. 6**]. Usually the author marks the planned cuts in the grafts with Bonney's Blue, while an assistant holds the hand and digits in the desired posture or stretch positions. The grafts are next cut to fit and are sewn in with multiple 4-0 plain gut sutures.

The dressing is now applied and is as important as any single part of the procedure described thus far. The hand is positioned in the safe ("intrinsic plus") position with the wrist extended about 20°. Tulle gauze followed by saline-soaked gauze, dry gauze, and then kling is applied. A palmar plaster of Paris splint is made to hold the hand and wrist in the safe position and secured with a tensor bandage. It is essential that the hand remain elevated through this part of the procedure and that, once dressed, the hand be immediately placed on a pillow or foam wedge to keep it elevated, even before the patient is moved off the operating table. The author believes that strict attention to this step

helps to reduce the chance of early hematoma formation under the sheet grafts.

Postoperative care

The hand remains dressed and within the plaster splint for 5 days, at which time the dressing is taken down and the grafts are inspected. The occupational therapist (OT) sees the patient at this time, and active ROM exercises are started. Gentle passive ROM exercises are added at the discretion of the OT, depending on the stability of the grafts and the progress of the patient. A thermoplastic safe-position resting splint may be made, depending on the patient's tendency to adopt the position of comfort hand posture. Generally this is done for the more severely ill patients who may not be able to comply with self-positioning and self-stretching. Most patients do not require a splint at this stage, especially when they are compliant and proceeding well with their exercises. All patients receive custom fitted compression gloves within 2 to 3 weeks following surgery [**Figs. 7A, B**], and these gloves are worn for a minimum of 6 to 12 months. Silicone gel sheeting and elastomer web-space inserts may be applied under the compression glove at the discretion of the OT. Outpatient hand therapy is arranged for virtually all patients, and patients are followed by the attending surgeon and OT at the multidisciplinary postburn clinic for at least 6 to 12 months.

The primary principles, interventions, and goals discussed here are summarized in Table 1.

Late outcomes

For the purposes of this article, the author has sought late follow-up data on all hand burns that he has treated surgically in the past 5 years and that have received the standardized approach to treatment described earlier. All data are reported as the mean ± standard deviation unless otherwise

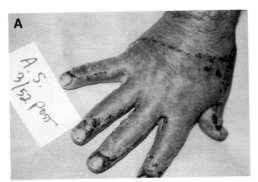

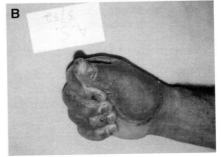

Fig. 7. Early postoperative result at 3 weeks in patient shown in **Figs. 5**A–D, F, demonstrating stable wound closure (A) and good early hand mobility (B). This hand is now ready to be fitted with a compression glove.

Table 1: Management of the burned hand

Intervention	Goals
Early evaluation of hand burn depth/distribution Emphasis on current and anticipated vascular status Escharotomies	Maintain or restore perfusion to the hand
Inpatient care for most of hand burns, (elevation, expert dressings, analgesia, hand therapy, safe-position splinting)	Optimization of early hand motion by effective edema reduction, wound care, pain control, and early hand therapist involvement
Early surgical excision and autografting for deep dermal and full-thickness hand burns	Stable wound closure by 14 days post burn
Early mobilization at 5 days post grafting, with safe-position splinting for patients unable to comply with self-positioning and stretching	Return to pregrafting range of motion within a few days of dressing take-down
Outpatient rehabilitation therapy, including compression gloves as soon as grafts can tolerate pressure, liberal use of silicone gel sheeting and inserts.	Return to preinjury strength and mobility

Summary of the major interventions and goals of each intervention, in chronologic order, for the management of the acutely burned hand.

indicated. Between April 6, 1999 and April 4, 2004, the author operated on 70 patients (113 hands) with deep partial- and full-thickness hand burns. Late follow-up data could not be obtained on 41 patients because of lost contact (23), refusal (16), or death (2). The large geographic region serviced by the author's regional burn center accounts for the large number of losses of contact. The vast majority of patients who declined follow-up were back at work, claimed to be happy with their hand function, and believed reassessment was unnecessary. Follow-up on the remaining 29 patients (48 hands) was at a mean of 32 months (range 12–60 months) postinjury. This group of patients had a mean age at follow-up of 40 ± 12 years and had sustained an original percentage of total body surface area burn of 22 ± 19 (range 1–70). Unilateral injuries occurred in 10 patients, with bilateral injuries in 19 patients, and 70% had involvement of the dominant hand. Surgery on these patients was performed at 6.5 ± 3.1 days postburn. Debridement and grafting of palmar burns (thenar and hypothenar borders only) was required in 8 of 48 hands (17%). There were no acute complications, and none of the patients required repeat debridement or grafting of their hands. Length of stay in the burn center was 40 ± 39 days (range 6–159 days).

Key pinch strength was 11 ± 3 kg (normal=11 kg) [26]. Grip strength was 45 ± 13 kg (normal=51 kg) [26]. Digital total active motion (TAM) was 217° ± 43° for the index, 236° ± 37° for the long finger, 227° ± 33° for the ring finger, and 222° ± 37° for the small finger, with an overall mean digital TAM of 225° ± 38°, which is within the accepted functional range of 220° to 230° [27]. Spread of the first web-space was 69° ± 19°, whereas mean spread of the second, third, and fourth webs was 47° ± 13°.

Patients also completed the Michigan Hand Questionnaire (MHQ) [28], which is a patient-based subjective evaluation of hand function, appearance, and pain. The six scales of the MHQ assess overall function, activities of daily living, pain, work performance, aesthetics, and satisfaction. Raw scores are normalized and range from 0 (worst) to 100 (best). Hence a higher score indicates a better subjective outcome, with the exception of pain, where a low score indicates minimal pain and a high score more severe pain. The author and colleagues have recently identified that scores on several categories of the MHQ (pain, work performance, satisfaction) correlate significantly with scores on the Test d'Evaluation des Membres Supérieurs des Personnes Agées, which is an objective detailed as-

Table 2: Michigan Hand Questionnaire results

Overall function	ADL	Work	Aesthetics	Satisfaction	Pain
71 ± 25	80 ± 19	63 ± 34	53 ± 24	70 ± 26	29 ± 26

Mean ± standard deviation Michigan Hand Questionnaire results for the domains of overall hand function, activities of daily living (ADL), work capacity, aesthetics, patient satisfaction, and degree of pain.

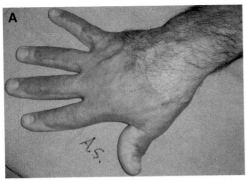
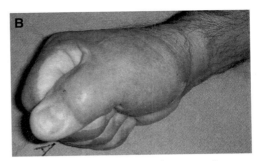

Fig. 8. Result at 8 months postinjury for patient shown in **Figs.** 5A–D, F and **Fig. 7**, demonstrating a smooth but slightly hyperpigmented graft, with an overall good aesthetic outcome on dorsum (*A*) and full digital range of motion (*B*).

sessment of hand function administered by an OT [29]. The MHQ scores, shown in Table 2, were moderate to good across all domains with the exception of aesthetics. Pain scores were low, indicating little residual pain.

The low aesthetic scores appeared somewhat unusual, because many patients had what the author considered good aesthetic outcomes with flat, evenly pigmented and supple grafts [Figs. 8–10]. However, in light of recent work the author and colleagues have done comparing a patient's assessment of the burn scar with their own objective evaluation of the scar, the low MHQ scores for aesthetics are perhaps not so surprising [30]. In a study involving burn patients, they showed that there was no relationship between the patient's subjective opinion of the scar quality and their own objective measurement of the scar using the Vancouver Scar Score, which is a validated and widely used tool for quantification of burn scar quality [30]. Because the hands are highly visible and not easily hidden under clothing, aesthetic concerns are important and should be considered

in the decision to proceed or not with surgery in the deep partial-thickness and indeterminate subset of hand burns. No study has compared aesthetic outcomes between the conservative and aggressive approaches, but the author's bias is that aesthetic results are better with grafting, especially when the skin is pigmented, because secondarily healed hand burns in these patients are prone to spotty and heterogeneous pigmentation.

Finally, among this group of patients, 76% had successfully returned to work at 9.4 ± 8.9 months (range 2–36 months), with 74% back at their original job, 15% on modified duties, and 11% at new employment.

These late outcomes are comparable to those of much larger studies, most notably that published by Sheridan and colleagues [6] on 1047 acute hand burns. In that study, the standardized approach used attention to acute splinting and elevation, with early ROM exercises, early excision and sheet grafting of deep partial- and full-thickness burns, and early motion initiated by day 7 postgrafting. Among patients with deep partial- and full-thick-

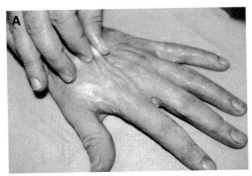
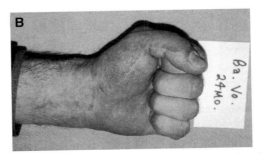

Fig. 9. (*A*) Result in a patient at 24 months postinjury, demonstrating loose, supple grafts on the dorsal surface. (*B*) Result in a patient at 24 months postexcision and grafting of dorsal hand burn, with full range of motion but slightly irregular graft surface on the thenar eminence.

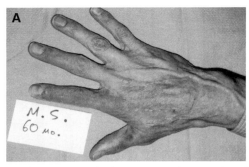
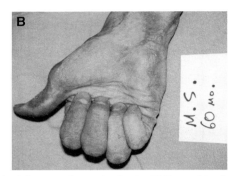

Fig. 10. Result at 60 months (5 years post–burn and grafting) for a patient who had a 60% total body surface area burn and underwent excision and grafting of full-thickness burns of the hands, demonstrating a good aesthetic outcome (*A*) and fully restored range of motion (*B*).

ness hand burns, 81% attained a normal functional result when assessed after a minimum of 6 months from their burn injury.

Summary

Good functional results may be reliably obtained for deep dermal and full-thickness burns of the hand when a standardized approach is used by an experienced team of burn surgeons, rehabilitation therapists, and nurses. The crucial aspects of this approach are (1) an emphasis on early inpatient care that focuses on wound care and dressings, strict hand elevation and splinting, and regular ROM exercises, (2) early excision and sheet grafting of deep partial- and full-thickness burns, with the goal being wound closure within 2 weeks postburn, and (3) aggressive and prolonged postoperative hand therapy and use of compression garments. These are not new concepts, but they are well worth repeating and emphasizing in view of the narrow margin of error in dealing with the burned hand.

Acknowledgments

The author thanks the nurses and rehabilitation therapists of the Ross Tilley Burn Centre for the skilled and dedicated care that they provide to our burn patients.

References

[1] Tredget EE. Management of the acutely burned upper extremity. Hand Clin 2000;16:187–203.
[2] Smith MA, Munster AM, Spence RJ. Burns of the hand and upper limb—a review. Burns 1998;24:493–505.
[3] Luce EA. The acute and subacute management of the burned hand. Clin Plast Surg 2000;27:49–63.
[4] Baker RA, Jones S, Sanders C, et al. Degree of burn, location of burn, and length of hospital stay as predictors of psychosocial status and physical functioning. J Burn Care Rehabil 1996;17:327–33.
[5] Greenhalgh DG. Management of acute burn injuries of the upper extremity in the pediatric population. Hand Clin 2000;16:175–86.
[6] Sheridan RL, Hurley J, Smith MA, et al. The acutely burned hand: management and outcomes based on a ten-year experience with 1047 acute hand burns. J Trauma 1995;38:406–11.
[7] Sheridan RL, Baryza MJ, Pessina MA, et al. Acute hand burns in children: management and long term outcomes based on a 10 year experience with 698 injured hands. Ann Surg 1999;229:558–64.
[8] Barillo DJ, Harvey KD, Hobbs CL, et al. Prospective outcome analysis of a protocol for the surgical and rehabilitative management of burns to the hands. Plast Reconstr Surg 1997;100:1442–51.
[9] Saffle J, editor. Practice Guidelines for Burn Care of the American Burn Association. J Burn Care Rehabil 2001;(Suppl):1S–69S.
[10] Salisbury RE. Acute care of the burned hand. In: McCarthy JG, May JW, Littler JW, editors. Plastic surgery. Philadelphia: WB Saunders; 1990. p. 5399–417.
[11] Van LB, Sicotte KM, Lassiter RR, et al. Digital photography: enhancing communication between therapists and nurses. J Burn Care Rehabil 2004;25:54–60.
[12] Goodwin CW, Maguire MS, McManus WF. Prospective study of burn wound excision of the hands. J Trauma 1983;23:510.
[13] Deitch EA, Wheelahan TM, Rose MP, et al. Hypertrophic burn scars: analysis of variables. J Trauma 1983;23:895–8.
[14] Burke JP, Bondoc CC, Quinby WC, et al. Primary surgical management of the deeply burned hand. J Trauma 1976;16:593–8.
[15] Magliacani G, Bormioli M, Cerutti V. Late results following treatment of deep burns of the hands. Scand J Plast Reconstr Surg 1979;13:137–9.
[16] Cole R, Shakespeare P, Rossi A. Conservative treatment of deep partial thickness hand burns—a long term audit of outcome. Br J Plast Surg 1992;45:12–7.

[17] Salisbury R, Wright P. Evaluation of early excision of dorsal burns of the hand. Plast Reconstr Surg 1982;69:670–5.

[18] Edstrom LE, Robson MC, Macchiaverna JR, et al. Prospective randomized treatments for burned hands: non operative vs operative. Scand J Plast Reconstr Surg 1979;13:131–5.

[19] Labandter H, Kaplan I, Shavitt C. Burns of the dorsum of the hand: conservative treatment with intensive physiotherapy vs. tangential excision and grafting. Br J Plast Surg 1976;29:352–4.

[20] Engrav L, Heimbach DM, Reus JL, et al. Early excision and grafting vs. non-operative treatment of burns of indeterminate depth: a randomized prospective study. J Trauma 1983;23: 1001–4.

[21] Edstrom LE, Robson MC, Macchiaverna JR, et al. Management of deep partial thickness dorsal hand burns: a study of operative vs. non-operative therapy. Orthop Rev 1979;8:27–34.

[22] Logsetty S, Heimbach DM. Modern techniques for coverage of the thermally injured upper extremity. Hand Clin 2000;16:205–14.

[23] Cartotto R, Musgrave MA, Beveridge M, et al. Minimizing blood loss in burn surgery. J Trauma 2000;49:1034–9.

[24] Mann R, Gibran NS, Engrav LH, et al. Prospective trial of thick vs standard split thickness skin grafts in burns of the hand. J Burn Care Rehabil 2001;22:390–2.

[25] Janzekovic Z. A new concept in the early excision and immediate grafting of burns. J Trauma 1970; 10:1103–8.

[26] Mathiowetz V, Kashman N, Vollard G, et al. Grip and pinch strength: normative data for adults. Arch Phys Med Rehabil 1985;66:69–72.

[27] Hunter JM, Mackin EJ, Callahan AD. Rehabilitation of the hand. 4th edition. St. Louis (MO): Mosby; 1995.

[28] Chung KC, Hamil JB, Walters MR, et al. The Michigan Hand Outcomes Questionnaire (MHQ): assessment of responsiveness to clinical change. Ann Plast Surg 1999;42:619–22.

[29] Umraw N, Chann Y, Gomez M, et al. Effective hand function assessment after burn injuries. J Burn Care Rehabil 2004;25:134–9.

[30] Martin D, Umraw N, Gomez M, et al. Changes in subjective vs objective burn scar assessment over time: does the patient agree with what we think? J Burn Care Rehabil 2003;24:239–44 [discussion: 238].

ELSEVIER
SAUNDERS

CLINICS IN
PLASTIC
SURGERY

Clin Plastic Surg 32 (2005) 529–536

Strategies for Nonrandomized Clinical Research in Hand Surgery

Brent Graham, MD, MSc

- Case-control studies
  Risk factors for scaphoid nonunion
- Cross-sectional study
  Risk factors for carpal tunnel syndrome
- Decision analysis
  Treatment options for cubital tunnel syndrome

- Health services research
  Complications of distal radius fractures
- Summary
- References

The randomized controlled trial is the gold standard for establishing best practice because of its capacity to neutralize the effect of both known and unknown sources of bias, which may remain uncontrolled in other research designs [1]. Although randomized trials have recently been increasingly used to answer clinical questions in surgery [2–6], issues of feasibility and, perhaps more importantly, generalizability continue to limit the routine use of this approach in hand surgery.

The cost of a properly designed and executed randomized clinical trial may be prohibitive. The costs in a randomized trial flow primarily from the process of subject recruitment, which usually takes much longer than anticipated [7]. Enrollment into a randomized trial that compares two treatments may be particularly slow, especially if one of the treatments under consideration is already well established. Although accrual into and retention in this type of study may vary depending on a number of factors, it should be assumed that only about 60% of individuals eligible for the study agree to participate after a full explanation of the nature of the trial. Of those who do agree to participate as many as 50% may drop out or be otherwise lost to follow-up. This means that only as few as 30% of

individuals initially eligible for enrollment complete the study. For planning purposes investigators may require access to a pool of potential participants about three times the size of their projected sample size. Identifying a large number of individuals who meet the inclusion criteria for the study may take an extended period of time, driving up the cost of the study. Significant costs may also be incurred from data collection, data security, and analysis [8,9].

A consideration of equal importance to that of cost is how well the results from the study generalize to other populations [10]. Generalizability is mainly affected by the composition of the study sample and the primary outcome measure of the study. The inclusion and exclusion criteria for enrolment into the study may result in the assembling of a cohort that is not representative of the population of interest [11]. Where the study population is narrowly defined, the results of the study may not be reproducible in other patients treated outside the context of the trial. The difference between outcomes observed in a randomized trial and those seen outside the trial setting is well recognized by clinical epidemiologists as the distinction between "efficacy" and "effectiveness." A treatment may be

University of Toronto/University Health Network Hand Program, Banting Institute, 100 College Street, M5G IL5 Toronto, Canada
E-mail address: brent.graham@utoronto.ca

0094-1298/05/$ – see front matter © 2005 Elsevier Inc. All rights reserved.
plasticsurgery.theclinics.com

doi:10.1016/j.cps.2005.06.001

shown to have efficacy in a trial where patients are closely supervised and side effects are recognized and treated but shown to have relatively lower effectiveness in a real world setting. This may result because patients discontinue or alter treatment or because other factors not accounted for in a trial (eg, comorbidities) may have an influence on the response to treatment.

The composition of the study sample may also be affected by a lack of consensus on any of a number of important issues related to the question under consideration. For example, the absence of widespread agreement on the diagnostic criteria for the condition of interest may result in a study sample that does not resemble the patient population treated by many clinicians. Unless there is agreement on the criteria for making the diagnosis of the condition of interest, the results of a methodologically sound study may not gain acceptance.

Similar issue must be considered in selecting an outcome measure. There must be general agreement that the outcome measured is meaningful [12]. A lack of consensus on which outcome is the most important may seriously reduce the impact of the study. Choosing multiple outcomes may result in ambiguous conclusions and also may reduce the feasibility of the study by necessitating the recruitment of a larger patient sample. This is frequently observed in studies in orthopedics where a number of impairment, radiographic, and patient-centered outcomes may be measured. When conflicting observations are made in these various domains the overall outcome of the study may be obscure and inconclusive.

Although often cited as an obstacle to a successful randomized trial, considerations related to ethical concerns [13,14] or the absence of equipoise in the surgical community [15] are actually smaller issues that can often be addressed in the design of a study with the assistance of the research ethics board in the sponsoring institution. Surgeons often have concerns about the standardization of procedures being tested in a randomized trial, but this is also frequently of lesser significance. In general, attempts at rigidly controlling technical aspects of a surgical trial should be avoided unless they are critical to the outcome of the trial. Excessive standardization may further reduce the generalizability of the study results. The important characteristics of prospective randomized trials are summarized in Box 1.

It is important to consider if the evidence resulting from a prospective randomized trial is sufficiently important to merit the cost or if the insight obtained using methods that are more susceptible to bias but which are more feasible and significantly less expensive is sufficient to address

Box 1: Summary of important characteristics of the prospective randomized trial

Advantages
  Controls for both known and unknown sources of bias
  Establishes cause and effect relationship
  Results are usually clearly understandable

Disadvantages
  Expensive
  Results may not generalize
  Usually limited to testing one variable

many, if not most, clinical issues. This has to be balanced against recognition of the sources, nature, and impact of bias within the various nonrandomized research methodologies that might be considered as an alternative to a randomized controlled trial.

Case-control studies

Many conditions encountered in hand surgery are relatively uncommon. Prospective cohort studies of any type are frequently unfeasible because of the length of time required to assemble the cohort. A case-control design is well suited to the study of rare or infrequently observed conditions. This is because this design starts with the condition of interest and then searches retrospectively for characteristics of the patient population that are more or less common than in the control group [16].

The main source of bias to be considered in a case-control method emanates from the process of identifying cases for inclusion in the study. Only cases that have been diagnosed and presented to the investigator are included. Individuals who have the condition but who remain undiagnosed or who may be referred to a different clinical setting may have some significant differences from the study sample; this may lead to some potentially important bias [17].

The choice of a control group is under the control of the investigators and represents another important potential source of bias in the case-control design. The objective is to choose controls that resemble the study sample except for the factors of interest. A poorly selected control group may have the effect of either increasing or decreasing the apparent importance of a particular characteristic of the study sample. The methods and assumptions used by the investigator in determining the controls should be made clear so that the reader of the study can decide where there may be bias. It is standard to identify at least two controls for every case.

The investigators have to recognize that case-control studies are retrospective. Because of their retrospective nature, case-control studies may also be biased by their reliance on predictor variables that are retrospectively measured in both the control group and the study sample [17]. These variables have been inaccurately or incompletely documented. The fact that the data have already been collected greatly reduces the cost of the study and, when carefully conducted, the case-control design represents a substantial improvement over a simple case series, mainly because of the comparison made with a control group.

The case-control design is often used to address questions of etiology. The results of a case-control study reflect the strength of an association between various factors and the condition of interest. As with many other nonprospective designs, a cause and effect relationship cannot be established but a strongly positive or negative association between the various factors and outcomes may allow some significant inferences to be made. Carefully designed, the case-control method may also be used to examine treatment. For example, one of the factors that may be linked to either a positive or negative outcome might be a specific treatment.

Risk factors for scaphoid nonunion

A case-control design could be used to study risk factors in the development of nonunion after fracture of the scaphoid, under most circumstances a relatively uncommon occurrence. Using this design the investigator assembles a sample of patients with a nonunion of the scaphoid and a control group of individuals who had successful healing of a scaphoid fracture. The control group might be matched with the study sample for a few variables that the investigators choose as important. In this instance these might include age and sex. The risk of bias in the control group is minimized if each case is matched against more than one control group. The potential predictor variables in this kind of study are such factors as mechanism of injury, fracture anatomy, various methods of treatment, or any other characteristic that the investigator believes is relevant.

Extraction of the data should occur without knowledge of the outcome (ie, without identifying if the case belongs to the study or the control group). Blinding the individual extracting the data from the cases minimizes the risk of bias in this part of the investigation. Frequently, the data extractor knows the outcome and this reduces the impact of the study because of the risk of bias this introduces. Where this is the case, the study is essentially reduced to two parallel cases series.

Once the data have been extracted, the cases can be attributed to either the case or control groups. The odds ratio is calculated for each of the variables of interest and the strength of association between each factor and the outcome of scaphoid nonunion is established. An association between any of these variables and the outcome of nonunion does not prove a cause and effect relationship; however, the demonstration of a strong relationship, for instance between fracture anatomy and outcome, suggests a linkage that can then be explored in a prospective study if sufficiently important.

Cross-sectional study

In a cross-sectional study the sample is examined at one point in time and without follow-up. The prevalence of the variable of interest can be estimated at the time of the study but, because there is no follow-up period, the incidence of the variables remains unknown.

Cross-sectional studies are usually relatively inexpensive because of the absence of any follow-up phase; however, they are only useful if the variable of interest is relatively common. Rare conditions require a large sample for a meaningful number of cases to be found. As a result, it may be difficult to find an association between the occurrence of interest and any potential predictor variables. Because of its retrospective nature, the cross-sectional study cannot establish a cause and effect relationship. Data from cross-sectional studies may be useful in demonstrating associations that can be studied in a prospective cohort to establish causality later.

The example of work relatedness and carpal tunnel syndrome was also cited in relation to the case-control design. In a case-control design, the diagnosis of carpal tunnel syndrome is identified in a group of workers and then their work history reviewed to search for specific exposures in comparison with a suitably selected control group without carpal tunnel syndrome. In contrast, study of this question in a cross-sectional study could take several forms. A study sample might be developed from among workers with a certain job description and the prevalence of carpal tunnel syndrome established in this group. A comparison could be made with the prevalence of carpal tunnel syndrome in one or more other samples taken from different work environments. Alternatively, a sample could be taken from the workforce of interest and the prevalence of carpal tunnel syndrome identified for each of the job descriptions within the sample. In either case a snapshot at one point in time is obtained. An association between a given particular work activity and carpal tunnel syndrome might be so strong that an etiologic link seems obvious or the association might be such that a prospective cohort, to establish whether carpal tunnel syndrome develops among workers with this job through time, might be warranted. Demonstration of a statistically significant association in the context of a prospective cohort study is evidence of an etiologic relationship.

Risk factors for carpal tunnel syndrome

A cross-sectional design could be used to explore the question of work-relatedness of a condition like carpal tunnel syndrome [18]. Carpal tunnel syndrome is considered a relatively common condition allowing it to be studied with a cross-sectional design.

The study group for a cross-sectional study could be drawn from a single workplace or from a larger cohort like workers within a particular industry. The investigators would identify the categories of work activity (eg, based on job description) and classify all the participants accordingly. The presence or absence of carpal tunnel syndrome would be determined in each participant according to criteria established by the investigators at the beginning of the study. These criteria might include self-reported symptoms, the judgment of a clinician, the results of electrodiagnostic tests, or some combination of these factors. Normally, prevalence studies are designed to maximize the sensitivity of the criteria used to identify the condition even though this is done at the expense of specificity.

The prevalence of carpal tunnel syndrome in each workplace category can be compared. If there seems to be a high prevalence of carpal tunnel syndrome associated with a particular work activity, a prospective cohort could be designed to determine whether exposure to this work resulted in development of the condition through time in comparison with a control group that was not exposed to the same work. This type of study is costly and time consuming but is necessary to prove causation. A prospective study is more likely to be successful to address a hypothesis generated by data from a cross-sectional design, however, than one resulting from anecdotal clinical experience alone.

Decision analysis

Clear evidence to guide decision-making is either absent or incomplete in most areas of medicine. There is usually uncertainty as to the best strategy for addressing a clinical problem because the potential approaches for dealing with the given problem often involve some type of trade-off. For example, one treatment may be considered more effective than an alternative treatment but is associated with more risk, discomfort, inconvenience, or expense. There may be a third treatment, which is intermediate between the other two with respect to some of these variables. A decision analysis is a quantitative method that can be used to help clinicians choose the best strategy under conditions of uncertainty [19]. Decision analyses are very inexpensive to perform and can also be very informative because of the explicit examination of all aspects of the question under consideration, which the decision analysis model requires. The key variables that influence the model and affect the decision can be fully explored in a sensitivity analysis [20]. In some instances, this characteristic of the decision analysis process may potentially provide more insight into the issue than is possible in the most carefully executed randomized trial.

There are three main steps in performing a decision analysis. First, the investigator develops a model of the clinical problem that includes all the relevant strategies for comparison. Obviously, there must be significant trade-offs in the use of any of the strategies under consideration. If one strategy is clearly the most effective and has the least downside with respect to cost, discomfort, morbidity, and complications, then a decision analysis is not required. Second, all of the potential outcomes for each strategy are also determined [21] together with the probability that each will occur. The third step is to establish the value of each of the potential outcomes. In decision analysis this value is usually expressed as the utility or desirability of the outcome. There are a number of methods that can be used to establish the utility of a health state but the two most important are the standard gamble and the time trade-off. A full discussion of these techniques is beyond the scope of this article but there are many articles in the literature that explore the value placed on different health states by patients and by normal healthy individuals [22–25]. The probability for any given outcome associated with each strategy, and the use of the various outcomes, can be estimated from the available literature [26]. The model uses this information to determine the best strategy for approaching the problem.

A potential weakness of the decision analysis concept is its dependence on data from the literature for the values given to the variables in the model. For example, for most instances where there is controversy about the best treatment for a given condition, a wide range of outcomes for each of the potential treatments have been reported in the literature. A decision analysis may be particularly useful in examining this type of problem because the uncertainty associated with each variable can be systematically explored using a sensitivity analysis [27,28]. In the sensitivity analysis each variable is varied throughout the entire range of plausible values to determine its effect on the choice of best strategy. This approach allows both an identification of the variables that have the most influence on the establishment of the best strategy and a quantification of the effect of each variable on the decision made by the model. For example, if a decision analysis comparing two treatments for a condition identifies the rate of a certain complication as the most important variable in establishing one of the treatments as the preferred strategy, the model can also determine at what level the preferred strategy changes to the alternative treatment. The clinician can decide whether the probability of the key complication is, in their hands, likely to be above or below this threshold value. This might lead to a decision to choose the alternative treatment.

Decision analysis has been used infrequently in clinical studies in surgery, although a few examples exist [29–32]. In hand surgery, decision analysis has been used to investigate treatment of early osteoarthritis of the wrist [33].

Treatment options for cubital tunnel syndrome

A randomized controlled trial to compare the potential surgical treatments for cubital tunnel is very difficult to carry out. Even if there is agreement on the diagnostic criteria for cubital tunnel syndrome and on the best outcome to measure to evaluate these treatments, the feasibility of carrying out a trial is limited. There are at least four surgical treatments that are all in common usage: (1) simple decompression, (2) medial epicondylectomy, (3) subcutaneous transposition, and (4) submuscular transposition. Even with an efficient outcome measure applied in a multicenter trial, a comparison of these four options is a substantial and costly undertaking.

In a decision analysis, a model comparing these four treatments is constructed by compiling all the published data on complications, perioperative morbidity, and outcome for each intervention. The model determines, based on these data, which treatment strategy is associated with the highest expected utility. The finding that one treatment has the highest expected use does not necessarily indicate that this is the best intervention under all circumstances but suggests which strategy is the best overall. The sensitivity analysis can indicate which variables have the largest impact on the model. This information can be used by clinicians to determine which treatment works best in their particular setting. Although the decision analysis does not provide as high a standard of evidence as a randomized trial, it is a methodologically sound approach to clinical controversies that are

not readily amenable to study in a randomized trial. In some ways, a decision analysis may be even more informative than a randomized trial because the sensitivity analysis is a unique dimension that may provide insights into the issue that are not possible in the context of a trial.

Health services research

Administrative databases that are assembled for purposes of administering expenditures for large health care entities often can be used to establish patterns of practice and associations of clinical importance [34–36]. These databases record important demographic information and general data relating to health services received by individuals included in the health care scheme. Although the data included are usually very general, observations made on such large datasets may be highly reliable. Administrative databases have been frequently used in the identification of regional variations in care [37], and recognition of these variations may provide interesting insights about the nature of and effect of medical services that prove to be clinically relevant. Like other methodologies capable of demonstrating associations, observations made on administrative databases usually cannot establish a cause and effect linkage between clinical phenomena. The size of most of these databases, however, means that the strength of association may be sufficiently large that causality may be strongly implied.

The key consideration when using administrative databases to address clinical research issues is to ask a question that can be answered using this methodology. It is important to understand the limitations of these databases.

Because most administrative databases are devised to monitor and record physician reimbursement, they are focused on interventions. As a result, codes for diagnoses may be less reliably recorded than those for operative procedures [38]. In some instances (eg, carpal tunnel syndrome) a surgical intervention is so directly linked to a diagnosis that the procedure may be considered a surrogate for the diagnosis. Cases that do not undergo an intervention, however, may not appear in the database, or be represented in a different area.

Administrative databases may also fail to distinguish bilateral conditions and repeated surgery for the same condition. This may be important in the study of conditions like carpal tunnel syndrome, where bilateral involvement is prevalent. If two codes for carpal tunnel release appear in the database for the same individual, it may not be possible to determine if this represents surgery for both limbs or repeated surgery on one hand where an initial release may have been unsuccessful. This may be less of a problem if there is a separate code for the revision procedure, and this has to be established by the researcher before conducting the study. The data may also be affected by errors in recording the codes for certain services; however, given the size of most databases, this is rarely a significant concern for most clinical research questions [38].

Given these considerations, researchers who use administrative databases require a good understanding of both patterns of care and the way in which a given database is assembled to develop an appropriate and informative research question. It is also important to be circumspect in interpreting the results of studies in this nature so that unwarranted conclusions are not made. With these provisos, however, important insights about the way care is administered and the effects of that care can be obtained, in most cases at relatively small expense, through the examination of large administrative databases.

Complications of distal radius fractures

One of the main complications of fracture of the distal radius is malunion. Treatment for a malunion of the distal radius requires surgical treatment in most instances where there are significant symptoms. The surgical procedures most likely to be performed for this problem include a corrective osteotomy of the radius, a shortening osteotomy of the ulna, or an excision of all or part of the distal ulna. In most payment systems, these procedures are associated with different payments and are identified by unique payment codes. These codes are likely be distinct from those associated with treatment of the acute fracture including open reduction and internal fixation, application of an external fixator, and treatment with closed reduction and cast immobilization.

An approach to investigating complications of fracture union in the distal radius using an administrative database starts with identifying all patients for whom a code has been entered for treatment of a distal radius fracture over a given time period. A unique numerical label identifies these patients so that confidentiality is very unlikely to be breached. Many administrative databases for physician reimbursement are linked to other databases that contain demographic information like date of birth, sex, location of residence and, in some cases, other diagnoses. From this information the composition of the study sample can be determined in moderate detail, including the presence of comorbid conditions. These cases can be classified by initial treatment because they are likely associated with codes to distinguish one treatment from another.

The next step is to determine the follow-up interval. Within this time frame the database is scanned for new codes associated with the corrective treatments identified at the beginning of the study. These data are compared with the initial study sample looking for the appearance of the same unique numerical labels, which identify individuals within the database, in both data pools. The implication is that the appearance of the patient within the second pool of data strongly suggests that they incurred a complication of the initial fracture that required treatment with one of the target procedures used to address malunion. In this way the overall rate of complication and the rate associated with each of the initial treatments can be established.

The main strength of this approach is that the number of cases might be very large. Even were the prevalence of distal radius fracture as little as 0.01%, in a health care system that serves millions of individuals there are thousands of cases to analyze. The problems to be considered are the inability of the database to distinguish between bilateral conditions, the possibility that subscribers left the system and were treated elsewhere, or that they did not come forward for treatment. Despite these shortcomings it might be possible to make some valuable observations based on the patterns of treatment for this condition among a large cohort of individuals.

Summary

Most clinical research questions in hand surgery may be effectively explored using a variety of nonrandomized study designs. The main advantage of any of these methods is that they are almost always more feasible than a prospective randomized, controlled trial. Although the level of evidence associated with nonrandomized designs is always lower than that of a randomized trial there are many instances in which the inferences based on these designs are sufficiently strong that important and meaningful conclusions can be made. Where the results dictate further study, data obtained in nonrandomized studies may establish a basis for a randomized trial that can be more effectively planned and performed. Table 1 summarizes the main characteristics and indications for various nonrandomized designs.

In making a decision about how a given clinical issue should be studied, it is important to consider whether a larger volume of lower-level evidence acquired reliably and at relatively low cost is preferable to the higher level of evidence obtainable in the context of an expensive randomized trial. The key considerations in using nonrandomized

Table 1: A summary of the characteristics and indications for various nonrandomized designs

Study design	Main advantage	Main disadvantage	Use this design to
Case control	Inexpensive	Control group is subject to substantial risk of bias	Study a condition that is a rare occurrence
Cross-sectional study	Inexpensive	Cannot establish cause and effect relationship	Find an association between factors
	Generates hypotheses for potential study with randomized trial		
Decision analysis	Inexpensive	Assumptions may not fit common clinical circumstances	Exploring multiple variables is required
Health services research	Results are usually reliable	Limited scope of potential research questions	Find an association between factors

designs are to frame the research question appropriately and to recognize and anticipate the limitations and biases that are inherent to each one of these approaches.

References

[1] McPeek B, Mosteller F, McKneally M. Randomized clinical trials in surgery. Int J Technol Assess Health Care 1989;5:317–32.

[2] McLeod RS. Issues in surgical randomized controlled trials. World J Surg 1999;23:1210–4.

[3] McLeod RS, Wright JG, Solomon MJ, et al. Randomized controlled trials in surgery: Issues and problems. Surgery 1996;119:483–6.

[4] Solomon MJ, Laxamana A, Devore L, et al. Randomized controlled trials in surgery. Surgery 1994;115:707–12.

[5] Solomon MJ, McLeod RS. Should we be performing more randomized controlled trials evaluating surgical operations? Surgery 1995;118:459–67.

[6] Solomon MJ, McLeod RS. Surgery and the randomised controlled trial: past, present and future. Med J Aust 1998;169:380–3.

[7] Rolnick SJ, Flores SK, Fowler SE, et al. Conducting randomized, controlled trials. Experience with the dysfunctional uterine bleeding intervention trial. J Reprod Med 2001;46:1–5 [discussion: 5–6].

[8] Pincus T, Stein CM. Why randomized controlled clinical trials do not depict accurately long-term outcomes in rheumatoid arthritis: some explanations and suggestions for future studies. Clin Exp Rheumatol 1997;15(Suppl 17):S27–38.

[9] Simon R. Randomized clinical trials in oncology. Principles and obstacles. Cancer 1994;74:2614–9.

[10] Kramer MS, Shapiro SH. Scientific challenges in the application of randomized trials. JAMA 1984;252:2739–45.

[11] Britton A, McKee M, Black N, et al. Threats to applicability of randomised trials: exclusions and selective participation. J Health Serv Res Policy 1999;4:112–21.

[12] Dellon AL, Coert JH. Results of the musculofascial lengthening technique for submuscular transposition of the ulnar nerve at the elbow. J Bone Joint Surg Am 2003;85:1314–20.

[13] Kanoti GA. Clinical research and ethics. Cleve Clin J Med 1983;50:28.

[14] Schafer A. The ethics of the randomized clinical trial. N Engl J Med 1982;307:719–24.

[15] Taylor KM, Margolese RG, Soskolne CL. Physicians' reasons for not entering eligible patients in a randomized clinical trial of surgery for breast cancer. N Engl J Med 1984;310:1363–7.

[16] Hayden GF, Kramer MS, Horwitz RI. The case-control study. A practical review for the clinician. JAMA 1982;247:326–31.

[17] Newman TB, Browner WS, Cummings SR, et al. Designing clinical research. Baltimore: Williams and Wilkins; 1988.

[18] Armstrong TJ, Foulke JA, Joseph BS, et al. Investigation of cumulative trauma disorders in a poultry processing plant. Am Ind Hyg Assoc J 1982;43:103–16.

[19] Detsky AS, Naglie G, Krahn MD, et al. Primer on medical decision analysis: Part 1-Getting started. Med Decis Making 1997;17:123–5.

[20] Krahn MD, Naglie G, Naimark D, et al. Primer on medical decision analysis: Part 4-Analyzing the model and interpreting the results. Med Decis Making 1997;17:142–51.

[21] Detsky AS, Naglie G, Krahn MD, et al. Primer on medical decision analysis: Part 2-Building a tree. Med Decis Making 1997;17:126–35.

[22] Card WI, Rusinkiewicz M, Phillips CI. Utility estimation of a set of states of health. Methods Inf Med 1977;16:168–75.

[23] Richardson J, Hall J, Salkeld G. The measurement of utility in multiphase health states. Int J Technol Assess Health Care 1996;12:151–62.

[24] Sackett DL, Torrance GW. The utility of different health states as perceived by the general public. J Chronic Dis 1978;31:697–704.

[25] Torrance GW, Boyle MH, Horwood SP. Application of multi-attribute utility theory to measure social preferences for health states. Oper Res 1982;30:1043–69.

[26] Naglie G, Krahn MD, Naimark D, et al. Primer

on medical decision analysis: Part 3-Estimating probabilities and utilities. Med Decis Making 1997; 17:136–41.

[27] Richardson WS, Detsky AS. Users' guides to the medical literature. VII. How to use a clinical decision analysis. A. Are the results of the study valid? Evidence-Based Medicine Working Group. JAMA 1995;273:1292–5.

[28] Richardson WS, Detsky AS. Users' guides to the medical literature. VII. How to use a clinical decision analysis. B. What are the results and will they help me in caring for my patients? Evidence Based Medicine Working Group. JAMA 1995;273:1610–3.

[29] Birkmeyer JD, Birkmeyer NO. Decision analysis in surgery. Surgery 1996;120:7–15.

[30] Leblanc R, Worsley KJ. Surgery of unruptured, asymptomatic aneurysms: a decision analysis. Can J Neurol Sci 1995;22:30–5.

[31] Pauker SG. Coronary artery surgery: the use of decision analysis. Ann Intern Med 1976;85:8–18.

[32] Richard CS, Nason RW, McLeod RS. Canadian Association of General Surgeons Evidence Based Reviews in surgery. 4. Decision analysis of total thyroidectomy versus thyroid lobectomy in low-risk, differentiated thyroid cancer. Can J Surg 2002; 45:450–2.

[33] Graham B, Detsky AS. The application of decision analysis to the surgical treatment of early osteoarthritis of the wrist. J Bone Joint Surg Br 2001; 83:650–4.

[34] Keller RB, Rudicel SA, Liang MH. J Bone Joint Surg Am 1993;75:1562–74.

[35] Kreder HJ, Wright JG, McLeod R. Outcome studies in surgical research. Surgery 1997;121: 223–5.

[36] Luft HS, Bunker JP, Enthoven AC. Should operations be regionalized? The empirical relation between surgical volume and mortality. N Engl J Med 1979;301:1364–9.

[37] Wennberg J, Gittelsohn A. Small area variations in health care delivery. Science 1973;182:1102–8.

[38] Fisher ES, Whaley FS, Krushat WM, et al. The accuracy of Medicare's hospital claims data: progress has been made, but problems remain. Am J Public Health 1992;82:243–8.

CLINICS IN
PLASTIC
SURGERY

Clin Plastic Surg 32 (2005) 537–547

Bone Challenges for the Hand Surgeon: From Basic Bone Biology to Future Clinical Applications

Birgit Weyand, MD, Herbert P. von Schroeder, MD, MSc*

- Vascular supply and neural innervation to bone
- Bone pathology and pathophysiology
- Bone challenges and clinical solutions
- Bone tissue engineering
- References

The osseous skeleton of the hand is composed of 27 single bones arranged in polyarticular chains that are connected by a sophisticated fibroligament system. Together with the musculotendinous system this assembly provides great flexibility and allows a unique range of fine coordinated movements required for the multifunctional use of the hand.

To accomplish the demands of stability and rigidity for the muscles and tendons, bone matrix consists mainly of hydroxyapatite, which is the "hard" mineral component consisting of an insoluble salt of calcium and phosphate (Ca_{10} [PO_4]$_6$ [OH]$_2$), but also contains magnesium, sodium, and bicarbonate. Hydroxyapatite comprises about 65% of the bone mass.

The hydroxyapatite mineralizes an organic scaffold consisting primarily of type I collagen fibers. Collagen fibrils are organized as triple helix chains that are stabilized by hydrogen bonds and cross-linked by covalent bonds [1]. Collagen fibrils aggregate into fibers, which form a network that supports the mechanical integrity of the mineral bone structure and account for the flexibility and tensile strength of the bone tissue [2]. The collagen network is very sensitive to its state of hydration because water makes up about 25% of the bone mass. Dehydrated bone specimens show decreased toughness, but an increase in strength and stiffness [1]. Together with small amounts of other collagen types, noncollagen proteins, and proteoglycans, the organic component comprises about 10% of the total bone mass.

The bone matrix is constantly remodeled by its cellular components according to mechanical, metabolic, regenerative, and hematopoietic demands [Fig. 1]. Mechanical loading of the skeleton is a major stimulus for bone remodeling [3,4]. Bone is also the major reservoir for calcium, containing about 99.5% to 99.9% of the body's calcium content [5]. The calcium homeostasis is controlled by three major hormones from the parathyroid glands, the thyroid gland, and the kidney: parathyroid hormone, calcitonin, and 1,25-dihydroxyvitamin D, which regulate calcium uptake, absorption, deposition, and release through bone, kidney, and gut [5]. Numerous other hormones, such as adrenal and gonadal steroids, thyroid and pituitary hormones, and additional factors including cytokines and growth factors also influence bone metabolism in various ways [see Fig. 1] [3,6].

The authors are grateful to the financial support of The Physicians' Services Incorporated Foundation and the German Research Foundation (DFG for BW, grant WE 2853/1-1).
University of Toronto Hand Program and Bone Laboratory, Faculty of Dentistry, University Health Network and University of Toronto, 399 Bathurst Street, Hand Clinic 2-East, Toronto M5T 2S8, Ontario, Canada
* Corresponding author.
E-mail address: herb.vonschroeder@uhn.on.ca (H.P. von Schroeder).

doi:10.1016/j.cps.2005.06.003

Factors:

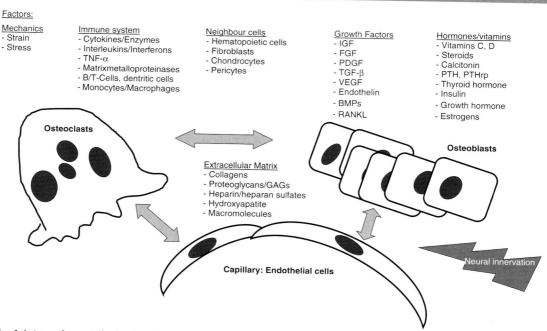

Fig. 1. Interactions at the basic multicellular unit that regulate net bone production or resorption. The production and maintenance of bone is the result of the coupled cellular interplay between bone-resorbing osteoclasts, bone-producing osteoblasts, vascular cells, and neural cells. These cells and their interactions are dependent on and controlled by the factors listed. See text for abbreviations.

The bone remodeling that occurs in response to metabolic demands, fracture healing, and mechanical stress is accomplished by the basic multicellular unit, which is composed of a group of bone-resorbing osteoclasts at its leading edge, followed by a group of bone matrix forming osteoblasts accompanied by vascular supply [7–9]. Osteoblasts originate from multipotential progenitor cells [6]. The progenitor cells, a subpopulation of mesenchymal stem cells, consist of fibroblasts that are capable of differentiating into various cell types including osteoblasts, chondrocytes, myoblasts, adipocytes, or fibroblasts, which form all of the connective tissue of the body [6–9].

Cell proliferation, differentiation, and migration of osteoblasts are influenced by a variety of hormones and growth factors, whose complex interactions are just beginning to be understood. The various factors act on preosteoblast cells by specific receptors that activate intracellular signaling cascades that induce the cells to differentiate into mature osteoblasts. Osteoblast-specific transcription factors (Runx2/core binding factor a 1 and Osterix) are at the end of the signaling paths and are required for osteoblast development and differentiation [6]. The activation of these transcription factors causes a further series of gene expression that results in the production of the extracellular matrix of bone that is characterized by collagen type I and osteoid (nonmineralized bone matrix)

and sequential expression patterns for enzymes like alkaline phosphatase, and bone-associated macromolecules including collagen type I, osteopontin, osteocalcin, and bone sialoprotein [6]. Moreover, osteoblasts can further differentiate into bone-lining cells covering the surfaces of cortical and cancellous bone, and also into osteocytes, which are located within lacunae of the cortical bone and are connected by their long, slender cytoplasmic processes through the lacuno-canalicular network [10]. Osteocytes can sense changes in mechanical and fluid shear stresses by nitric oxide synthetase and take part in regulation of the calcium homeostasis and bone remodeling [11–13].

Osteoclasts are derived from hematopoietic stem cells and are mononucleated or multinucleated cells that have receptors for the calcium-regulating hormone calcitonin and are able to resorb mineralized bone matrix by the production of acid and specific enzymes [14,15]. Osteoblasts produce receptor activator of nuclear factor-kappa B ligand, which acts on specific preosteoclast receptors, and induce osteoclast differentiation [6,14].

Vascular supply and neural innervation to bone

The blood supply of the bone tissue plays a major role during bone growth but also for bone maintenance and remodeling. The diaphysis of the long bones of the hand receive their main supply by principal nutrient arteries, which transverse the cortex into the medullary cavity and give separate terminal branches for supply of the cortex and the bone marrow cavity [**Fig. 2**] [16,17]. Within the cortex these arterioles branch into vessels supplying the transverse Volkmann's and the horizontal Haversian canals, whereas the short arterioles for the bone marrow distribute into the marrow sinusoids [**Fig. 3**]. Blood flow is centrifugal from the medulla to the periosteum [16]. Periosteal vessels provide venous drainage in the cortex, whereas the medullary sinusoidal network drains into a large medullary sinus and from there into emissary veins, which cross the cortex. The metaphysis gets additional supply from the periarticular plexus [16,17]. Interestingly, during growth the epiphyseal capillaries near the resting zone of chondrocytes in the growth plate seem to retract and leave channels, which are used by the capillaries from the diaphysis that invade the zone and initiate ossification [17] that results in growth of the bone. The coupling of vascular events with osteoblast and osteoclast activity is just being understood as an important concept in bone biology. Incorporation of this concept is required for the successful implementation of bone substitutes.

The irregular bones of the carpus are supplied by nutrient vessels arising from a network of dorsal and palmar arches from the radial artery, the anterior interosseous artery, and the ulnar artery. The nutrition depends on the availability of nonarticular surfaces for the entrance of the nutrient arteries, on the reliance of a single artery or branches from different arteries or vascular arches, and on the presence or absence of intraosseous anastomoses [16,18]. The distal 20% to 30% of the scaphoid, for example, receives blood supply from palmar branches of the radial artery [18,19]. The proximal 70% to 80% of the scaphoid receives its vascular supply mainly from the radial artery by vessels entering the bone on its dorsal ridge of the scaphoid [18]. The tenuous blood supply to the proximal pole is thought to contribute to the >50% rate of nonunions of proximal pole fractures [20].

Neural innervation of bone also plays significantly on bone metabolism and remodeling [21–23]. Anatomic studies have shown nerve fiber bundles inside the Haversian system and within cartilage channels accompanying blood vessels. The neuropeptides calcitonin gene–related peptide, vascular intestine peptide, and substance P have been detected in bone [24–27]. The presumed interactions between neural, vascular, osteogenic, and osteolytic factors in bone physiology are also a relatively new area of research.

Bone pathology and pathophysiology

Any disturbance of metabolism, nutrition, and blood flow, remodeling and growth, or stability and integrity of bone results in impairment of its

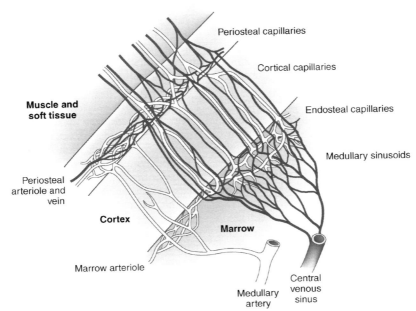

Fig. 2. Bone is a highly vascularized tissue. Cortical bone receives its blood supply from medullary arteries and an arteriolar system within the bone and from a periosteal network at the perimeter of the bone.

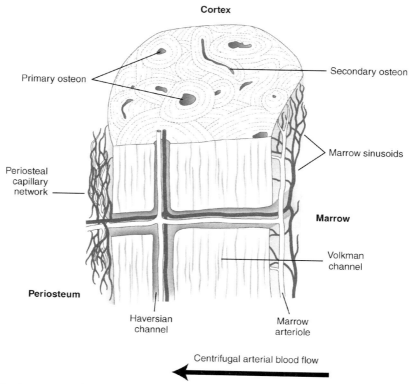

Fig. 3. Within the bone arterioles branch into vessels supplying the transverse Volkmann's and the horizontal Haversian canals. The Haversian canals are the center of the osteons that are the basic unit of bone. All osteons are vascularized. Blood flow is primarily centrifugal from the medulla to the periosteum as shown. Periosteal vessels provide venous drainage in the cortex, whereas the medullary sinusoidal network drains into a large medullary sinus and from there into emissary veins, which cross the cortex.

physiologic functions. Alterations in metabolism can be caused by changes in levels of hormones, vitamin C and D, cytokines, mechanical load, or genetic defects [4,5,14,17]. These perturbations can affect bone perfusion and the activity of the different cell types found in bone, which ultimately changes bone structure, density, growth, and remodeling. If external loads exceed the flexibility and elasticity of the weakened bone, pathologic fractures or subluxations occur. Common examples in the hand include osteoporotic distal radius fractures and mallet fractures in the elderly, and fractures into enchondromas in younger individuals. Changes in bone composition are also seen in rapid-forming so-called "woven" bone in bone metastasis or in Paget's disease where collagen fibrils are laid down in a disorderly fashion leading to impaired elasticity and susceptibility for spontaneous fractures [17].

The two essential parameters of successful fracture healing are blood supply and stabilization. In the event that these requirements cannot be fulfilled, delayed healing and pseudoarthrosis can occur. Disruption of the arterial blood supply and blockade of the venous drainage can cause osteonecrosis of the bone [16]. If the injury involves the vascularization of the metaphysis in children or damages the growth plate itself, impairment or arrest of the bone growth can take place [16,17]. Fortunately, these outcomes are rare considering the high incidence of childhood upper extremity trauma.

There are two ways that fractures heal: primary (direct) or secondary fracture healing. In primary fracture healing the sides of the fracture are in direct contact, and the basic multicellular unit and osteon of one fragment can directly cross the fracture line to the other fragment (Haversian remodeling). Here the bridging leads to deposition of already mature, axially orientated bone [17]. During fracture healing the osseous blood flow dramatically increases in the first 2 weeks following a fracture with a peak at day 10, and returns to an almost normal vascular pattern with typical internal medullary circulation at 5 weeks after the event if there was little displacement of the fracture.

In secondary fracture healing, the gap must be bridged by callus to heal. The disruption of the fracture results in hematoma formation. Within the hematoma a fibrin network is established that converts into granulation tissue with capillary sprouts. An inflammatory response occurs characterized by chemotaxis for leukocytes, mononuclear cells, and fibroblasts and fibrocytes. Fibroblasts and endothelial cells secrete growth factors and cytokines including vascular endothelial growth factor, basic fibroblast-like growth factor, and platelet-derived growth factor-β, which stimulate migration of pluripotential cells from the endosteum, periosteum, and bone marrow cavity. These cells differentiate and lay down soft callus (around day 5 after fracture) that has a vascularized fibrocartilaginous matrix, which is subsequently transformed into hard bone callus and remodeled into new bone. The amount of cartilage within the callus depends on the rate of growth and vascularization: if vascular ingrowth is high there is less cartilagenous tissue (and vice versa).

Callus forms in the medullary, intercortical, and periosteal regions. Periosteal callus is visible radiologically when its calcium content reaches about 40%. The softness of the callus allows it to be sharply dissected off of a healing bone for at least 3 weeks following injury in the hand. As such, late treatment of fractures with anatomic reduction is achievable despite radiographic evidence of healing. Increased amounts of callus are an attempt to stabilize a fracture; however, excessive motion at a fracture site is one factor that prevents the callus from bridging the site, hence resulting in a delayed union or nonunion. Inflammation and infection of the bone can also induce production of periosteal callus. Callus does increase the initial strength of the repair site and is then resorbed, at least in part, as remodeling of the site occurs. In contrast, cases of internal fixation and primary healing are dependent on the hardware to maintain the stability and initial strength of the repair site until healing is complete [28].

The mineralization process of the fibrocartilaginous callus is similar to endochondral bone formation in the growth plate. Ingrowing capillaries, pericytes, and osteoblast progenitor cells migrate into the callus. The endothelial cells stimulate proliferation of osteoblasts by secretion of growth factors. The osteoblasts differentiate and deposit osteoid (unmineralized bone matrix) on their side that is away from the vascular buds. The osteoid is subsequently mineralized, and in accordance with the mechanical loads and stresses, osteoblasts and osteoclasts then remodel the bone.

Invasion of new vessels into the fracture site starts immediately after the event and comes predominately from the surrounding soft tissues. Initially, the fracture ends are often less perfused, and hence develop a degree of osteonecrosis. Resorbing osteoclasts begin to remove some of the devascularized bone; however, some of this bone is incorporated into new bone and becomes revascularized slowly over time [17]. The cortical bone directly underneath minimally traumatized periosteal or fascial attachments can still remain viable, but the vascular supply is limited and may reduce healing.

The neurohumoral regulation of blood perfusion of bone may also contribute to the changes seen during fracture healing [29–31]. Besides fracture healing, increased bone perfusion is also found in Paget's disease and bone metastases, whereas blood flow becomes impaired during avascular osteonecrosis, osteomyelitis, antiphospholipid syndrome, and lupus [32,33]. Changes in perfusion lead to increased intraosseous pressure during inflammation, stress fractures, and osteonecrosis, resulting in pain [32]. The secondary inflammation and eventual arthritic effects on adjacent cartilage surface results in further pain.

Bone pain differs from other types of pain, such as skin pain, with respect to its quality (often described as aching rather than sharp, pricking, stabbing, or burning) and also with respect to its response to treatment with opioids or prostaglandin inhibitors [32]. Central sensitization mechanisms seem to be involved in bone nociception [34]. Peripheral mechanisms involve substance P, calcitonin gene–related peptide, and prostaglandins. In osteoid osteoma, a very painful bone tumor that often presents in the hand, myelinated nerve fibers accompanying blood vessels have been found at the nidus [35]. In osteoarthritis, sensory fibers of the joint can become responsive to sympathetic activity, and the same may happen to adrenergic fibers present in the haversian canals in bone. Calcitonin or sympathetic blockade is used for treatment of the early stages of chronic regional pain syndrome, a condition that occasionally presents after hand injuries and must be recognized early by the hand surgeon for referral for intense interdisciplinary pain treatment [36].

Bone challenges and clinical solutions

The hand surgeon is exposed to various clinical challenges in respect to bone repair, reconstruction, or replacement. Because the hand consists of multiple elements including a complex skeleton, tendons, ligaments, muscles, nerves, vessels, and skin coverage, any disturbance of a single part entails the function of the whole complex and requires special attention to gain or maintain function. Treatment of the hand skeleton needs assessment of the deficit, a strategy for repair, and ideally an objective for rehabilitation after trauma and surgical procedures. Because rehabilitation is highly dependent on the healing process, physiotherapy, and certainly the motivation of the patient, it is not always predictable. Complications of trauma and surgery, such as infection, osteomyelitis, complex regional pain syndromes, delayed union or nonunion of fracture healing, or "fracture disease" with muscle atrophy and stiff joints, can lead to severe loss of hand function.

Challenges in treatment of fractures of the hand skeleton are manifold. Stable closed fractures can be treated by closed reduction and splinting. Unstable or open fractures require osteosynthesis to restore bone stability, length, and integrity of the skeletal chain, and to permit early rehabilitation to minimize stiffness. The decision for any type of osteosynthesis is made based on the location and type of fracture, the degree of soft tissue injury, age, occupation and gender of the patient, any accompanying diseases, and the experience of the surgeon [37,38]. Percutaneous fragment fixation by Kirschner wires minimizes soft tissue and blood supply disturbances but may delay start of active physiotherapy compared with the use of plates or screws for fracture stabilization. Although generally considered a simple method of fixation, Kirschner wires are associated with a high complication rate [39]. New devices like bioabsorbable screws, plates, and pins have been successfully introduced in selected clinical cases; however, their high production costs still need to be balanced with saving the costs for secondary surgical removal of a metal implant if required [37,40,41]. Innovative approaches for intra-articular fractures include fixation of osteochondral fragments with fibrin glue [42]. Highly comminuted fractures, or those with a missing bone, can be treated with an external distraction device [43]. This method also has advantages for lengthening of shortened phalanges or metaphalanges by distraction osteosynthesis, which was originally introduced by Codivilla [44] in 1905 and extensively studied by Ilizarov [45] for long bones. Distraction techniques involve lengthening through continuously produced fracture callus. This is followed by a consolidation period when the new-formed bone remodels. As an alternative to bone grafting, this method has been used to restore length of a digital ray in certain congenital deformities, cases of growth impairment, or traumatic amputations [46–48].

The scaphoid remains a common problem in hand practices. Unstable fractures of the scaphoid waist or particularly the proximal pole are prone to delayed healing or nonunion [49,50]. To date, research of the fracture kinetics or the underlying anatomic characteristics of the extraosseous and intraosseous blood supply of this bone has not been able to answer comprehensively the question as to why this bone is so often destined to healing difficulties [19]. Multiple factors likely contribute

to this problem including prolonged hypoxia caused by interrupted intraosseous vascular supply, especially for the proximal pole. Low numbers of osteoprogenitor cells including periosteal progenitors, the inhibitory effects of synovial fluid on cell proliferation, and micromotion caused by insufficient fracture stabilization are all potential factors that may delay healing and require investigation.

The development of microsurgery in the 1960s has revolutionized the field of hand surgery. It has now become possible to transplant bone together with its main vascular bundle as in vascularized bone grafts. Roy-Camille [51] described the first pedicled vascularized bone graft for the carpus in 1965 by using the scaphoid tubercle on an abductor pollicis brevis muscle to assist in healing of a scaphoid waist fracture [52]. Beck [53] used the pedicled vascularized pisiform for treatment of osteonecrosis of the lunate (Kienböck's disease). Various techniques for harvesting a vascularized bone graft from the palmar and dorsal side of the distal radius have been reported for the carpal bones [52,54,55]. Free vascularized bone grafts from other anatomic sides (fibula, iliac crest) for reconstruction of the hand and wrist have also been described [38]. Hori and coworkers [56] described the transplantation of a vascular loop for successful revascularization in cases of osteonecrosis of carpal bones. Finally, microvascular transfer of toes for joint or finger replacement in traumatic amputations or developmental defects has been successfully performed [37,57,58]. Isolated cases of the transplantation of a whole hand are met with the obstacles of immunogenic rejection; failed functionality (stiffness and insensibility); and the acceptance by the recipient of lifelong immunosuppressive medication and related complications [59]. Future techniques like the concept of tissue engineering aim to minimize morbidity and overcome the problems associated through composite tissue allograft transplantation.

Bone tissue engineering

Tissue engineering describes the application of principles of life sciences and engineering to regenerate natural tissues or to create biologic substitutes to restore, maintain, or improve the function of any tissue or organ [Fig. 4]. Bone substitutes must fulfill a range of requirements to replace bone tissue and its function. Ideally they should have osteoconductive, osteoinductive, and osteogenic properties. An osteoconductive material allows bone ingrowth from an osseous bed. An osteoinductive material provides a biologic stimulus for the migrated undifferentiated mesenchymal progenitor cells to differentiate into osteoblasts. Osteogenesis is defined as the capacity to form new bone and is usually

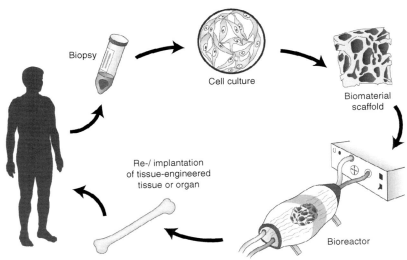

Fig. 4. Schematic representation of the basic steps of tissue engineering. Cells are harvested and grown in vitro within a scaffold. Further growth is promoted within a bioreactor that allows appropriate proliferation and differentiation of cells within a three-dimensional matrix. Treatment of the original defect or disease is achieved by implantation of the engineered tissue, which is followed by a healing and rehabilitation phase.

achieved by a material that contains cells capable of differentiation into bone-forming osteoblasts.

Synthetic biomaterials for clinical use have to be sterile, safe, and nontoxic in the human environment. Safety is paramount and sterilization must minimize the possibility of infections from bacteria, viruses including HIV and hepatitis C, and prions. Degradation of the synthetic biomaterials can release toxic intermediate products or end products. Preferably, the biomaterials should be resorbable in a time-dependant manner and be replaced by bone in the long term; ingrowth of vessels from surrounding tissue and migration of cells should be permitted and promoted. The immune response must be minimized to reduce any adverse inflammatory response or even rejection or rapid absorption of an implant. Finally, for the surgeon the material should be easy to store and to handle, applicable to different shapes as needed, and provide the stability required for early rehabilitation of the function of the injured hand. Several biomaterials for bone replacement and reconstruction have been approved for clinical or investigational use, and there are numerous ongoing research studies of newly synthesized biomaterials and composite materials in vitro and in vivo [60].

Natural materials, such as bone autografts or bone marrow stromal cells, have osteoinductive and osteogenic properties. Although bone autografts have been tried since beginning of the nineteenth century (1810 Merrem in dog skull; 1825 von Walther reimplantation in human skull; 1875 Nussbaum first successful human limb autograft), autografts from the red marrow have been known for its osteogenic potency since the work of Goujon (1869) [61]. Based on animal studies with bone allografts seeded with red marrow autografts, Urist and coworkers proposed that precursor cells from the vascular sinusoids of the marrow differentiate into osteogenic cell [61]. Clinical trials have introduced bone marrow stromal cells alone and in combination with synthetic bone substitutes of bovine collagen and porous calcium phosphate ceramics. Bone marrow stromal cells have been expanded ex vivo, seeded on a scaffold, and then implanted for bone replacement in humans [62]. It is probable that similar techniques will be routinely available in the future for reconstructing bone defects in the hand and possibly for complex tissue reconstructions.

Bone allografts, such as demineralized or freeze-dried bone, are both osteoconductive and osteoinductive. Bone banks process cadaver bone to reduce surface antigenicity, ensure sterility, and preserve stability for storage and future use. Demineralized bone matrix is also commercially available in combination with glycerol, porcine gelatin, hyaluronate, or calcium sulfate.

Various synthetic biomaterials with mainly osteoconductive properties have been introduced for clinical applications and many are still being tested in animals. Structural features, such as porosity, pore size, interconnectivity, and pore-wall microstructure, and surface quality (properties) are important for uniform cell seeding. The ability for cellular migration and adhesion into the synthetic matrix, and the diffusion of nutrients and metabolites throughout the scaffolds, are technical challenges in biomaterial design that still have to be worked out [63–65].

An important class of biomaterials for bone repair are calcium phosphate ceramics, which are osteoconductive and resemble the mineral component of natural bone. Processing these materials, however, is difficult. Although they are hard and strong, they tend to be brittle, and are difficult to shape. The two major substitutes are hydroxyapatite and tricalcium phosphate, but other substances, such as carbonated apatite or calcium sulfate, are also being used. Problematic is their rate of degradation, which should ideally follow the rate of new bone formation. Tricalcium phosphate is rapidly resorbed within days and weeks, whereas hydroxyapatite is relatively inert with a resorption rate of years or none at all [61]. An alternative natural material, calcium carbonate, is derived from coral and a composition and pore size that is similar to bone. New trials combine nanoparticles of hydroxyapatite or tricalcium phosphate either with an organic carrier like collagen type I or with synthetic polymers [66]. Injectable bioactive cements based on carbonated apatite or bioglass are also on the market [67].

Biodegradable synthetic polymers include a wide spectrum of different materials including polyesters (polyglycolic acid, polylactic acid, and copolymers); polyanhydrides; tyrosine-based polycarbonates; polyorthoesters; polyphosphazenes; and polyurethranes [65,68]. Advantages of polymers are a better control of stability, morphology, shape, and degradation rate compared with naturally derived materials, such as fibrin or collagen. Polyglycolic acid, polylactic acid, and their copolymers have been used for resorbable screws, pins, and plates in hand surgery. Resorption rates range from a few months to several years. These biomaterials showed good biocompatibility and minor or no associated inflammation and can save a second surgery for removal of the osteosynthesis material [37]. Only a few studies describe complications, however, such as considerable inflammatory responses or refractures caused by rapid hydrolysis and loss of stability of the implant [69,70].

Some of the materials, such as polypropylene fumarate or hydrogels, can even be used as an injectable scaffold, which offers great benefits in some surgical applications [78]. In addition, polymers can be coupled with chemical functional groups that can induce tissue ingrowth [65]. Problematic issues are insufficient material strength and toxic by-products during degradation. These can lead to hyperacidity followed by cell death and rapid matrix breakdown and an immunologic or foreign body reaction. There are various fabrication techniques for polymer scaffolds (solvent-casting and particulate leaching technique, gas-foaming process, emulsion freeze drying, electrospinning, rapid prototyping, thermally induced phase separation), but not all of them are able to avoid a closed porous structure without interconnectivity that is a critical parameter for cell and vascular ingrowth in vivo [65]. New approaches use computer-aided manufacturing devices for three-dimensional printing of polymeric or fibrin-based scaffolds using stereolithography, rapid prototyping, or solid freeform fabrication processes [71–73].

Rapid vascularization of the biomaterials is essential for subsequent osteogenesis and survival of osteoblasts and progenitor cells seeded in these scaffolds to promote the ossification process. Several approaches are currently being tried to improve vascularization of the constructs. New efforts combine calcium ceramic components with polymers or organic substrates and try to enhance angiogenesis and osteoinduction by additional incorporation of growth factors that ideally are gradually released from the matrix [71,74,75]. The incorporated growth peptides, such as bone-morphogenic protein, fibroblast growth factor, vascular endothelial growth factor, platelet-derived growth factor, insulin-like growth factor, or transforming growth factor-β stimulate migration of endothelial cells or mesenchymal progenitor cells and some of them also support cell proliferation, differentiation, or survival within the scaffold. These growth factors can be loaded into microspheres; mixed into polymeric hydrogels with reactive polyethylene glycol chains; or cross-linked enzymatically by transglutaminase to polysaccharides (alginate, chitosan, hyaluronate, agarose) or proteins like collagen or fibrin [75]. Scaffolds with combination of two growth factors have already been shown to exceed those with a single factor in their in vivo performance with respect to neoangiogenesis and osteogenesis in initial trials [76–78]. Alternatively, an injectable polypropylene fumarate mixed with polylactic-co-glycolic acid and polyethylene glycol microparticles loaded with an osteogenic peptide has been developed and allowed tissue ingrowth and showed controlled release when implanted into a bone defect [74]. Recombinant human bone-morphogenic proteins-2 and -7 have been approved for certain orthopedic procedures (eg, spinal fusion) in human trials [79]. Their use for scaphoid fractures or other problematic hand fractures has not yet been performed.

Tissue engineering by transplantation of genetically modified cells combines the osteogenic properties of the cell with the osteoinductive potential of genes encoding for bone growth factors. Transfection is done by vectors, such as liposomes, polymers, or different virus forms, achieving variable transfection efficiencies depending on the method used [80,81]. The transcribed gene product is produced by the cells to create a stimulatory microenvironment that promotes angiogenesis and bone production. Mesenchymal stromal cells and cells of nonosteogenic origin, such as fibroblastic and myoblastic cells, have been used for this purpose [80,82]. An alternative approach is the so-called "gene-activated matrix," where plasmids encoding a certain gene are incorporated into a biomatrix (eg, collagen or fibrin) [83]. These methods, however, are still far from clinical application.

As alternatives to joint arthrodesis and prosthetic arthroplasty, engineering of composites for joint replacement requires the combination of layers of cartilage and bone to mimic biology. Such an implant must fit the basic shape of the joint to ensure proper function and hold the prerequisites for stress and strength for this particular part of the bone. In addition to the engineering challenges, the immune system is still a major obstacle in maintaining the integrity of such a multipart implant in vivo.

Vacanti and coworkers [84] described a case where an amputated thumb was replaced by a tissue-engineered composite phalanx. Critics claimed that conventional therapies, such as replacement by an autologous bone graft, bone lengthening, or microvascular toe-to-thumb transfer, are superior because they can be less time consuming and have a more reliable outcome. The case, however, demonstrates the current potential, and the limitations of the evolving new materials and techniques of tissue engineering.

The field of tissue engineering requires an understanding of the basic biology of bone including signaling mechanisms between different cell types during the different stages of bone repair, the influence of external stress forces on those cells, and the interaction with the immune system with respect to transplanted cells and matrices. The requirement for angiogenesis is paramount and the concept of coupling between blood vessels and bone cells is a part of the complex milieu of bone biology. Modeling of composites of vascularized bone and joint replacements, and their growth and differentiation in bioreactors, may enable clinicians to grow full bone and more complex structures in vitro for transplantation into the body. Until then, the complexities, controlling factors, and adaptive remodeling of bone are challenges that require ongoing basic research.

References

[1] Wang X, Puram S. The toughness of cortical bone and its relationship with age. Ann Biomed Eng 2004;32:123–35.

[2] Burr DB. The contribution of the organic matrix to bone's material properties. Bone 2002;31: 8–11.

[3] Basso N, Heersche J. Characteristics of in vitro osteoblastic cell loading models. Bone 2002;30:347–51.

[4] Eastell R, Baumann M, Hoyle NR, et al. Bone markers: biochemical and clinical perspectives. London: Martin Dunitz; 2001.

[5] Greger RF. Physiology and pathophysiology of calcium homeostasis. Z Kardiol 2000;89(Suppl 2): II/4–II/8.

[6] Aubin JE, Heersche JN. Bone cell biology: osteoblasts, osteocytes, and osteoclasts. In: Glourieux FH, Pettifer JM, Hüppner H, editors. Pediatric bone. San Diego: Elsevier Science; 2002.

[7] Jilka RL. Biology of the basic multicellular unit and the pathophysiology of osteoporosis. Med Pediatr Oncol 2003;41:182–5.

[8] Parfitt A. Targeted and nontargeted bone remodeling: relationship to basic multicellular origination and progression. Bone 2002;30:5–7.

[9] Parfitt AM. Osteonal and hemi-osteonal remodeling: the spatial and temporal framework for signal traffic in adult human bone. J Cell Biochem 1994;55:273–86.

[10] Menton DN, Simmons DJ, Chang SL, et al. From bone lining cell to osteocyte: an SEM study. Anat Rec 1984;209:29–39.

[11] Burr D. Targeted and nontargeted remodeling. Bone 2002;30:2–4.

[12] Caballero-Alias AM, Loveridge N, Lyon A, et al. NOS isoforms in adult human osteocytes: multiple pathways of NO regulation? Calcif Tissue Int 2004;75:78–84.

[13] Klein-Nulend J, Semeins CM, Ajubi NE, et al. Pulsating fluid flow increases nitric oxide (NO) synthesis by osteocytes but not periosteal fibroblasts: correlation with prostaglandin upregulation. Biochem Biophys Res Commun 1995;217:640–8.

[14] Helfrich MH. Osteoclast diseases. Microsc Res Tech 2003;61:514–32.

[15] Rousselle A-V, Heymann D. Osteoclastic acidification pathways during bone resorption. Bone 2002;30:533–40.

[16] Brookes M, Revell WJ. Blood supply of bone. 2nd edition. London: Springer; 1998.

[17] Sumner-Smith G. Bone in clinical orthopedics. 2nd edition. New York: Thieme; 2002.

[18] Freedman DM, Botte MJ, Gelberman RH. Vascularity of the carpus. Clin Orthop Rel Res 2001; 383:47–59.

[19] Büchler U, Nagy L. The issue of vascularity in fractures and non-union of the scaphoid. J Hand Surgery [Br] 1995;20:726–35.

[20] Segalman KA, Graham TJ. Scaphoid proximal pole fractures and nonunions. J Am Soc Surg Hand 2004;4:233–49.

[21] Hukkanen M, Konttinen YT, Santavirta S, et al. Rapid proliferation of calcitonin gene-related peptide-immunoreactive nerves during healing of rat tibial fracture suggests neural involvement in bone growth and remodelling. Neuroscience 1993;54:969–79.

[22] Imai S, Matsusue Y. Neuronal regulation of bone metabolism and anabolism: calcitonin gene-related peptide-, substance P- and tyrosine hydroxylase-containing nerves and the bone. Microsc Res Tech 2002;58:61–9.

[23] Konttinen Y, Imai S, Suda A. Neuropeptides and the puzzle of bone remodeling: state of the art. Acta Orthop Scand 1996;67:632–9.

[24] Ahmed M, Srinivasan GR, Theodorsson E, et al. Extraction and quantitation of neuropeptides in bone by radioimmunoassay. Regul Pept 1994; 51:179–88.

[25] Bjurholm A. Neuroendocrine peptides in bone. Int Orthop 1991;15:325–9.

[26] Bjurholm A, Kreichberg A, Schultzberg M. Fixation and demineralization of bone tissue for immunohistochemical staining of neuropeptides. Calc Tissue Int 1989;45:227–31.

[27] Strange-Vognsen HH, Arnbjerg J, Hannibal J. Immunocytochemical demonstration of pituitary cyclase activating polypeptide (PACAP) in the porcine epiphyseal cartilage canals. Neuropeptides 1997;31:137–41.

[28] Kostopoulos V, Vellios L, Fortis AP, et al. Comparative study of callus performance achieved by rigid and sliding plate osteosynthesis based upon dynamic mechanical analysis. J Med Eng Technol 1994;18:61–6.

[29] Briggs PJ, Moran CG, Wood MB. Actions of endothelin-1, 2, and 3 in the microvasculature of bone. J Orthop Res 1998;16:340–7.

[30] Brinker MR, Lippton HL, Cook SD, et al. Pharmacological regulation of the circulation of bone. J Bone Joint Surg Am 1990;72:964–75.

[31] Gross PM, Heistad DD, Marcus ML. Neurohumoral regulation of blood flow to bone and marrow. Am J Phys 1979;237:H440–8.

[32] Haegerstam GAT. Pathophysiology of bone pain. Acta Orthop Scand 2001;72:308–17.

[33] Laroche M. Intraosseous circulation from physiology to disease. Joint Bone Spine 2002;69: 262–9.

[34] Mercadante S. Malignant bone pain: pathophysiology and treatment. Pain 1997;69:1–18.

[35] Greco F, Tamburrelli F, Laudati A, et al. Nerve fibers in osteoid osteoma. Ital J Orthop Traumatol 1988;14:91–4.

[36] Appelboom T. Calcitonin in reflex sympathetic dystrophy syndrome and other painful conditions. Bone 2002;5:84S–6S.

[37] Brüser P, Gilbert A. Finger bone and joint injuries. London: Martin Dunitz; 1999.

[38] Saffar P, Amadio PC, Foucher G. Current practice in hand surgery. London: Martin Dunitz; 1997.

[39] Botte MJ, Davis JL, Rose BA, et al. Complications of smooth pin fixation of fractures and dislocations in the hand and wrist. Clin Orthop 1992; 276:194–201.

[40] Ambroise CG, Clanton TO. Bioabsorbable implants: review of clinical experience in orthopedic surgery. Ann Biomed Eng 2004;32:171–7.

[41] Waris E, Ninkovic M, Harpf C, et al. Self-reinforced bioabsorbable miniplates for skeletal fixation in complex hand injury: three case report. J Hand Surg [Am] 2004;29:452–7.

[42] Shah MA, Ebert AM, Sanders WE. Fibrin glue fixation of a digital osteochondral fracture: case report and review of the literature. J Hand Surg [Am] 2002;27:464–9.

[43] Pennig D, Gausepohl T, Mader K. Die Anwendung des Minifixateurs bei Frakturen des Handskelettes. Osteosynthese Intern 1997;5:158–65.

[44] Codivilla A. On the means of lengthening in the lower limb the muscle and tissues which are shortened through deformity. Am J Orthop Surg 1905;2:353–69.

[45] Ilizarov G. Clinical application of the tension-stress effect for limb-lengthening. Clin Orthop Rel Res 1990;250:8–26.

[46] Matev I. Reconstructive surgery of the thumb. Orthop Trauma 1966;3:126–32.

[47] Minguella J, Cabrera M, Escolá J. Techniques for small-bone lengthening in congenital anomalies of the hand and foot. J Pediatr Orthop 2001; 10B:355–9.

[48] Rudolf K-D, Preiser P, Partecke B-D. Callus distraction of the hand skeleton. Injury Int J Care Injured 2000;31:113–20.

[49] Merrell GA, Wolfe SW, Slade JF. Treatment of scaphoid nonunions: quantitative meta-analysis of the literature. J Hand Surg [Am] 2002;27: 685–91.

[50] Sauerbier M, Germann G, Dacho A. Current concepts in the treatment of scaphoid fractures. Eur J Trauma 2004;2:80–92.

[51] Roy-Camille R. Fractures et pseudarthroses du scaphoide moyen: utilisation d'un greffo pedicule. Actual Chir Ortho Hopital Raymond Poincare 1965;4:197–214.

[52] Shin AY, Bishop AT. Vascular anatomy of the distal radius: implications for vascularized bone grafts. Clin Orthop Rel Res 2001;383:60–73.

[53] Beck E. Die Verpflanzung des Os pisiforme am Gefaessstiel zur Behandlung der Lunatummalazie. Handchirurgie 1971;3:64–7.

[54] Boyer MI, von Schroeder HP, Axelrod TS. Scaphoid nonunion with avascular necrosis of the proximal pole: treatment with a vascularized bone graft from the dorsum of the distal radius. J Hand Surg [Br] 1998;23:686–90.

[55] Roux JL. Les transferts osseoux vascularisés au poignet et à la main. Chir Main 2003;22:173–85.

[56] Hori Y, Tamai S, Okuda H, et al. Blood vessel transplantation to bone. J Hand Surg 1979;4: 23–33.

[57] Chung KC, Kotsis SV. Outcomes of multiple microvascular toe transfers for reconstruction in 2 patients with digitless hands: 2- and 4-year follow-up case report. J Hand Surg [Am] 2002; 27:652–8.

[58] Tan B-K, Wei F-C, Lutz BS, et al. Strategies in multiple toe transplantation for bilateral type II metacarpal hand reconstruction. Hand Clin 1999; 15:607–62.

[59] Siemionow M, Ozer K. Advances in composite tissue allograft transplantation as related to the hand and upper extremity. J Hand Surg [Am] 2002;27:565–80.

[60] Bauer TW, Smith ST. Bioactive materials in orthopaedic surgery: overview and regulatory considerations. Clin Orthop Rel Res 2002;395:11–22.

[61] Urist MR, O'Connor BT, Burwell RG. Bone grafts, derivates and substitutes. Oxford: Butterworth-Heinemann; 1994.

[62] Quarto R, Mastrogiacomo M, Cancedda R, et al. Repair of large bone defects with the use of autologous bone marrow stromal cells. N Engl J Med 2001;344:385–6.

[63] Green D, Walsh D, Mann S, et al. The potential of biomimesis in bone tissue engineering: lessons from the design and synthesis of intervertebrate skeletons. Bone 2002;30:810–5.

[64] LeGeros RZ. Properties of osteoconductive biomaterials: calcium phosphates. Clin Orthop Rel Res 2002;395:81–98.

[65] Liu X, Ma PX. Polymeric scaffolds for bone tissue engineering. Ann Biomed Eng 2004;32:477–86.

[66] Wei G, Ma PX. Structure and properties of nano-hydroxyapatite/polymer composite scaffolds for bone tissue engineering. Biomaterials 2004;25:4749–57.

[67] Larsson S, Bauer TW. Use of injectable calcium phosphate cement for fracture fixation: a review. Clin Orthop Rel Res 2002;395:23–32.

[68] Gunatillake PA, Adhikari R. Biodegradable synthetic polymers for tissue engineering. Europ Cells Materials 2003;5:1–16.

[69] Bostman O, Hirvensalo E, Makinen J, et al. Foreign-body reactions to fracture fixation implants of biodegradable synthetic polymers. J Bone Joint Surg Br 1990;72:592–6.

[70] Lionelli GT, Korentager RA. Biomechanical failure of metacarpal fracture resorbable plate fixation. Ann Plast Surg 2004;49:202–6.

[71] Calvert JW, Weiss LE, Sundine M. New frontiers in bone tissue engineering. Clin Plast Surg 2003;30:641–8.

[72] Cooke MN, Fisher JP, Dean D, et al. Use of stereolithography to manufacture critical-sized 3D biodegradable scaffolds for bone ingrowth. J Biomed Mater Res 2002;64:65–9.

[73] Landers R, Hubner U, Schmelzeisen R, et al. Rapid prototyping of scaffolds derived from thermoreversible hydrogels and tailored for applications in tissue engineering. Biomaterials 2002;23:4437–47.

[74] Hedberg EL, Tang A, Crowther RS, et al. Controlled release of an osteogenic peptide from injectable biodegradeble polymeric composites. J Control Release 2002;84:137–50.

[75] Zisch AH, Lutolf MP, Hubbell JA. Biopolymeric delivery matrices for angiogenic growth factors. Cardiovasc Pathol 2003;12:295–310.

[76] Cao R, Brakenhielm E, Pawliuk R, et al. Angiogenic synergism, vascular stability and improvement of hind-limb ischemia by a combination of PDGF-BB and FGF-2. Nat Med 2003;9:604–13.

[77] Richardson TP, Peters MC, Ennet AB, et al. Polymeric system for dual growth factor delivery. Nat Biotechnol 2001;19:1029–34.

[78] Simmons C, Alsberg E, Hsiong S, et al. Dual growth factor delivery and controlled scaffold degradation enhance in vivo bone formation by transplanted bone marrow stromal cells. Bone 2004;35:562–9.

[79] Issack PS, DiCesare PE. Recent advances toward the clinical application of bone morphogenetic proteins in bone and cartilage repair. Am J Orthop Surg 2003;32:429–36.

[80] Blum JS, Barry MA, Mikos AG. Bone regeneration through transplantation of genetically modified cells. Clin Plast Surg 2003;30:611–20.

[81] Gamradt SC, Lieberman JR. Genetic modification of stem cells to enhance bone repair. Ann Biomed Eng 2004;32:136–47.

[82] Peng H, Usas A, Gearhart B, et al. Converse relationship between in vitro osteogenic differentiation and in vivo bone healing elicited by different populations of muscle-derived cells genetically engineered to express BMP4. J Bone Miner Res 2004;19:630–41.

[83] Bonadio J. Tissue engineering via local gene delivery. J Mol Med 2000;78:303–11.

[84] Vacanti CA, Bonassar LJ, Vacanti MP, et al. Replacement of an avulsed phalanx with tissue-engineered bone. N Engl J Med 2001;344:1511–4.

CLINICS IN
PLASTIC
SURGERY

Clin Plastic Surg 32 (2005) 549–561

Closed Reduction of Hand Fractures

Alan E. Freeland, MD

Management of closed simple displaced extra-articular hand fractures with stable configurations by closed reduction and splinting has gradually and almost imperceptibly become passé, whereas operative treatment has become increasingly popular. Why has this occurred? Physicians and patients have become more aware of the correlation between anatomic restoration and fracture stability and outcome in terms of fracture healing, correction or subsequent avoidance of deformity, and recovery of digital motion [1–5]. Reliable implants and fixation techniques are now available and present attractive alternatives. The ease and maintenance of anatomic restoration with secure fracture stability are relative benefits of an open procedure. When one opens the fracture, attains a perfect or nearly perfect reduction, and stabilizes it with an implant, there is substantially less risk of the patient's returning with a displaced fracture reduc-

tion and requiring a second procedure. There is also less likelihood of the noncompliant patient's returning with a malunion, nonunion, or other complication [6]. Plaintiff attorneys may more easily persuade lay juries to vote *convicto* rather than *absolvo* in instances of poor outcomes or complications when fracture reduction is less than anatomic, even when the position of the fracture is within acceptable parameters. Stable fracture fixation enhances pain management, allows earlier and more intensive rehabilitation, and may consequently offset some of the menace of stiffness and fragment devascularization posed by the surgical procedure [4,7]. Consequently, open reduction and internal fixation has increasingly become a first option for many closed and even marginally displaced extra-articular simple fractures of stable configuration.

Perhaps hand surgeons individually and collectively have lost sight of the travails of operative

No funding was received for this article. The author receives departmental and institutional support from AO North America and royalties from Elsevier Publishing Company.
Department of Orthopaedic Surgery and Rehabilitation, University of Mississippi Medical Center, Jackson, MS 39216-4505, USA
E-mail address: afreeland@orthopedics.umsmed.edu

doi:10.1016/j.cps.2005.05.010

treatment, which may include the generation of additional fibroplasia (scar tissue) and an increased risk of consequent stiffness [8–15]. Although there are many instances in which operative management is justified and indicated, nonoperative methods, including manipulative reduction, remain a cornerstone of the management of simple hand fractures [16–38]. When stable anatomic or near-anatomic position is initially present or can be achieved by closed reduction, the risks of additional stiffness and fragment devascularization from surgery may be avoided. This article details indications and techniques for closed reduction, splinting, and rehabilitation of simple hand fractures of stable configuration and adds some commentary on other treatment choices for unstable fractures.

Evaluation

Hand fractures present with a history of trauma. Demographic information, such as age, hand dominance, occupation, avocations, date of injury, and any previous treatment, should be solicited and recorded. Demographic information may influence treatment selection. The hand and involved digit or digits are assessed for posture, deformity, swelling, tenderness, discoloration, heat, wounding, functional and sensory deficit, and stability. Digital or wrist anesthetic block followed by observation of digital motion may assist the physician in determining whether fractures with mild deformity on radiograph have any critical visible clinical deformity or inherent instability [5]. Plain radiographs alone are generally adequate for the evaluation of hand fractures [3–5]. The accumulated information assists the physician and patient in establishing a dialogue and forming a treatment plan that considers options, potential risks and benefits, expectations, possible problems and complications, individual patient considerations, and a timetable for rehabilitation and recovery.

Anatomic fracture reduction parameters

Functional restoration follows the restitution of form. Alterations of bone anatomy may affect functional outcome commensurate with their severity [39]. Although a perfect reduction is, of course, ideal, tolerable allowances may be made for minor

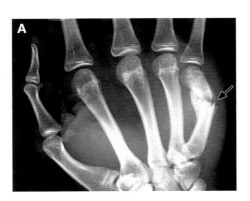
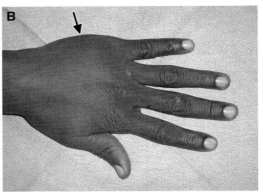
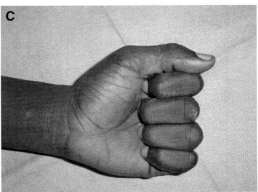

Fig. 1. (*A*) Radiograph of a patient initially presenting with a healed malunion of a fifth metacarpal fracture. (*B, C*) The patient had an apparent deformity (*arrows*) but had full digital motion, no finger impingement, nearly full strength, and no pain or tenderness. The result was accepted and no surgery was performed.

anatomic deficits seen on radiograph without serious clinical deformity or significant functional loss. The hand and digits have a capacity for functional adaptation to and tolerance of small degrees of anatomic deformity.

Shortening, angulation, and rotation may be seen individually or in combination. The physician must weigh the risk-to-benefit ratio of operative versus nonoperative fracture management for each patient. The risk of postoperative digital stiffness may outweigh the benefit of small gains in anatomic fracture restoration in instances of minor deformities. This is particularly true of inveterate fractures and nascent malunions, with or without radiographic evidence of callus formation that cannot be manipulated into position [Fig. 1].

Anatomic parameters and functional correlations

Metacarpal fractures

The intrinsic hand muscles may contribute as much as 40% to 90% of grip strength [40,41]. As much as 8% loss of grip power may result from every 2 mm of metacarpal shortening [42,43]. The ring and little fingers may be less affected than the index and middle fingers owing to their increased carpometacarpal flexibility. Approximately 7° of extensor lag may develop for each 2 mm of residual finger metacarpal shortening after fracture healing [44]. The intermetacarpal ligaments usually prevent more than 3 to 4 mm of shortening of finger metacarpal fractures [45]. Internal metacarpals (third and fourth metacarpals) have more restraint than border metacarpals (second and fifth metacarpals), because they are anchored by intermetacarpal ligaments on both sides of the metacarpal head. Hence finger metacarpals may tolerate as much as 3 to 4 mm of shortening with only minimal clinical deformity and functional loss.

Metacarpal shaft fractures tend to angulate dorsally, owing to the unbalanced pull of the interosseous muscles and extrinsic finger flexors on the distal fragment. The fracture gap tends to be wider dorsally and narrower volarly. Altered intrinsic muscle tension dynamics lead to measurable progressive correlative grip weakness after 30° of dorsal metacarpal angulation [43,46]. There may be loss of knuckle contour, pseudoclawing, and a palpable metacarpal head in the palm corresponding to the degree of residual metacarpal angulation. Dorsal metacarpal angulation may be compensated by carpometacarpal joint motion. Dorsal angulation of 10° to 15° greater than the carpometacarpal joint motion may be tolerated. The ring and small finger metacarpals are more tolerant of dorsal angulation

than those of the index and middle fingers, owing to their greater carpometacarpal flexibility. Satisfactory results have been reported with as much as 70° of dorsal angulation in subcapital metacarpal (Boxer's) fractures [47].

Lateral metacarpal angulation of as much as 10° may be tolerated, provided that there is no finger impingement during motion [4]. Border metacarpals may allow even slightly greater than 10° lateral angulation. Clinical deformity from lateral metacarpal angulation is usually best observed with the fingers straight.

Metacarpal rotational deformity greater than approximately 5° may result in finger impingement or "scissoring" (overlap) [48,49]. Rotational deformity of the fingers, other than fingernail malalignment, may not be apparent with full digital extension, but it becomes progressively more pronounced as the collateral ligaments tighten with finger flexion. The intermetacarpal ligaments provide some rotational stability to the distal fragment. Again, internal metacarpals (third and fourth) have more restraint than border metacarpals (second and fifth), because they are anchored by intermetacarpal ligaments on both sides of the metacarpal head.

Phalangeal fractures

Displaced fractures of the proximal phalangeal shaft characteristically display an apex palmar angulation with the fracture gap wider volarly and narrower dorsally. The intrinsic muscles flex the proximal fragment, whereas the attachment of the central slip to the dorsal lip of the middle phalanx extends the distal fragment. The axis of rotation of proximal phalangeal fractures lies on the fibro-osseous border of the flexor tendon sheath [50]. The moment arm from the rotational axis of the fracture site to the extensor tendons is greater than that between the axis and the flexor tendons, further contributing to apex palmar angulation. When volar fracture angulation is greater than 15°, the dorsal gliding surface of the proximal phalanx starts to become significantly shortened relative to the length of the extensor mechanism [50]. As palmar angulation incrementally shortens the fractured proximal phalanx, the extensor mechanism may have 2 to 6 mm of reserve, owing to its viscoelastic adaptive properties, before the sagittal bands tighten to produce a progressive extensor lag at the proximal interphalangeal joint. This lag may average 12° for every millimeter of bone–tendon discrepancy [51]. Pseudoclawing of the finger may occur [52]. Persistent volar angulation of greater than 25° may also progressively limit the ability of the flexor pad of the involved finger to touch the distal palmar crease of the hand [53].

Simple articular fractures

Operative treatment of articular fractures must be prudently considered, because devascularization may place articular fragments in danger of avascular necrosis and the joint in danger of future stiffness, instability, and arthritis [18,26,28,54–57]. An additional risk exists of growth disturbance in epiphyseal fractures in children. Incongruity or displacement of as much as 2 mm may be acceptable in articular fractures, provided that there is no joint subluxation and early motion is initiated [Fig. 2] [28,54–57]. Fractures with greater displacement may require reduction and internal fixation, especially if they involve more than 20% of the articular surface. Articular fractures with accompanying joint subluxation should be restored to correct joint deformity and instability [28,54–57]. Articular fractures occasionally heal with fibrous rather than osseus union. This healing may be acceptable provided that the fracture is stable and asymptomatic or minimally symptomatic.

Fracture management principles

Hand fracture management should be principle driven. Fracture management principles include the attainment of anatomic or near-anatomic position and sufficient stability to control pain and facilitate reliable fracture healing and early progressive soft tissue response guided active digital

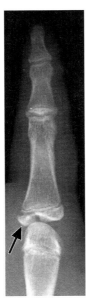

Fig. 2. Epiphyseal fracture of an index finger (*arrow*) with minimal displacement and a well-aligned joint in an adolescent. There was no clinical deformity or finger impingement on the adjacent middle finger during digital flexion.

motion [3–5,7]. In assessing the risk-to-benefit ratio of operative versus nonoperative treatment, the physician must consider that additional operative soft tissue damage may disrupt circulation at the fracture site and create more potentially adherent scar tissue [3–18,20,21,28]. Ideally, the goals of fracture restoration and stability and early digital motion should be pursued with the least possible degree of additional soft tissue trauma.

Many factors, including an intangible called judgment, may affect the decision-making process. Although acceptable anatomic reduction parameters and fracture management principles guide us, they are relative rather than absolute, allowing the management of each patient to remain an individual consideration. The judgment of the physician remains paramount in the decision-making process and may vary among patients who have similar fracture configurations and soft tissue injuries. More than one permissible treatment method may exist for any specific fracture configuration. Physicians' treatment choices are often influenced by their personal background, training, judgment, and experience.

Stability

A fracture is considered stable when it does not displace spontaneously or with gentle, active, unresisted range of motion exercises in the "safe" midrange of motion [4]. Fracture configuration, impaction, periosteal disruption, muscle forces, and external forces may influence stability. Simple (ie, two fragments) transverse and short oblique extra-articular fracture configurations are considered stable. Oblique and comminuted fractures and those with bone loss have unstable configurations. Periosteal disruption correlates with the degree of fracture displacement. Fractures with stable configurations may be unstable if they are severely displaced owing to periosteal disruption, whereas fractures with unstable configurations may be stable when undisplaced or minimally displaced, because the periosteum remains relatively intact. Unbalanced muscle forces or external forces, such as an impact, may cause fracture displacement during the course of treatment, especially in fractures of unstable configuration.

The spectrum of closed simple hand fracture management

Undisplaced closed simple hand fractures

Most hand fractures are closed, simple, undisplaced or minimally displaced, and stable [Fig. 3] [23,33]. Such fractures of stable configuration simply require dynamic splinting (allowing early motion)

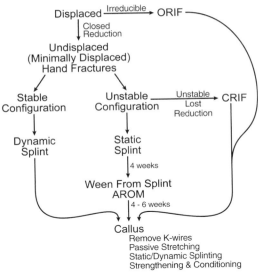

Fig. 3. Algorithm for the treatment of closed simple hand fractures. AROM, active range of motion; CRIF, closed reduction and internal fixation; ORIF, open reduction and internal fixation.

or buddy-taping or splinting to an adjacent finger. Indeed, some physicians may elect to treat impacted fractures of this nature without splinting or taping in reliable patients, particularly when there is minimal swelling and tenderness [25].

Undisplaced or minimally displaced extra-articular fractures with unstable configuration require static protective splinting (no motion allowed) for a brief period (approximately 4 weeks). Simple, closed, undisplaced articular fractures should be considered unstable, owing to their oblique configuration and thin adjacent periosteum, and may be most

safely treated with 3 to 4 weeks of static splinting before initiation of rehabilitation. Some reports recommend Kirschner wire or miniscrew fixation of unicondylar proximal phalanx fractures adjacent to the proximal interphalangeal joint to minimize the risk of spontaneous displacement [26,56,57].

Minimally displaced closed simple hand fractures

Minimally displaced stable closed hand fractures that fall within the parameters of acceptable reduction, initially or following closed reduction, may be treated similarly to undisplaced fractures [**Fig. 4**] [16–38]. Nonoperative treatment may be acceptable for fractures with borderline displacement to avoid the risk of increased digital stiffness posed by surgery. Later corrective osteotomy remains an option, although it is seldom necessary. However, some physicians may believe that the risk-benefit ratio favors the use of traction or percutaneous, internal, or external fixation reduction.

Displaced simple hand fractures with a stable configuration

Simple extra-articular diaphyseal hand fractures of stable configuration displaced beyond acceptable parameters may be treated by closed manipulative reduction [16–28]. Fractures of transverse and short oblique configuration tend to be stable following closed reduction and may be managed thereafter similarly to closed undisplaced fractures of like kind. Fractures with simple angulation often are easily reduced and will maintain their reduction when splinted in a functional position with the muscles balanced. The cortices on the angulated side of the fracture act as a hinge to implement

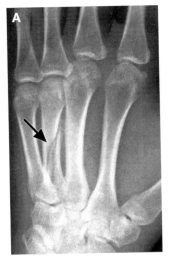
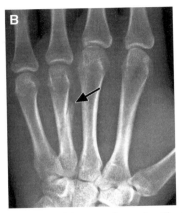

Fig. 4. (A) Oblique undisplaced (unstable configuration) metacarpal fracture (*arrow*) with minimal displacement and no clinical deformity. (B) Fracture callus (*arrow*) apparent 5 weeks after injury.

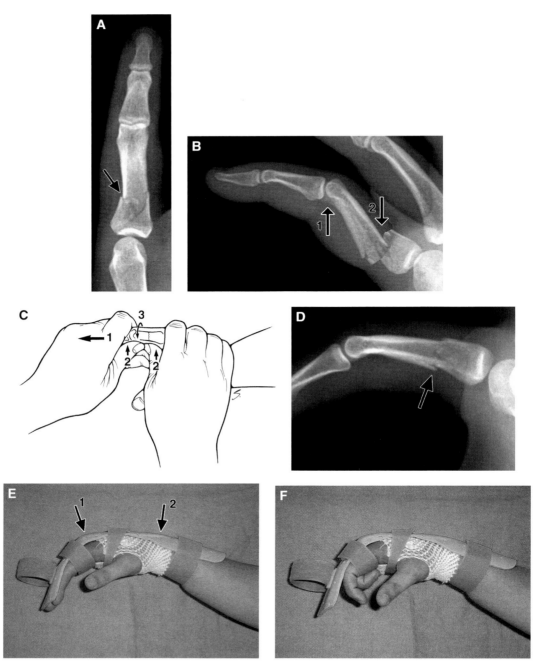

Fig. 5. (*A*) Posterior-anterior view of a transverse extra-articular fracture (*arrow*) of an index finger. (*B*) Lateral view. Arrow 1 demonstrates condylar rotation of the proximal phalanx and pseudoclawing of the proximal interphalangeal joint, owing to an extensor tendon lag. Arrow 2 points to the palmarly angulated fracture hinged on the palmar cortices. (*C*) Fracture reduction is accomplished by traction (*arrow 1*), compression at the apex of the fracture (*arrows 2*), and flexion and rotation of the distal fragment into a reduced position (*arrow 3*). (*D*) The fracture immediately after reduction (*arrow*). Dynamic thermoplastic splint allowing finger extension (*E*) and flexion (*F*). Arrow 1 demonstrates the mold for metacarpophalangeal joint flexion. Arrow 2 displays the mold for slight wrist flexion. (*G*) Posterior-anterior and (*H*) lateral views of the healed fracture. Arrows point to periosteal fracture callus.

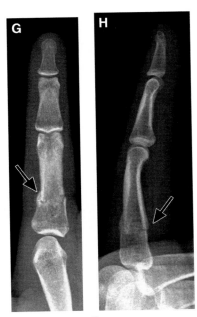

Fig. 5 (continued).

reduction. The periosteum may be sufficiently intact to contribute to stability in the reduced position.

Case 1

A 19-year-old woman was thrown from her horse and sustained a displaced closed transverse extra-articular fracture of the proximal phalanx of her dominant right hand [**Figs. 5A, B**]. She had an abrasion on the dorsum of the hand proximal to the fracture site. A closed reduction was performed [**Figs. 5C, D**]. She was treated in a static splint for 2 weeks and then converted to a dynamic functional splint [**Figs. 5E, F**]. A poor extensor tendon moment arm and weak extensor power at the proximal interphalangeal joint compared with the flexion moment arm and muscle power predispose this joint to extensor lag and the risk of contracture. Consequently, the metacarpophalangeal joints were flexed to balance muscle forces at the fracture site and facilitate proximal interphalangeal joint extension. The wrist was placed in slight flexion to improve the digital extensor contribution to proximal interphalangeal joint extension [52]. An exercise program was initiated. Six weeks after injury, the patient's fracture was healed [**Figs. 5G, H**]. Eight weeks after injury, she had no pain, tenderness, or swelling and had recovered full digital motion. She subsequently returned to work as a waitress.

Case 2

A 22-year-old man sustained a closed subcapital (Boxer's) fracture of his dominant hand in an alter-

cation [**Fig. 6A**]. A Jahss maneuver was performed to accomplish a closed reduction [**Fig. 6B**] [58]. The fracture was first immobilized in a static plaster ulnar gutter splint for 2 weeks. A molded thermoplastic splint was worn for 4 additional weeks [**Figs. 6C, D**]. Exercises were started 4 weeks after injury. Six weeks after injury, the fracture was healed [**Fig. 6E**]. Eight weeks after injury, the patient had no pain, tenderness, or swelling and had recovered full digital motion. He returned to work as a surgical technician.

Case 3

Displaced closed simple fractures of stable configuration with shortening (bayoneting) may be difficult to reduce and maintain, owing to swelling, muscle shortening, and extensive periosteal disruption. Nevertheless, an effort at closed reduction is sometimes rewarded.

A 17-year-old football player sustained a closed displaced transverse fracture of the right fifth metacarpal with shortening (bayonet apposition) and slight dorsal angulating of the fragments [**Fig. 7A**]. A closed reduction was performed on the night of injury [**Fig. 7B**]. A molded static ulnar gutter splint was applied. Four weeks after injury, the patient was placed in a molded thermoplastic splint, which he wore for 3 additional weeks, removing it only for exercises. He did not return to competition for the remainder of the season. When the patient was seen 4 months after injury, the fracture had healed; he had no complaints, swelling, or tenderness and was cleared for baseball season [**Fig. 7C**].

Displaced simple hand fractures with an unstable configuration

Displaced simple long oblique closed diaphyseal and articular fractures that may be manipulated into an acceptable position require some form of stabilization. The application of percutaneous Kirschner wire or miniscrew fixation has been termed "closed reduction and internal fixation" [1–5,18,26,59,60]. Static traction or mini–external fixation, with or without percutaneous pinning of the principal fragments, has also been successful as an alternative method of minimally invasive treatment [61–67]. Closed fracture reduction with or without percutaneous Kirschner wire, miniscrew fixation, traction, or mini–external fixation is atraumatic compared with open operative procedures; it is accompanied by less risk for adherent scar formation and minimal risk for fragment devascularization. Fracture healing is usually sufficiently advanced at 4 to 6 weeks that Kirschner wires and mini–external fixators may be removed or traction discontinued. When fracture callus is apparent, the

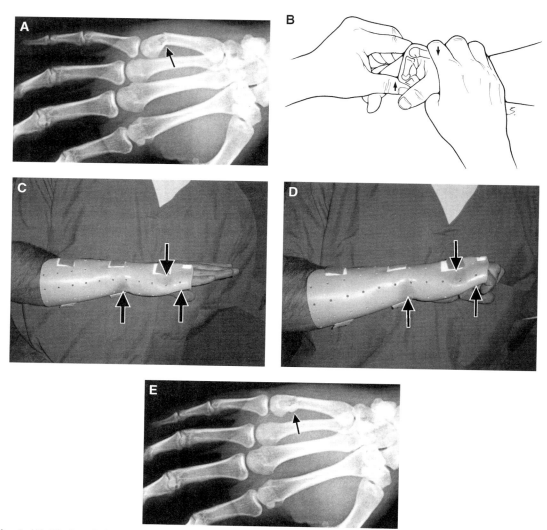

Fig. 6. (*A*) Displaced closed transverse subcapital ("Boxer's") fracture (*arrow*) of a fifth metacarpal. (*B*) Jahss reduction maneuver. Arrows demonstrate the direction of the physician's digital compression at the proximal and distal fragment sites. A functional thermoplastic splint is molded (*arrows*) to support the fracture and balance the muscle forces at the fracture site while allowing finger interphalangeal extension (*C*) and flexion (*D*). (*E*) Healed fracture with apparent external palmar fracture callus (*arrow*).

physician is reasonably assured that the fracture will remain stable after removal of Kirschner wire, mini–external fixator, or traction. Miniscrews and plates in adults and more mature adolescents are usually removed only if they become symptomatic. The rare miniscrew or plate inserted in a growing child or adolescent should be considered for removal after fracture healing to avoid embedding in new bone growth.

Irreducible simple fractures

If a simple closed displaced hand fracture cannot be satisfactorily reduced by nonoperative methods,

open reduction is indicated [1–6]. Operative dissection should be minimized and adequate internal or external minifixation applied. Open simple fractures that cannot be reduced satisfactorily may be treated likewise, with extension of the wound by incision or by separate incision when necessary [1–7]. Treatment thereafter is similar to that of reducible unstable displaced simple fractures.

Loss of closed fracture reduction

If fracture reduction is lost at any time during the nonoperative treatment process, the fracture should be considered unstable regardless of its configu-

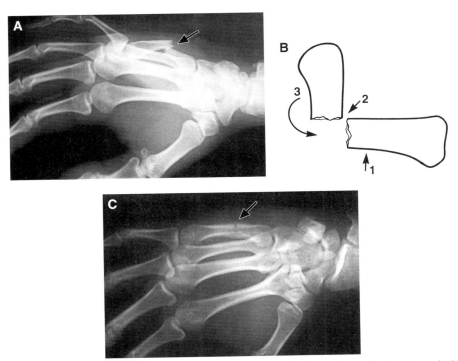

Fig. 7. (*A*) Closed transverse midshaft fifth metacarpal fracture with shortening and dorsal angulation (*arrow*). Note the pseudoclaw deformity of the small finger. (*B*) Reduction maneuver. The proximal fragment is stabilized (*arrow 1*). The distal fragment is extended and the dorsal cortices are engaged to create a "hinge" (*arrow 2*). The distal fragment is flexed to complete the reduction. (*C*) Healed fracture with periosteal callus (*arrow*).

ration [4]. Although a second attempt at closed manipulative reduction without fixation may be considered, it may be prudent to secure the fracture to avoid a second failure of treatment. This option is especially prudent when one must take the patient to the operating room, because it permits one to avoid the embarrassment of a second loss of reduction and a second trip to the operating room for the same fracture.

Comminuted fractures

Although this article primarily addresses the treatment of low-energy closed simple fractures with a limited zone of injury, a few words should be said about higher-energy comminuted fractures that have a more expanded zone of injury. Comminuted fractures are inherently unstable and are more frequently compounded by wounding and tendon, nerve, and vascular injury than are simple fractures. Ultimate digital stiffness correlates with severity of initial injury to bone and soft tissue. Comminuted fractures tend to lead to a higher risk for stiffness than simple fractures. This is especially true of articular fractures as contrasted with extra-articular fractures. The injured finger's proximal interphalangeal

joint is especially vulnerable. Open reduction and internal fracture fixation, even when essential, may significantly increase the risk of digital stiffness. Closed manipulation and careful splinting sometimes provide reasonable positioning and avoid surgically upsetting a collection of minute bone bits. Comminuted pilon fractures of the proximal articular surface of the middle phalanx have been most successfully managed with dynamic traction or external fixation carefully calibrated to maintain fracture reduction without distraction [67–71]. Ancillary Kirschner wires or miniscrews may be added to secure major fracture fragments. This principle may be extended to the treatment of other comminuted joint fractures in the hand, whether closed or open. Comminuted diaphyseal hand fractures may be treated with miniplates, mini–external fixators, Kirschner wires, or static traction. Miniplates have the advantage of permanency, maintaining fracture support throughout healing and allowing earlier and more intensive rehabilitation; they also have the disadvantage of requiring operative dissection. Kirschner wires, mini–external fixators, and static traction are less invasive, but premature loosening or removal may lead to fracture settling or collapse. No clear solution to this dilemma exists.

Surgeons must use their best judgment based on individual fracture considerations.

Rehabilitation

Recovery of motion is the fundamental goal of rehabilitation [4,26,27]. Progressive exercises initiated as early as safely possible may be crucial to the recovery of motion [72,73]. No penalty in final outcome is likely in closed fractures so long as exercises are initiated within 4 weeks of injury, but morbidity may be lessened when exercises can be started early (within 21 days) [74]. Once fracture healing is assured and motion has been recovered, strength, power, and endurance can be recouped.

Fracture stability limits pain and allows more rapid implementation of exercises. Progressive active range of motion exercises may be gradually initiated from the outset in undisplaced, reduced, and especially impacted fractures of stable configuration, in fractures with internal fixation, and after 4 weeks in fractures of unstable configuration that have not been fixed. Continuous static splinting should ordinarily not exceed 4 weeks [14].

Kirschner wire and mini–external fixator pins often skewer the extensor apparatus. They may limit tendon excursion and joint motion and even lead to adhesions. In patients treated with these devices, the therapist should strive gently and progressively to help the patient regain 60° of midrange motion in the hand before their removal. This degree of motion correlates with the 4 to 5 mm of flexor and extensor tendon excursion considered necessary to prevent permanent adhesions [75]. It is also "safe" enough to protect the Kirschner wires and mini–external fixator pins from any serious loosening, provided the patient does not exceed the point of subjective aggravation.

Closed unoperated hand fractures heal through a process of forming a collar of external endosteal callus, first involving the outer cortices and then gradually involving the medullary cortex and cancellous bone. During this process, calcium deposition in the fracture callus escalates at 10 to 21 days after injury [76,77]. At 4 weeks after injury, fracture callus is sufficiently developed and pain, swelling, and tenderness are sufficiently improved or resolved so that splints may be removed for therapy sessions consisting of gentle progressive active range of motion exercises. The splints are worn protectively between sessions until fracture callus is visualized on radiograph (usually at 4 to 6 weeks after injury). Once callus is visualized on radiograph, the fracture is "locked." At this point, Kirschner wires may be removed, patients may be weaned from protective splinting, and strengthening and conditioning exercises may safely be initiated. Pas-

sive stretching exercises and static joint blocking and dynamic splints designed to overcome tendon and joint adhesions may also be applied.

Complications

Stiffness is the most common complication of hand fractures [8–15]. The risk for developing stiffness is primarily related to initial fracture severity and the extent of the zone of injury, although even justifiable operative treatment slightly increases this risk [1–7]. Implants alone do not substantially increase the risk of stiffness. The primary culprit is the operative trauma necessary to apply them. Nonoperative treatment, when applicable, minimizes this risk. Operative tenolysis and capsulectomy are reserved for the most severe and recalcitrant instances of tendon and joint contracture [8,9].

Nonunion of hand fractures, especially closed simple fractures, is rare [78]. Malunion of consequence also rarely occurs in simple fractures, provided the fracture parameters described here are followed. Articular fragments are at risk for devascularization and subsequent avascular necrosis and joint arthritis. Nevertheless, symptomatic postoperative arthritis of hand fractures requiring further surgery, even in articular fractures, is uncommon [22,29–32,79]. Every effort is made to treat children's fractures by closed methods to minimize the risk of epiphyseal plate injury and future growth disturbances.

Summary

Stiffness is the most frequent consequence of open hand fracture treatment [8–15]. Although initial injury severity and occurrence adjacent to the flexor tendon sheath are the most highly correlated determinants of hand fracture outcome, operative intervention accentuates the ultimate risk of stiffness [1–5,7]. Closed treatment may minimize this risk. Articular fractures are at greater risk for stiffness than extra-articular fractures, and among these finger proximal interphalangeal joint fractures are the most susceptible.

Functional tolerance for small amounts of variation from perfect anatomic restoration gives us increased latitude for closed hand fracture management [40–53]. Rehabilitation of stable simple closed fractures may start early (within 21 days), and rehabilitation of unstable fractures with the expectation of good-to-excellent functional recovery may start after 4 weeks [16–38]. Operative treatment may be justified for simple closed fractures when they are unstable, irreducible, or open, or when the surgeon believes that the risk-to-benefit ratio is favorable [1–7].

References

[1] Pun WK, Chow SP, So YC, et al. A prospective study on 284 digital fractures of the hand. J Hand Surg 1989;14A(3):474–81.

[2] Ip WY, Ng KH, Chow SP. A prospective study of 924 digital fractures of the hand. Injury 1996; 27(4):279–85.

[3] Kozin SH, Thoder JJ, Lieberman G. Operative treatment of metacarpal and phalangeal shaft fractures. J Am Acad Orthop Surg 2000;8(2): 111–21.

[4] Freeland AE, Geissler WB, Weiss APC. Operative treatment of common displaced and unstable fractures of the hand. J Bone Joint Surg 2001; 83A(6):928–45.

[5] Stern PJ. Management of fractures of the hand over the last 25 years. J Hand Surg 2000;25A(5): 817–23.

[6] Hall RF. Treatment of metacarpal and phalangeal fractures in noncompliant patients. Clin Orthop 1987;214:31–6.

[7] Duncan RW, Freeland AE, Jabaley ME, et al. Open hand fractures: an analysis of the recovery of active motion and complications. J Hand Surg 1993;18A(3):387–94.

[8] Creighton JJ, Steichen JB. Complications in phalangeal and metacarpal fracture management. Results of extensor tenolysis. Hand Clin 1994;10(1):111–6.

[9] Green DP. Complications of phalangeal and metacarpal fractures. Hand Clin 1986;2(2):307–28.

[10] Kuczynski K. The proximal interphalangeal joint: anatomy and causes of stiffness in the fingers. J Bone Joint Surg 1968;50B(3):656–63.

[11] Merritt WH. Written in behalf of the stiff finger. J Hand Ther 1998;11(2):74–9.

[12] Page SM, Stern PJ. Complications and range of motion following plate fixation of metacarpal and phalangeal fractures. J Hand Surg 1998; 23A(5):827–32.

[13] Stern PJ, Wieser MJ, Reilly DG. Complications of plate fixation in the hand skeleton. Clin Orthop 1987;214:59–65.

[14] Strickland JW, Steichen JB, Kleinman WB, et al. Phalangeal fractures: factors influencing digital performance. Orthop Rev 1982;11(8):39–50.

[15] Fusetti C, Meyer H, Borisch N, et al. Complications of plate fixation in metacarpal fractures. J Trauma 2002;52(3):535–9.

[16] Barton N. Fractures of the phalanges of the hand. Hand 1977;9(1):1–10.

[17] Barton NJ. Fractures of the shafts of the phalanges of the hand. Hand 1979;11(2):119–33.

[18] Barton NJ. Fractures of the hand. J Bone Joint Surg 1984;66B(2):159–67.

[19] Bloem JJ. The treatment and prognosis of uncomplicated dislocated fractures of the metacarpals and phalanges. Arch Chir Neerl 1971;23(1): 55–65.

[20] Burkhalter WE. Hand fractures. Instr Course Lect 1990;39:249–53.

[21] Burkhalter WE. Closed treatment of hand fractures. J Hand Surg 1989;14A(2):390–3.

[22] Cannon SR, Dowd GS, Williams DH, et al. A long-term study following Bennett's fracture. J Hand Surg 1986;11B(3):426–31.

[23] Corley Jr FG, Schenck Jr RC. Fractures of the hand. Clin Plast Surg 1996;23(3):447–62.

[24] Ebinger T, Erhard N, Kinzl L, et al. Dynamic treatment of displaced proximal phalangeal fractures. J Hand Surg 1999;24A(6):1254–62.

[25] Ford DJ, Ali MS, Steel WM. Fractures of the fifth metacarpal neck: is reduction or immobilization necessary? J Hand Surg 1989;14B(2):165–7.

[26] Freeland AE, Sennett BJ. Phalangeal fractures. In: Peimer CA, editor. Surgery of the hand and upper extremity, Vol. 1. New York: McGraw-Hill; 1995. p. 921–37.

[27] Freeland AE, Torres J. Extraarticular fractures of the phalanges. In: Berger RA, Weiss APC, editors. Hand surgery. Philadelphia: Lippincott, Williams and Wilkins; 2004. p. 121–37.

[28] Freiberg A, Pollard BA, MacDonald MR, et al. Management of proximal interphalangeal joint fractures. J Trauma 1999;46(3):523–8.

[29] Kahler DM. Fractures and dislocations of the base of the thumb. J South Orthop Assoc 1995;4(1): 69–76.

[30] Kjaer-Petersen K, Langhoff O, Andersen K. Bennett's fracture. J Hand Surg 1990;15B(1):58–61.

[31] Konradsen L, Nielsen PT, Albrecht-Beste E. Functional treatment of metacarpal fractures. One-hundred randomized cases with or without fixation. Acta Orthop Scand 1990;61(6):531–4.

[32] Livesley PJ. The conservative management of Bennett's fracture dislocation: a 26-year follow-up. J Hand Surg 1990;15B(3):291–4.

[33] Maitra A, Burdett-Smith P. The conservative management of proximal phalangeal fractures of the hand in an accident and emergency department. J Hand Surg 1992;17B(3):332–6.

[34] McNemar TB, Howell JW, Chang E. Management of metacarpal fractures. J Hand Ther 2003;16(2): 143–51.

[35] McKerrell J, Bowen V, Johnston G, et al. Boxer's fractures—conservative or operative management? J Trauma 1987;27(5):486–90.

[36] Reyes FA, Latta LL. Conservative management of difficult phalangeal fractures. Clin Orthop 1987; 214:23–30.

[37] Timmenga EJ, Blokhuis TJ, Maas M, et al. Long-term evaluation of Bennett's fracture. A comparison between open and closed reduction. J Hand Surg 1994;19B(3):373–7.

[38] Viegas SF, Tencer A, Woodard P, et al. Functional bracing of fractures of the second through fifth metacarpals. J Hand Surg 1987;12A(1): 139–43.

[39] Seitz Jr WH, Froimson AI. Management of malunited fractures of the metacarpal and phalangeal shafts. Hand Clin 1988;4(3):529–36.

[40] Schreuders TA, Stam HJ. Strength measurements of the lumbrical muscles. J Hand Ther 1996;9(4): 303–5.

[41] Kozin SH, Porter S, Clark P, et al. The contribution of the intrinsic muscles to grip and pinch strength. J Hand Surg 1999;24A(1):64–72.

[42] Low CK, Wong HC, Low YP, et al. A cadaver study of the effects of dorsal angulation and shortening of the metacarpal shaft on the extension and flexion force ratios of the index and little fingers. J Hand Surg 1995;20B(5):609–13.

[43] Meunier MJ, Hentzen E, Ryan M, et al. Predicted effects of metacarpal shortening on interosseous muscle function. J Hand Surg 2004; 29A(4):689–93.

[44] Strauch RJ, Rosenwasser MP, Lunt JG. Metacarpal shaft fractures: the effect of shortening on the extensor tendon mechanism. J Hand Surg 1998; 23A(3):519–23.

[45] Eglseder Jr WA, Juliano PJ, Roure R. Fractures of the fourth metacarpal. J Orthop Trauma 1997; 11(6):441–5.

[46] Birndorf MS, Daley R, Greenwald DP. Metacarpal fracture angulation decreases flexor mechanical efficiency in human hands. Plast Reconstr Surg 1997;99(4):1079–83 [discussion: 1084–5].

[47] Hunter JM, Cowen NJ. Fifth metacarpal fractures in a compensation clinic population. A report on one-hundred and thirty-three cases. J Bone Joint Surg 1970;52A(6):1159–65.

[48] Opgrande JD, Westphal SA. Fractures of the hand. Orthop Clin North Am 1983;14(4): 779–92.

[49] Royle SG. Rotational deformity following metacarpal fracture. J Hand Surg 1990;15B(1):124–5.

[50] Agee J. Treatment principles for proximal and middle phalangeal fractures. Orthop Clin North Am 1992;23(1):35–40.

[51] Vahey JW, Wegner DA, Hastings III H. Effect of proximal phalangeal fracture deformity on extensor tendon function. J Hand Surg 1998; 23A(4):673–81.

[52] Freeland AE, Hardy MA, Singletary S. Rehabilitation for proximal phalangeal fractures. J Hand Ther 2003;16(2):129–42.

[53] Coonrad RW, Pohlman MH. Impacted fractures in the proximal portion of the proximal phalanx of the finger. J Bone Joint Surg 1969;51A(7): 1291–6.

[54] Hastings II H. Unstable metacarpal and phalangeal fracture treatment with screws and plates. Clin Orthop 1987;214:37–42.

[55] Stern PJ, Roman RJ, Kiefhaber TR, et al. Pilon fractures of the proximal interphalangeal joint. J Hand Surg 1991;16(5):844–50.

[56] Freeland AE, Benoist LA. Open reduction and internal fixation method for fractures at the proximal interphalangeal joint. Hand Clin 1994;10(3):239–50.

[57] Freeland AE, Sud V. Unicondylar and bicondylar proximal phalanx fractures. Journal of the American Society of the Hand 2001;1(1):14–24.

[58] Jahss SA. Fractures of the metacarpals. A new method of reduction and immobilization. J Bone Joint Surg 1938;20B(3):486–90.

[59] Green DP, Anderson JR. Closed reduction and percutaneous pin fixation of fractured phalanges. J Bone Joint Surg 1973;55A(8):1651–4.

[60] Belsky MR, Eaton RG, Lane LB. Closed reduction and internal fixation of proximal phalangeal fractures. J Hand Surg 1984;9(5):725–9.

[61] Rooks M. Traction treatment for unstable proximal phalangeal fractures. Southern Orthopaedic Journal 1(1):15–9.

[62] Collins AL, Timlin M, Thornes B, et al. Old principles revisited—traction splinting for proximal phalangeal fractures. Injury 2002;33(3):235–7.

[63] Nagy L. Static external fixation of finger fractures. Hand Clin 1993;9(4):651–7.

[64] Schuind F, Cooney WP, Burny F, et al. Small external fixation devices for the hand and wrist. Clin Orthop 1993;293:77–82.

[65] Pennig D, Gausepohl T, Mader K, et al. The use of minimally invasive fixation in fractures of the hand—the minifixator concept. Injury 2000; 31(Suppl 1):102–12.

[66] Fricker R, Thomann Y, Troeger H. AO external minifixateur for the hand bones. Surgical technique and initial experiences. Chirurgy 1996; 67(7):760–3.

[67] Drenth DJ, Klausen HJ. External fixation for phalangeal and metacarpal fractures. J Bone Joint Surg 1998;80(2):227–30.

[68] Fahmy NR. The Stockport Serpentine Spring System for the treatment of displaced comminuted intraarticular phalangeal fractures. J Hand Surg 1990;15B(3):303–11.

[69] Schenck RR. The dynamic traction method. Combining movement and traction for intraarticular fractures of the phalanges. Hand Clin 1994;10(2):187–98.

[70] Johnson D, Tiernan E, Richards AM, et al. Dynamic external fixation for complex intraarticular phalangeal fractures. J Hand Surg 2004; 29(1):76–81.

[71] Sarris I, Goitz RJ, Sotereanos DG. Dynamic traction and minimal internal fixation for thumb and digital pilon fractures. J Hand Surg 2004; 29(1):39–43.

[72] Crosby CA, Wehbe MA. Early motion in hand and wrist rehabilitation. Hand Clin 1996;12(1): 31–41.

[73] Margles SW. Early motion in the treatment of hand fractures and dislocations in the hand and wrist. Hand Clin 1996;12(1):65–72.

[74] Feehan LM, Bassett K. Is there evidence for early mobilization following an extraarticular hand fracture? J Hand Ther 2004;17(2):300–8.

[75] Duran RS, Houser RG. Controlled passive motion following flexor tendon repair in zones two and three. In: AAOS Symposium on Flexor Tendon Surgery in the Hand. St. Louis (MO): CV Mosby; 1975. p. 105–11.

[76] Einhorn TA, Hirschman A, Kaplan C, et al. Neutral protein-degrading enzymes in experimental fracture callus: a preliminary report. J Orthop Res 1989;7(6):792–805.

[77] Buckwalter JA, Einhorn TA, Bolander ME, et al.

Healing of musculoskeletal tissues. In: Rockwood Jr CA, Green DP, Bucholz RW, et al, editors. 4th edition. Fractures in adults, Vol. 1. Philadelphia: Lippincott-Raven; 1996. p. 261–304.

[78] Jupiter JB, Koniuch MP, Smith RJ. The management of delayed union and nonunion of the metacarpals and phalanges. J Hand Surg 1985; 10A(4):457–66.

[79] O'Rourke SK, Gaur S, Barton NJ. Long-term outcome of articular fractures of the phalanges: an eleven-year follow-up. J Hand Surg 1989; 14B(2):183–93.

ELSEVIER
SAUNDERS

CLINICS IN
PLASTIC
SURGERY

Clin Plastic Surg 32 (2005) 563–573

Challenges in Creating a Good Randomized Controlled Trial in Hand Surgery

Achilleas Thoma, MD, MSc, FRCSC, FACS[a,b,*]

- Consolidated Standards of Reporting Trials statement
- Specific challenges in the design and execution of randomized controlled trials in hand surgery
  The surgical learning curve
  Randomization
  Concealment and blinding
  Loss to follow-up
  Intention-to-treat analysis

Surgical equipoise
Differential care
Treatment effect and implications for sample size
- The use of economic analysis in hand surgery
- Changing the "hand surgeons' *culture*"
- Acknowledgments
- References

Although a number of study designs are frequently used in clinical research, the randomized controlled trial (RCT) is generally regarded as the most scientifically rigorous study design to evaluate the effect of a surgical intervention. This type of study offers the maximum protection against selection bias [1,2].

In the 1970s and early 1980s, neurosurgeons frequently performed extracranial–intracranial bypass surgeries in which the superficial temporal artery was anastomosed to the middle cerebral artery, believing that this prevented strokes. Comparisons of outcomes among nonrandomized cohorts of patients who for various reasons did or did not undergo this procedure appeared to show that the bypass procedure had a salutary effect on these patients. However, when a large, multicenter RCT was undertaken, in which patients were randomly allocated to surgical or medical treatment, the study demonstrated that the only effect of surgery was to increase adverse outcomes in the immediate post-surgical period [3]. Another instance in which an RCT provided a contrary finding to prevailing practice is the discovery that steroid injections do not mitigate facet-joint back pain [4].

Readers of hand surgery literature are constantly bombarded with articles claiming the superiority of the "novel" technique over the "traditional" technique. The positive outcomes frequently achieved in hand surgery studies in which physicians' or patients' choice determined whether a patient received the experimental surgical treatment may have several causes. The true effect of the experimental treatment is just one of the multiple factors that can account for the outcome. Such studies are called observational studies, and, unfortunately, they are the most commonly encountered studies in the hand surgery literature.

[a] Department of Surgery, McMaster University, Hamilton, Ontario, Canada
[b] Surgical Outcomes Research Centre, St. Joseph's Healthcare, 101-206 James Street South, Hamilton, Ontario L8P 3A9, Canada
* Surgical Outcomes Research Centre, St. Joseph's Healthcare, 101-206 James Street South, Hamilton, Ontario L8P 3A9, Canada.
E-mail address: athoma@mcmaster.ca

doi:10.1016/j.cps.2005.05.002

Table 1: **Checklist of items to include when reporting a randomized trial (2003 Revised CONSORT Statement)**

	Item number	Descriptor	Reported on page number
Title and abstract	1	How participants were allocated to interventions (eg, "random allocation," "randomized," or "randomly assigned")	
Introduction Background	2	Scientific background and explanation of rationale	
Methods Participants	3	Eligibility criteria for participants and the settings and locations where the data were collected	
Interventions	4	Precise details of the interventions intended for each group and how and when they were actually administered	
Objectives	5	Specific objectives and hypotheses	
Outcomes	6	Clearly defined primary and secondary outcome measures and, when applicable, any methods used to enhance the quality of measurements (eg, multiple observations, training of assessors)	
Sample size	7	How sample size was determined and, when applicable, explanation of any interim analyses and stopping rules	
Randomization Sequence generation	8	Method used to generate the random allocation sequence, including details of any restriction (eg, blocking, stratification)	
Allocation concealment	9	Method used to implement the random allocation sequence (eg, numbered containers or central telephone), clarifying whether the sequence was concealed until interventions were assigned	
Implementation	10	Who generated the allocation sequence, who enrolled participants, and who assigned participants to their groups	
Blinding (masking)	11	Whether or not participants, those administering the interventions, and those assessing the outcomes were aware of group assignment. If not, how the success of masking was assessed	
Statistical methods	12	Statistical methods used to compare groups for primary outcome(s); methods for additional analyses, such as subgroup analyses and adjusted analyses	
Results Participant flow	13	Flow of participants through each stage (a diagram is strongly recommended). Specifically, for each group, report the numbers of participants randomly assigned, receiving intended treatment, completing the study protocol, and analyzed for the primary outcome. Describe protocol deviations from study as planned, together with reasons.	
Recruitment	14	Dates defining the periods of recruitment and follow-up	
Baseline data	15	Baseline demographic and clinical characteristics of each group	
Numbers analyzed	16	Number of participants (denominator) in each group included in each analysis and whether the analysis was by "intention to treat." State the results in absolute numbers when feasible (eg, 10 of 20, not 50%).	

(continued on next page)

Table 1: **(continued)**

	Item number	Descriptor	Reported on page number
Results			
Outcomes and estimation	17	For each primary and secondary outcome, a summary of results for each group, and the estimated effect size and its precision (eg, 95% confidence interval).	
Ancillary analyses	18	Address multiplicity by reporting any other analyses performed, including subgroup analyses and adjusted analyses, indicating those prespecified and those exploratory.	
Adverse events	19	All important adverse events or side effects in each intervention group	
Discussion			
Interpretation	20	Interpretation of the results, taking into account study hypotheses, sources of potential bias or imprecision, and the dangers associated with multiplicity of analyses and outcomes	
Generalizability	21	Generalizability (external validity) of the trial findings	
Overall evidence	22	General interpretation of the results in the context of current evidence	

From Moher D, Schulz KF, Altaman DJ. The CONSORT statement: revised recommendations for improving the quality of reports of parallel-group randomized trials. Clin Oral Invest 2003;7:4; with permission.

Hand surgical trials attempt to determine the impact of the surgical intervention on such outcomes as grip strength, control of pain, ability to return to activities of daily living, and ability to return to work. These events are often referred to as the trial's target outcomes or primary events. A number of factors, however, can determine the frequency with which the trial's target outcomes occur. These prognostic factors may include the age and sex of the patient, the severity of the condition before the patient entered the study, and current treatment. Diabetes and cardiac conditions are examples of comorbid conditions that can affect the frequency of the trial's target outcomes. It is fair to say that the Workers Compensation status of a patient can also affect the return to work target outcome.

If a particular study does not take into consideration the prognostic factors, both those we do and do not know about (ie, if these factors are not balanced in the experimental and control groups), then there is a good chance the study's outcomes will be biased. The study will either over- or underestimate the true effect of the surgical intervention.

The prognostic factors usually influence surgeons' recommendations and patients' decisions about submitting themselves to surgical interventions. As a result, observational studies often yield misleading results. It is well recognized that observational studies tend to show larger treatment effects than do RCTs [5–8]. Although, in theory, one can balance prognostic factors in observational studies, the methods of doing this have limitations. Only in the properly designed RCT are the investigators certain that there is a balance of prognostic factors between the experimental and control groups, minimizing bias and maximizing the chance that the results are valid.

Although the RCT is considered the best of all research designs or "the most powerful tool in modern clinical research" [9], it is not a panacea for all clinical questions. The popular belief that only the RCT produces trustworthy results and that all observational studies are misleading does disservice to patient care, clinical investigation, and the education of health care professionals [10]. In many situations an RCT is not feasible, necessary, or appropriate. For example, in a hypothetical question of harm, we cannot use a suspected teratogenic drug versus placebo in an RCT to see if in fact the drug produces phocomelia in newborns. In such a scenario, a case-control study design is the most appropriate and ethical design to answer the question.

Nevertheless, the RCT is the ideal study design to answer questions related to the effects of hand surgery interventions that are small to moderate. A hierarchy of strength of evidence for surgical treatment decisions follows:

Systematic review of RCTs (meta-analysis)
Single RCT
Systematic review of observational studies addressing patient-important outcomes

Single observational study addressing patient-important outcomes

Physiologic studies (eg, rodent experiments on nerve regeneration and bone healing)

Unsystematic clinical observations

Unfortunately, the hand surgery community has not embraced the RCT to the same degree as our colleagues from various medical subspecialties. In addition, when hand-related surgical RCTs are reported in the literature, their validity is often questionable because of faulty methodology. The mere reporting of a hand surgical study as "randomized" does not allow hand surgeons to infer validity. Thoma and colleagues [11] recently presented a review of all the randomized controlled trials that compared endoscopic carpal tunnel release (ECTR) with open carpal tunnel release (OCTR) and found serious methodologic flaws in the reporting of those studies. These RCTs gave conflicting conclusions. Because the reporting was found to be flawed, one must question the validity of these studies. It is surprising that these "randomized controlled trials" made it through the various journals' editors despite the fact that guidelines for the reporting of RCTs have existed since the mid-1990s.

In this article, the author begins by discussing the application of the Consolidated Standards of Reporting Trials, or the CONSORT statement. This statement is a formal list of items that editors of journals expect investigators to report in any RCT. The precondition for a successful RCT in hand surgery is that investigators include the items of the CONSORT in the study's design. The author then discusses the unique challenges in the execution of an RCT in hand surgery, including (1) the surgical learning curve, (2) randomization, (3) concealment and blinding, (4) loss to follow-up, (5) intention-to-treat analysis, (6) surgical equipoise, (7) differential care, and (8) treatment effect and implications for sample size. In the following section, the author discusses the use of economic analysis in RCTs in hand surgery. The article concludes with a discussion of changing the hand surgeons' research culture and with a look at the bigger picture.

Consolidated Standards of Reporting Trials statement

In the mid-1990s, two independent initiatives to improve the reporting of RCTs were undertaken by a group of international epidemiologists, clinical trialists, biostatisticians, and biomedical editors. These initiatives led to the publication of the CONSORT statement [12]. The CONSORT statement comprises a checklist and a flow diagram to be used by investigators in reporting an RCT. It has recently been upgraded: the revised version includes a 22-item checklist [Table 1] and the flow diagram [**Fig. 1**] [13].

When reading a report of an RCT in hand surgery, one should know the quality of the methodology used. The RCT report should convey to the reader why the study was undertaken, how it was conducted, and how data were analyzed. All this should be reported in a clear and transparent fashion. Are these requirements important? Definitely. Evidence suggests that inadequately reported randomization has been associated with bias in estimating the effectiveness of interventions [2,14]. As a consequence, the execution of an RCT in hand

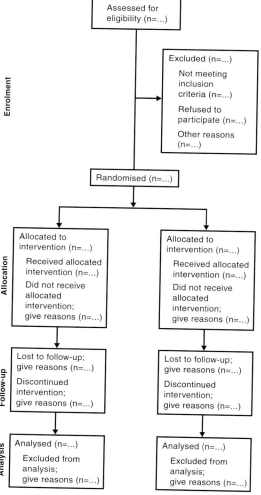

Fig. 1. Flow diagram of progress through the phases of a randomized trial. (*From* Moher D, Schulz KF, Altaman DG. The CONSORT statement: revised recommendations for improving the quality of reports of parallel-group randomized trials. Clin Oral Investig 2003;7:5; with permission.)

surgery must consider the items included in the CONSORT statement.

Specific challenges in the design and execution of randomized controlled trials in hand surgery

In contrast to medical studies that may compare a new pill to a placebo pill or an experimental pill to a standard pill, the execution of a hand surgery RCT poses some specific challenges. In this section, the author discusses particular challenges to the execution of an RCT in hand surgery.

The surgical learning curve

In most pharmaceutic clinical trials, a new drug is compared with a placebo, and no special skills are necessary to administer the different pills. In hand surgery, by contrast, when we compare the "novel" to the "usual" intervention, we need to account for the learning curve in the surgical technique. The learning curve refers to the accumulated experience a surgeon gains in performing a new intervention, in which there is an element of continuous refinement of patient selection, operative technique, and postoperative care. It is inappropriate to compare familiar with unfamiliar surgical procedures, because mistakes and adverse outcomes are more likely to occur with the unfamiliar procedure, and, as a result, this approach will bias results against the novel technique [15–17].

For example, consider the ECTR versus OCTR debate. An investigator has been performing OCTR for the first 10 years of her practice and now would like to compare this technique to the newly introduced ECTR in an RCT. If she does not master the learning curve, a number of possibilities exist, including (1) the investigator may damage more nerves, (2) the investigator may inadequately release the carpal ligament, and (3) the investigator may transect the palmar arch. If, in this hypothetical RCT, the outcome measured is pain and numbness, a good chance exists that the greater proportion of patients with persisting pain and numbness after the intervention will be in the ECTR group. Therefore, we would incorrectly conclude that the ECTR is a useless innovation.

An RCT should only be considered when the participating surgeons are equally capable of performing the novel and the comparator interventions. Failure to control for the learning curve may underestimate the effect size of the novel intervention.

Randomization

Unfortunately, the methods of allocation in trials described as "randomized" are poorly and infrequently reported, even when these are published in prominent journals [18,19]. Although randomization seems like a simple step in the execution of an RCT, this crucial step has often been performed in a faulty manner that invalidates the entire study. In a systematic review of the RCTs that compared ECTR with OCTR, Thoma et al [11] found that 73% of the studies used faulty or inadequate methods of randomization. This step is so crucial to the validity of the study that it needs to be done correctly and to be transparent. The randomization is faulty if investigators use such methods as even or odd birth year or alternate chart number, because these are prone to selection bias [6]. The correct way is for investigators to use random number tables or computer programs to generate the sequences.

Concealment and blinding

It is important that those making the decision about patient eligibility not be aware of the arm of the study to which a particular patient will be allocated (ie, OCTR or ECTR). This measure ensures concealment of the allocation. If investigators fail on the concealment, then they run a risk of enrolling patients with more severe conditions or perhaps lower-risk patients with mild conditions; this selection bias of patient recruitment has been shown to lead to biased results [2,14]. In other words, selection bias may be introduced when some potentially eligible individuals are selectively excluded from the study because of prior knowledge of the group to which they would be allocated if they participated [20]. If this exclusion were to occur, the assignment to treatment would still be random, but the randomization would not be concealed.

A separate issue is the method of allocation. For example, even or odd birth year is a method of allocation that is not randomized. In addition, it is not concealed, and investigators may consciously or unconsciously select patients to enter the study based on knowledge of the group to which they are allocated. True randomization means that each patient has a 50:50 chance of being allocated to one or the other treatment arm in a trial.

Using opaque sealed envelopes is one method of concealing patient allocation. However, there are reports of investigators previewing envelope codes by using a bright light or steaming the envelope open and then resealing it, or simply using the allocation for the next patient or discarding the envelope [20]. The strongest safeguard of concealed randomization is for the hand surgeon to call the randomization center after consent has been obtained, as the patient enters the operating room. This way, the surgeon is unable to exclude the patient based on the treatment allocation the patient receives.

In pharmaceutic randomized trials, the randomization concealment and masking of treatment can be carried to the end of the study. In contrast, in surgical trials, the concealment and masking can only take place until the surgeon opens the opaque envelope or calls the randomization center to find out to which surgical technique the next patient has been assigned.

Studies that are reported as single, double, or triple blinded may be misleading when they do not indicate exactly who was blinded. Blinding may be implemented at six different levels in an RCT: (1) the patients, (2) the clinicians who administer the treatment, (3) the clinicians who take care of patients during the trial, (4) the individuals who assess the patients throughout the trial and collect the data, (5) the data analyst, and (6) the investigators who interpret and write up the results of the trial [20].

In pharmaceutic trials, the investigators, the patients, and the assessors of the outcome may all be blinded, because the placebo may look, smell, and taste exactly like the investigated pill. In hand surgery, the hand surgeons cannot be blinded, because they know whether they have performed an ECTR or OCTR. In addition, the patients know whether they have undergone ECTR or OCTR from the shape of the suture line and eventual scar. The literature acknowledges that a patient who knows the treatment and believes it is efficacious may feel better than patients who do not, even if the treatment is no different from the comparative technique. This phenomenon has been called the placebo effect [21]. The same applies to the occupational therapist who may be the designated assessor for the study. Even if the two surgical groups have been kept prognostically balanced, the study may still introduce bias if the assessors of the outcomes have not been blinded. If either surgical arm of the study receives more frequent or thorough measurement of outcome or cointervention (eg, additional physiotherapy, positive interpretation of marginal findings, or an offer of differential encouragement during performance tests), the results may be distorted [22] in favor of the surgical group that received additional attention. Theoretically, one may blind the assessor of the outcome by covering the scar on the patient's hand before the grip or pinch measurements, if this is the primary outcome of the study.

In many situations, blinding the patient and the outcome assessors is possible; this is the case in procedures where the scars are similar. Examples of these include carpal tunnel release versus carpal tunnel release accompanied by synvovectomy and comparison of various arthroplasy techniques of the carpo-metacarpal joint of the thumb. In most RCTs in hand surgery, it is possible to blind the data analyst and the investigators who interpret and write the results. In an ideal comparative hand surgery RCT, the investigators should consider these issues before embarking on the study.

Loss to follow-up

A major threat to the validity of an RCT in hand surgery is failure to account for all patients at the end of the study [23]. Even the best-designed RCTs suffer when patients are lost to follow-up [24]. Incomplete follow-up biases the results of a trial when patients who drop out are different from those for whom follow-up is completed, and this effect is exaggerated further by differential dropout rates between study groups [24]. Only by striving to achieve a 0% loss to follow-up rate can we be certain that this type of bias does not affect the results of an RCT in hand surgery.

Some patients who are lost to follow-up may have had a bad outcome or died, and it is also possible that some patients had a satisfactory outcome and did not bother to return for follow-up appointments [23]. Only a 0% loss to follow-up ensures the benefits of randomization, although it is unrealistic to expect perfect follow-up in all RCTs [25]. Some researchers suggest that less than 5% loss probably leads to little bias, whereas greater than 20% loss potentially poses serious threats to validity, and intermediate levels lead to intermediate levels of problems [26–28]. The type of hand surgery (chronic versus acute), the outcome event rates, and the length of the follow-up all affect loss to follow-up rates [25].

A large loss to follow-up rate can reduce the study power. The occurrence of the event of interest among patients is uncertain after a specified time when follow-up data collection ends. It is unknown when or whether the event of interest occurred subsequently. Such patients are described as censored or lost to follow-up [29,30]. These patients still contribute to the study up to the time at which their outcome status was last known. One way to examine the data for censoring effect entails the use of appropriate analytic methods, such as survival analysis (application of life-table method to data) [28,31].

Sprague and colleagues [24] suggest a number of primary, secondary, and tertiary strategies for reducing loss to follow-up in surgical RCTs [Box 1]. These measures require the research staff to be highly organized, to allocate time for contacting patients who are at risk for becoming lost to follow-up, and to be committed to the study and reducing loss to follow-up [24]. These innovative techniques

Box 1: Primary, secondary, and tertiary strategies for reducing loss to follow-up

Primary strategies: trial design

- Exclude individuals who are unlikely to complete follow-up (eg, patients with no fixed address, those who report a plan to move out of town in the next year, those who are intellectually challenged without adequate family support, those who are uncertain about their willingness to complete follow-up).
- Fully inform patients of the burden of the study before randomization.
- Provide patients with information on their injuries, the risk for complications, potential treatment effects, and expectations for personal benefit from study participation; provide motivation for adherence with follow-up visits and research protocols.
- At the time of randomization, obtain contact information for the patient, primary care physician, and alternate contacts.
- Before hospital discharge, have the attending surgeon take time with the patient to emphasize how the study will help future patients who have the same problem and to discuss the importance of returning for all follow-up visits.
- Design the study's follow-up schedule to coincide with normal surgical follow-up visits.
- Have study staff at the methods center contact the clinical sites regularly to discuss and to help locate any patients with overdue visits.

Secondary strategies: innovative designs to minimize losses

- Schedule follow-up appointment times around patient preferences.
- Provide patients with reminders for upcoming follow-up visits, maintain regular contact, and obtain information on any planned change in residence.
- Minimize the amount of time patients spend waiting at a follow-up visit and encourage patients to complete questionnaires while waiting.
- Reduce the demands of participation in the study for patients who have a language barrier, cognitive impairment, or as a last resort for patients who do not want to complete the quality of life questionnaires by following for primary events only.
- Closely monitor data for missed and overdue follow-up visits.
- Have methods center staff develop strategies with the clinical staff to locate patients with overdue follow-up appointments.
- Contact patients or alternate contacts by telephone for follow-up, even during evenings and weekends if necessary.

Tertiary strategies: locating patients who are labeled lost to follow-up

- If the methods center receives an early withdrawal form, have methods center staff contact the clinical center immediately to discuss the patient's situation.
- If a patient finds it difficult to continue, have study staff negotiate with the patient to encourage him or her to continue with the study and perhaps offer to reduce the demands of study participation.
- Continue trying to contact lost patients and all alternate contacts until you are able to reach someone to determine the patient's status, unless the telephone lines have been disconnected.
- Have clinical staff watch for patients reappearing in their clinic for other reasons.
- Have staff at the methods center help the clinical centers contact patients they are having a difficult time reaching.

From Sprague S, Leece P, Bhandari M, et al, on behalf of the SPRINT investigators. Limiting loss to follow up in a multi-centre randomized controlled trial in orthopaedic surgery. Control Clin Trials 2003;24:723; with permission.

require a substantial amount of time, increased personnel resources, and, consequently, funding [24]. Many previous surgical trials have been conducted with limited funding, which may explain the high numbers of patients lost to follow-up [32]. Through planning, organization, and committing time and resources to minimizing this loss, it is possible to achieve high rates of follow-up in surgical patients.

Intention-to-treat analysis

Randomization can accomplish the goal of balancing groups with respect to both known and unknown determinants of outcomes only if patients are analyzed in the groups to which they are randomized [27]. It is possible for hand surgeons to corrupt randomization if not all patients receive their assigned surgery. Take for example the scenario of a patient who was assigned to undergo ECTR. As the surgeon makes the incision the charge nurse alerts him that the endoscopic instrument is not functioning properly or has failed the sterilization test. Now the surgeon is in the uncomfortable position of carrying on with the OCTR technique. Another, more likely scenario is that the surgeon has been informed that the next patient has been allocated to the ECTR, but during surgery he finds that he cannot negotiate the endoscope through a very tight carpal tunnel. Because he believes that further attempts run the real risk of damaging the median nerve, he prudently decides to convert to the OCTR. Yet another scenario is that of an RCT comparing single- with double-strand flexor tendon repair. Suppose that during surgery the surgeon recognizes that the quality of the tendon is such that he believes that single strand will in all probability rupture, and therefore he decides to use double-strand closure.

If hand surgeons include such poorly destined patients in one surgical treatment group and not the other, then even a suboptimal surgical procedure may appear to be effective. Intention-to-treat analysis is the principle that avoids this potential bias [27,33]. The analysis of the outcomes is based on the treatment arm to which patients were randomized and not on which surgical treatment they received. The intention-to-treat analysis includes all patients, regardless of whether they actually satisfied the entry criteria, received the treatment to which they were randomly allocated, or deviated from the protocol. Analyzing patients based on the treatment they actually receive can destroy the prognostic balance of randomization, because the reasons for which patients do not take their medication or do not receive a particular surgical intervention are often related to prognosis [34]. With this method of analysis, both the prognostic factors we know and do not know about are equally distributed in the two surgical groups [23].

Surgical equipoise

Another important yet unappreciated precondition to undertaking an RCT in hand surgery is the state of equipoise. Equipoise is defined as a state of genuine uncertainty about the benefits or harms that may result from each of two or more regimens [30]. A state of equipoise is an indication for an RCT, because it implies that there are no scientific or ethical concerns about one regimen's being better for a particular patient [30,35,36].

Instances in hand surgery where recent research has identified equipoise despite a number of small RCTs are the ongoing controversies between ECTR and OCTR [37,38] and among the numerous arthroplasty techniques of the carpo-metacarpal joint of the thumb [39].

Differential care

In hand surgery RCTs, the concept of randomization is fairly straightforward; however, the understanding of concealment remains problematic. A pharmaceutic investigator can conceal the experimental pill and the placebo pill until the end of the study. In hand surgery the concealment usually disappears once the incision is made. A hand surgeon who participates in an RCT may bias the results while the patient is in the operating room or during follow-up encounters by providing a little extra care, such as better hemostasis, extra care with the suturing or dressing, or more frequent visits with the patient for the technique toward which he may be biased. Moreover, the surgical intervention may include additional procedures that influence the postoperative results and overestimate the effect size.

In contrast to pharmaceutic RCTs, the standardization of surgical procedures is difficult, and the investigators need to be careful and aware. Methods of standardizing the surgical procedures include (1) ensuring that all participating surgeons agree on how the procedure should be performed before the trial begins, (2) holding teaching sessions before the trial, (3) auditing surgical performance throughout the trial, and (4) stratifying patients by surgeon at the time of randomization [40]. Stratifying by surgeon will not eliminate the variation in how a procedure is performed, but it may reduce the imbalance between groups [20]. Investigators need to standardize the surgical protocol before initiating an RCT and report on how the surgical protocol was standardized in their final report.

In addition to standardizing the protocol for the different surgical techniques, it is necessary to standardize the protocol for patients following their surgery. Items that can be standardized in the trial protocol include perioperative treatment, postoperative treatment, medications, physiotherapy, and number of follow-up visits with the hand surgeon.

Treatment effect and implications for sample size

One common mistake identified in reported RCTs in hand surgery is the choice of sample size. Investigators arbitrarily choose a convenient sample size from their practice and then conduct an RCT. The usual finding is no difference between the experimental and the standard technique. This is called a type II error. This result should be no surprise to anyone, because a study with a small sample size can only identify a statistically significant difference if the expected effect size is large. For example, the effect size between the competing techniques ECTR and OCTR is very small. Although such a small effect difference may appear of no consequence, in fact when such a procedure is common it carries clinically important economic consequences and is thus highly relevant. To perform an RCT when the effect size is thought to be small or moderate, the investigators need to estimate the baseline risk of the outcome event in the control group, estimate an expected relative risk reduction, and calculate the sample size. Depending on these variables, the sample size will vary. In many instances, the sample size is in the thousands rather than the usual hundreds. The inadequacy of the sample size in a meta-analysis of RCTs that compared ECTR and OCTR was recently reported [38].

All these considerations imply that, if hand surgery is to advance in a quantum leap, it has to adopt well-established methodologic principles from clinical trialists and epidemiologists. Small RCTs are often underpowered and highly unlikely to provide the answers we are seeking. They confuse the issue in that they usually conclude no difference (type II error). At the same time, small studies also capitalize on the play of chance, in that they may factitiously identify a difference (type I error). Large studies are generally needed to detect clinically important differences between surgical interventions. Hand surgeons should consult a biostatistician to perform a sample-size calculation while planning an RCT. The formal sample-size calculation will determine which sample size is required to show a true difference.

In addition, hand surgeons need to learn to collaborate with their colleagues at other centers and conduct large multicenter trials to achieve the recruitment of the large sample sizes that are necessary. Because few hand surgeons are knowledgeable in research methodology, it is imperative that they collaborate with clinical trialists and biostatisticians from university epidemiology departments in the design of an RCT. It is also important to ensure that the CONSORT checklist is followed carefully [see Table 1 and **Fig. 1**]. The hand societies need to play a key role in this regard by identifying hand problems that meet the criteria of equipoise and actively encouraging members to participate in such studies to maintain membership [41].

The use of economic analysis in hand surgery

In the last 2 decades, the cost of medical care has come under scrutiny by third party payers in many jurisdictions [42]. When claims are made in the hand surgery literature that a "new" surgical technique is superior to the "old" technique, surgeons should consider the validity of the evidence in support of the claim. Consideration should be given to the value of the benefits that are forgone because the resource is not available for its best alternative use. Health economists term this the "opportunity cost" [43]. It behooves the hand surgeon to weigh not only the benefits and risks of the "novel" surgical technique but also whether the benefits provided by this technique warrant spending scarce health care dollars.

To make informed decisions, hand surgeons can use economic analyses to decide whether the "novel" surgical procedure should be adopted. Economic analysis is a set of formal, quantitative methods used to compare alternative strategies with respect to their resource use and their expected outcomes [44,45]. Although various types of economic evaluations are reported in the literature, the basic principle of an economic analysis is that choices must be made between alternative uses of resources, and these decisions must consider both cost and outcome [44,46]. Therefore, studies can only be considered formal economic evaluations when the cost and outcomes are compared among two or more treatment options. All types of evaluation that fail to satisfy these criteria should be designated partial evaluations; they do not allow us to answer efficiency questions based on the study results [47]. In general, four types of economic evaluation are commonly described in the literature: (1) cost-minimization analysis, (2) cost-effectiveness analysis (CEA), (3) cost-utility analysis, and (4) cost-benefit analysis [43,48].

Economic analyses, although admittedly rare in hand surgery, can help to inform surgeons and health care decision makers about the best allocation of limited health care resources. Unfortunately, only rarely do hand surgeons consider economic analysis in their studies, despite the tremendous usefulness of such studies to the society. For example, despite the nearly 2-decade controversy between ECTR and OCTR, only two economic analyses have been performed, and these used a deterministic analysis based on secondary rather than primary data [49,50]. Problems with the use of secondary data are related to the use of accurate data on the various complications (health pathways) that are fitted into the decision analytic model. For example, the CEA performed by Chung and colleagues [49] using a decision analytic model of the probabilities of the complications of two early RCTs [51,52], estimating the costs of the different pathways and using utilities from experts, reached the conclusion that the ECTR is cost-effective if the probability of nerve injury is 1% less in the ECTR than in the open technique. The evidence from recent systematic overviews, however, has shown that irreversible nerve damage is uncommon in either technique [37,38]. Only one such injury occurred in the OCTR group [52]. The other problem is the accuracy of the costs used in the analyses, which are limited to the perspective of third party payers and do not reflect those of the society [53].

The ideal cost-effectiveness study would consist of a large, multicenter RCT study that recruits a few thousand patients (based on a formal sample-size calculation) to compare ECTR and OCTR. Costs would then be collected along with the sampled data. Unfortunately, no such study has been performed to date, so there is no definitive answer on which treatment (ECTR or OCTR) is more cost-effective. When designing and conducting an economic analysis, such as the one described above, the hand surgeon should collaborate with a health economist to ensure that the correct methodology is followed.

Changing the "hand surgeons' culture"

Traditionally, surgeons have worked and published in solitary or small-group fashion. Rarely do we see large, multicenter trials. Recent evidence suggests that the sample size required to carry out the definitive study for our example, ECTR versus OCTR (in which the effect size is small), requires the recruitment of some 5000 patients [54]. To conduct such a "megarandomized controlled trial" requires collaboration, as well as resources far beyond the means of a single surgeon or even a group of surgeons. It requires the involvement of a whole society, such as the American Society for Surgery of the Hand, the American Association for Hand Surgery, or even both. An economic analysis can be "piggy-backed" to such a "megatrial," which in addition to determining the efficacy of the "novel" procedure can also provide the definitive evidence of its cost-effectiveness from the patients', third party payers', and society's perspective [38]. Hand surgeons with a few exceptions are not familiar with the complexities of conducting and successfully executing large RCTs. Collaboration with biostatisticians, health economists, epidemiologists, and clinical trialists is vital to carrying a study to successful completion.

Acknowledgments

The author would like to thank Dr. Deborah Cook and Sheila Sprague, MSc for review of this chapter.

References

[1] Coditz GA, Miller JN, Mosteller F. How study design affects outcomes in comparisons of therapy. I: Medical. Stat Med 1989;8:411–54.

[2] Schultz KF, Chalmers I, Hayes RJ, et al. Empirical evidence of bias: dimensions of methodological quality associated with estimates of treatment effects in controlled trials. JAMA 1995;273:408–12.

[3] Haynes RB, Mukherjee J, Sackett DL, et al. Functional status changes following medical or surgical treatment for cerebral ischemia: results in the EC/IC Bypass Study. JAMA 1987;257:2043–6.

[4] Carette S, Marcoux S, Truchon R, et al. A controlled trial of corticosteroid injections into facet joints for chronic low back pain. N Engl J Med 1991;325:1002–7.

[5] Sacks HS, Chalmers TC, Smith Jr H. Sensitivity and specificity of clinical trials: randomized v historical controls. Arch Intern Med 1983;143:753–5.

[6] Chalmers TC, Celano P, Sacks HS, et al. Bias in treatment assignment in controlled clinical trials. N Engl J Med 1983;309:1358–61.

[7] Colditz GA, Miller JN, Mosteller F. How study design affects outcomes in comparisons of therapy. I: Medical. Stat Med 1989;8:441–54.

[8] Emerson JD, Burdick E, Hoaglin DC, et al. An empirical study of the possible relation of treatment differences to quality scores in controlled randomized clinical trials. Control Clin Trials 1990;11:339–52.

[9] Silverman WA. Gnosis and random allotment. Control Clin Trials 1981;2:161–4.

[10] Concato J, Shah N, Howitz RI. Randomized controlled trials, observational studies, and hierarchy of research designs. N Engl J Med 2000;342:1887–92.

[11] Thoma A, Chew TC, Veltri K. Application of the CONSORT statement to randomized controlled trials comparing endoscopic carpal tunnel release (ECTR) and open carpal tunnel release (OCTR). Presented at the American Association for Hand Surgery Annual Meeting. Palm Springs (CA), January 16, 2004.

[12] Begg CB, Cho MK, Eastwood S, et al. Improving the quality of reporting of randomized controlled trials: the CONSORT statement. JAMA 1996;276:637–9.

[13] Moher D, Schulz KF, Altaman DG. The CONSORT statement: revised recommendations for improving the quality of reports of parallel-group randomized trials. Clin Oral Investig 2003;7:2–7.

[14] Moher D, Pham B, Jones A, et al. Does the quality of reports of randomized trials effect estimates of intervention efficacy reported in meta-analyses? Lancet 1998;352:609–13.

[15] Bonenkamp JJ, Songun I, Hermans I, et al. Randomized comparison of morbidity and mortality after DI and D2 dissection for gastric cancer in Dutch patients. Lancet 1995;345:745–8.

[16] Ramsay CR, Grant AM, Wallace SA, et al. Statistical assessment of the learning curves of health technologies. Health Technol Assess 2001;5:1–79.

[17] Mohammed MA, Cheng KK, Rouse A, et al. Bristol, Shipman, and clinical governance: Shewhart's forgotten lessons. Lancet 2001;357:463–7.

[18] Altman DG, Dore CJ. Randomization and baseline comparisons in clinical trials. Lancet 1990;335:149–53.

[19] Moher D, Fortin P, Jadad AR, et al. Completeness of reporting of trials in languages other than English: implications for the conduct and reporting of systematic reviews. Lancet 1996;347:363–6.

[20] Jadad A. Randomized controlled trials. London: BMJ Books; 1998.

[21] Kaptchuk TJ. Powerful placebo: the dark side of

the randomized controlled trial. Lancet 1998; 351:1722–5.

[22] Guyatt GH, Pugsley SO, Sullivan MJ, et al. Effect of encouragement on walking test performance. Thorax 1984;39:818–22.

[23] Thoma A, Farrokhyar F, Bhandari, et al, for the Evidence-Based Surgery Working Group. Users' guide to the surgical literature. How to assess a randomized controlled trial in surgery. Can J Surg 2004;47:200–8.

[24] Sprague S, Leece P, Bhandari M, et al. on behalf of the SPRINT investigators. Limiting loss to follow up in a multi-centre randomized controlled trial in orthopaedic surgery. Control Clin Trials 2003;24:719–23.

[25] Schultz KF, Grimes DA. Sample size slippages in randomised trials: exclusions and the lost and wayward. Lancet 2002;359:781–5.

[26] Sackett DL, Richardson WS, Rosenberg W, et al. Evidence-based medicine: how to practice and teach EBM. New York: Churchill Livingstone; 1997.

[27] Evidence-based Medicine Working Group. Users' guides to the medical literature: a manual for evidence-based clinical practice. In: Guyatt G, Rennie D, editors. JAMA & Archives Journals. Chicago: American Medical Association; 2002.

[28] Harrell Jr FE. Regression modeling strategies, with application to linear models, logistic regression, and survival analysis. New York: Springer-Verlag; 2001.

[29] Elwood M. Critical appraisal of epidemiological studies and clinical trials. New York: Oxford University Press; 1998.

[30] Last MJ. A dictionary of epidemiology. 3rd edition. New York: Oxford University Press; 1995.

[31] Armitage P, Berry G. Statistical methods in medical research. London: Blackwell Scientific Publications; 1994.

[32] Solomon MJ, McLeod RS. Surgery and the randomized controlled trial: past, present, and future. Med J Aust 1998;169:380–3.

[33] Hollis S, Campbell F. What is meant by intention to treat analysis? Survey of published randomized controlled trials. BMJ 1999;319:670–4.

[34] Bhandari M, Guyatt GH, Swiontowski MF. Users' guide to the orthopaedic literature: how to use an article about a surgical therapy. J Bone Joint Surg 2001;83A:916–26.

[35] Schafer A. The ethics of the randomized clinical trial. N Engl J Med 1982;307:719–24.

[36] Pocock SJ. Ethical issues. In: Pocock SJ, editor. Clinical trials. Toronto: John Wiley & Sons; 1984. p. 100–9 [reprinted 1993].

[37] Thoma A, Veltri K, Haines T, et al. A systematic review of reviews comparing endoscopic and open carpal tunnel decompression. Plast Reconstr Surg 2004;113:1184–91.

[38] Thoma A, Veltri K, Haines T, et al. A meta-analysis of randomized controlled trials comparing endoscopic and open carpal tunnel decompression. Plast Reconstr Surg 2004;114:1137–46.

[39] Martou G, Veltri K, Thoma A. Surgical treatment of osteoarthritis (OA) of the carpometacarpal (CMC) joint of the thumb: a systematic review. Plast Reconstr Surg 2004;114(2):421–32.

[40] McLeod RS. Issues in surgical randomized trials. World J Surg 1999;23:1210–4.

[41] Thoma A. Evidence-based hand surgery. ASSH Correspondence Newsletter 2003;2:2.

[42] Russell LB, Gold MR, Siegel JE, et al. The role of cost-effectiveness analysis in health and medicine. Panel on cost-effectiveness in health and medicine. JAMA 1996;276:1172–7.

[43] Drummond MF, O'Brien BJ, Stoddart GL, et al. Methods for the economic evaluation of health care programmes. 2nd edition. New York: Oxford University Press; 1997.

[44] Eisenberg JM. Clinical economics: a guide to the economic analysis of clinical practices. JAMA 1989;262:2879–86.

[45] Detskey AS, Nagie IG. A clinician's guide to cost-effectiveness analysis. Ann Intern Med 1990;113: 147–54.

[46] Jefferson T, Demicheli V, Mugford M. Elementary economic evaluation in health care. London: BMJ Publishing Group; 1996.

[47] Drummond MF, Richardson WS, O'Brien BJ, et al, for the Evidence-Based Medicine Working Group. Users' guide to the medical literature XIII. How to use an article on economic analysis in clinical practice: A. Are the results of the study valid? JAMA 1997;277:1552–7.

[48] Krieger LM. The new medical marketplace. II. Cost and outcome studies. Plast Reconstr Surg 1996;98:1102–7.

[49] Chung KC, Walters MR, Greenfield MLVH, et al. Endoscopic versus open carpal tunnel release: a cost-effectiveness analysis. Plast Reconstr Surg 1998;102:1089–99.

[50] Thoma A, Veltri K, Duku E. Decompression of the carpal tunnel with the open and the endoscopic method: a cost-utility analysis. Can J Plast Surg 2001;9:109.

[51] Brown RA, Gelberman RH, Seiler JG, et al. Carpal tunnel release: a prospective randomized assessment of open and endoscopic methods. J Bone Joint Surg Am 1993;75:1265–75.

[52] Agee JM, McCarroll Jr HR, Tortosa RD, et al. Endoscopic release of the carpal tunnel: a randomized prospective multicenter study. J Hand Surg [Am] 1992;17:987–95.

[53] Thoma A, Sprague S, Tandan V. Users' guide to the surgical literature: how to use an article on economic analysis. Can J Surg 2001;44: 347–54.

[54] Thoma A, Haines T, Goldsmith C, et al. Design of a randomized controlled trial comparing endoscopic carpal tunnel release (ECTR) and open carpal tunnel release (OCTR): Canadian collaborative initiative. Can J Plast Surg 2003; 11:96.

CLINICS IN
PLASTIC
SURGERY

Clin Plastic Surg 32 (2005) 575–604

ELSEVIER
SAUNDERS

The Challenge to Manage Reflex Sympathetic Dystrophy/Complex Regional Pain Syndrome

Wyndell H. Merritt, MD

- Definitions, classifications, and terminology
- Difficulty assessing the literature, incidence, true prognosis, and causes
  Incidence
  Prognosis
  Inciting events (causes)
- Clinical manifestations
  Characteristic pain
  Physical findings and stages
  Myofascial dysfunction and reflex sympathetic dystrophy
  Clinical forms of reflex sympathetic dystrophy
- Biologic mechanisms causing trophic changes
  Neurogenic inflammation: the role of substance P and other neuropeptides
  Role of the sympathetic nervous system
  Role of the opioid pain control system
- Psychologic findings
- Psychophysiologic etiology

- Diagnostic techniques
  Radiography and bone scan
  MRI
  Thermography
  Other diagnostic tests
  Functional assessment
- Treatment techniques
  Surgical treatment
  Stellate ganglion and other nerve blocks
  Intravenous regional pharmacologic infusion
  Acupuncture
  Biofeedback therapy
  Transcutaneous nerve stimulation
  Pharmacologic medical treatment
  Hand therapy
  Psychotherapy
- Ten practical principles in the treatment of reflex sympathetic dystrophy
- Summary
- References

The challenge to understand and successfully manage reflex sympathetic dystrophy (RSD) and complex regional pain syndrome (CRPS) is unparalleled among disorders confronting plastic surgeons, because of ignorance of cause, pathophysiology, and proper treatment. As such, it is frustrating and controversial with an unpredictable incidence and course developing with little or no warning. Consequently, the unsuspecting plastic surgeon can easily underrate a patient's severe pain complaints after minor injury or operation only later to be confronted by a dystrophic, functionless hand or chronically painful face, now easily diagnosed as RSD-CRPS. Unfortunately, once

Department of Surgery, Virginia Commonwealth University School of Medicine, 2002 Bremo Road, Suite 202, Richmond, VA 23226, USA
E-mail address: wyndell@hotmail.com

0094-1298/05/$ – see front matter © 2005 Elsevier Inc. All rights reserved.
plasticsurgery.theclinics.com

doi:10.1016/j.cps.2005.07.002

diagnosis is easy, treatment is not, because the dystrophic changes and chronic pain are difficult to reverse, and often result in litigation. It is imperative to develop the sensitivity needed for early recognition, in hopes that early intervention may prevent progression. Such early recognition is difficult because there is no one definitive diagnostic test, and etiology, pathophysiology, and even definition of the disorder remain obscure and controversial.

The challenge to understand RSD-CRPS is one that requires a better understanding of the complex relationship between the central nervous system (CNS) and peripheral nervous system. To date, there is no comprehensive hypothesis that clearly explains the etiology and no uniformly successful treatment method. This brief summary of the challenge reviews some of what is known, hypothesizes a possible etiologic mechanism, and proposes 10 common-sense principles for management that recognizes the handicap of limited knowledge.

Definitions, classifications, and terminology

It is difficult to define a clinical entity without standardized diagnostic clinical criteria and no clear understanding of origin. In this disorder controversy began with its name, with more than 60 medical disorders describing symptoms that include disproportionate pain and inflammatory or autonomic system-type dysfunction [1].

In 1991, Amadio [2] reported the consensus of an American Association for Hand Surgery committee appointed to define better this disorder. This committee selected three basic criteria for diagnosis:

1. Disproportionate pain
2. Interference with function
3. Autonomic-type abnormality (eg, skin discoloration, sweating, dryness, edema, temperature change, osteoporosis)

Although other disorders, such as scleroderma with sclerodactyly and severe Raynaud's disease, may fulfill these criteria, RSD-CRPS can be distinguished by the peculiar nature of the disproportionate pain with hyperpathia (prolonged pain after stimulation) and allodynia (marked pain from a usually nonpainful simulation), and the pain is usually constant. Although the inciting event may seem minor, the amount of distress is profound and should never be underestimated or belittled. Confusion is increased by the fact that authors vary widely in their diagnostic criteria, with no single test that consistently diagnoses early RSD. Some authors require only the unique hyperpathia and allodynia pain and associated distress to justify diagnosis [3–5], and this approach

recognizes that earlier treatment might improve the prognosis [1,6–11]. Most patients are symptomatic more than 6 months before diagnosis, often previously misdiagnosed as malingerers or psychoneurotics [12]. The opportunity to classify any undiagnosed pain as RSD-CRPS, however, has created cynicism about its overuse and many clinicians believe RSD has lost usefulness as a designation because of indiscriminate use. Furthermore, controversy now exists as to the role of the sympathetic nervous system. This led the International Pain Nomenclature Group task force to introduce the term "complex regional pain syndrome" in 1996 to replace RSD [13,14]. One should be aware that this new designation, CRPS, is also defined on purely clinical grounds, with no new diagnostic tests or improved understanding of the etiology of this disorder [Box 1] [3].

The advantage of this new classification is to emphasize that chronic pain syndromes exist that do not respond to sympathetic blocks, and this new nomenclature avoids the prejudicial designation of an RSD diagnosis, with its historic legal and administrative connotations. However, the criteria for CRPS do not clarify how one classifies patients who have variable response to sympathetic block, as do many RSD-CRPS patients, and they have no designation for the 10% to 30% of patients who spontaneously develop RSD and do not fulfill the criterion of an "initiating noxious event." In many ways, the new designation adds to the confusion by implying a new understanding and there remains a need for better definition, classification, and clarification. A standardized criterion was initially proposed for CRPS, based on use of phentolamine blocks [15]. Phentolamine is presently not approved for this intravenous test in the United States, however, and studies have questioned whether phentolamine block has any effect other than placebo [3,16]. At present, RSD remains the most frequent designation in the English literature (often "algodystrophy" is found in the European literature) [1,7]. More than 30 years ago, Sunderland [17] stated his objection to defining any disorder on the basis of a response to a treatment: "To define a certain type of pain by reference to its response to one form of treatment, namely sympathetic interruption, is artificial…and unreasonable." Such definition is "circular," with the definition of sympathetically maintained pain (CRPS type I) made by being relieved by blocks; it follows then that any pain relieved by sympathetic blocks is then sympathetically maintained [3]. This circular logic implies a perfectly sensitive test, clearly an unrealistic expectation [18].

An older classification system, suggested by Lankford [9], used inciting cause as a means of classifying RSD. This classification by precipitating factors has offered no prognostic or therapeutic benefit. It is important, however, to separate Lankford's classic major causalgia from other causative factors leading to RSD.

Mitchell and coworkers [19] coined the term "causalgia" to identify patients with peculiar disproportionate pain during the American War of Northern Aggression in 1864 following gunshot wounds, which caused partial injury to major mixed peripheral nerves, such as the femoral nerve in the thigh or median nerve in the arm. His careful description of the peculiar symptoms in Yankee soldiers remains unparalleled. He described a "burning, constant, unremitting pain that could be aggravated by soft touch, loud noises and even emotional stress." He observed that despite cold weather, some soldiers filled their boots with water and placed their injured feet in them or wrapped their upper extremities in moist cool cloths to relieve constant burning pain. He coined the term causalgia from the Greek kausis (heat) and algos (pain) to denote this peculiar pain in these patients. Years later, Evans [20] coined the term "reflex sympathetic dystrophy" specifically to distinguish patients with identical symptoms but without specific injury to a major peripheral nerve. It is important to distinguish between these two because, whereas the causalgia patients generally respond to sympathetic blocks or sympathectomy, a significant proportion of RSD patients do not.

Difficulty assessing the literature, incidence, true prognosis, and causes

Incidence

It is impossible to know the true incidence of RSD-CRPS because the diagnosis remains clinical, with variable diagnostic criteria used among differing authors. For example, Sunderland [17] found that reports of causalgia varied from less than 1% to as high as 16%. Plewes [21] estimated that RSD occurred in 1 of every 2000 accidents, whereas Hartley [22] reported 1 in 20. Overall, it seems most reports average about a 5% incidence after an inciting cause, such as a sprain or elective surgery. The more common injuries and surgery, such as Colles fracture and carpal tunnel syndrome, have the highest frequency of cause. In many reports, however, 10% to 30% of patients have spontaneous occurrence with no evident precipitating cause or condition [23–26]. Although RSD-CRPS is most commonly found in the upper and lower extremities, orofacial RSD is reported after maxillofacial surgery [27], head injury [12], dental procedures [28,29], and vascular surgery in the neck [30]. These patients do not characteristically develop the dystrophic change commonly seen in the extremities [30,31]. Many reports suggest a greater frequency in women [32,33], although this is controversial [30], and most age ranges are 30 to 60 years, with the mean in the late 40s. Children are not exempt from this disorder [34–36], however, with the disturbing observation that there is as high as a 30% recurrent pain syndrome in these children [35,36]. RSD-CRPS is a polymorphic condition that may occur more frequently than it is reported, and may be present in all ages, all races, and both sexes, either spontaneously or precipitated by a wide variety of inciting causes.

Prognosis

There is a widespread misconception that RSD-CRPS always spontaneously improves and "burns out" with time. This probably derives from observation of causalgia patients who have partial injury to a major mixed peripheral nerve that usually develops spontaneous improvement and may occasionally completely resolve [17]. Numerous authors, however, have observed that in other forms of RSD-CRPS, complete remission is rare [33,37–40]. The prognostic result of surgical efforts to treat RSD were well summarized by Sunderland [17] as having an initial interval of seeming success, only later to have "a disheartening tendency for the pain to recur."

Nath and coworkers [41] provided an excellent overview of RSD treatment results among three popular management methods, and the findings seemed bizarre. Results from stellate sympathetic block, intravenous sympathetic block, and surgical sympathectomy had an astonishing variation in reported results within each category. For example, results of 25 reports using sympathetic block varied from 100% failure rate in one study [42] to 100% success rate in another [43]. Intravenous regional sympathetic block in 15 studies showed results varying from a 100% good [41] to a 93% failure rate [44]. Surgical sympathectomy in 19 different reports had results ranging from 99% good [42] to 95% failure [45,46]. Such a spectrum seems inexplicable until Nath and coworkers noted that among the 59 studies reviewed, only seven had 1 year or longer follow-up, and only seven were prospective randomized studies (not the same seven). Most reports were retrospective and non-randomized by design, with no definitive length of follow-up.

In a provocative review of diagnosis and treatment techniques for RSD-CRPS, Tanelian [47] studied more than 30 treatment methods, with most reporting 70% to 100% success rate. He noted, however, that most of these were uncontrolled and provided inadequate numbers of patients. Using data from Zar [48], Tanelian [47] pointed out that at least 36 patients are needed in a randomized, double-blind, placebo-controlled study to prove 80% efficiency. Without these controls, more than 200 patients are needed to prove a 75% treatment effect. Of his reports, only four met these criteria, and these four showed success of only 0% to 30%.

Subbarao and Stillwell [49] provide further insight into these reported discrepancies by a survey of 125 patients greater than a year following RSD treatment. They noted that the treating physicians described a 77% success rate (good to excellent results) 3 months after treatment. Their questionnaire a year or more later, however, revealed 87% of these patients still complaining bitterly of pain or stiffness and only 25% resuming full activity, and only one patient completely relieved. Successful treatment reports should be regarded with suspicion unless followed for more than 1 year. Overall, review of the literature gives the impression that most treatment methods result in approximately one third of patients with excellent to good relief, one third with some improvement, and one third with no improvement or worsening of symptoms. Wang's and coworkers study [50] of long-term response to sympathetic block 3 years after treatment found only 40% of patients reported good to excellent results and 38% reported poor results. When patients received their sympathetic blocks within 6 months of the onset of symptoms, however, 70% of patients reported long-term good to excellent results, implying that early treatment might result in better prognosis. Finally, the incidence of recurrent or migratory RSD is reported to be as high as 15% to 75% [36,45,46,51–54] and often occurs at a different site.

Given this prognostic knowledge, one should expect that most patients with this disorder continue to suffer some degree of chronic pain and are likely to have recurrent syndromes. When physicians can help them cope with their pain and resume function and activity, this is an adequate and realistic goal.

Inciting events (causes)

There is an incredible array of reported precipitating causes for reflex dystrophy, so widely varied that there seems to be no common feature. Traumatic causes vary from a paper cut on the finger to spinal cord injury, and nontraumatic conditions are as varied as ovarian carcinoma, shingles, myocardial infarction, stroke, and use of phenobarbital. This spectrum is so vast that it is more appropriate to call these "inciting events," rather than "precipitating causes," although the medical (and legal) profession prefers the latter term.

Apparently any trauma or incident can lead to RSD-CRPS, with the most common hand operations (eg, carpal tunnel surgery) and common injuries (eg, Colles fracture) sharing blame as the most common precipitating causes. RSD is reported to occur in 2% [55] to 5% [56] of carpal tunnel operations and as many as 11% [7] to 37% [57–59] of Colles fractures. In most reports, soft tissue trauma is the most common precipitating cause, with fractures a close second.

Other traumatic and nontraumatic causes represent a puzzling spectrum, with cardiac origin common in 5% to 20% of cases and elective surgery in 11% to 16% [55]. Less frequent causes include dental extractions [28,29,60], ovarian [61] and pancreatic carcinoma [62], stroke [12], myocardial infarction [63], spinal cord injury [25,64–67], myelogram [68], diabetic neuropathy [25], herpes zoster [12,69], facial fracture [27], carotid surgery [30], degenerative disk disease [70], meningococcal meningitis [71], cervical rib resection [38], phenobarbital [25,72–74], antituberculosis medications and cyclosporine [75], syringomyelia [76], amyotrophic lateral sclerosis [77], lymphoma and recurrent breast carcinoma [78], bladder cancer [62], and venipuncture and intramuscular injection of pain medications [38]. In many reports, no apparent cause for onset was seen in as many as 30% of cases [23–26].

Because this disorder can have any type of precipitating cause, or no apparent cause at all, it seems patently unfair that physicians are so frequently held liable for a disorder with such ubiquitous and sometimes spontaneous onset. It is more appropriate to identify these as inciting events rather than causes. Certainly, the remarkable variety of precipitating events, which include CNS disorders, suggests that cortical function may play a major role in the etiology of RSD-CRPS.

Clinical manifestations

Characteristic pain

The most characteristic clinical feature of RSD is the peculiar disproportionate unremitting pain. Distinguishing characteristics are hyperpathia (persistent pain after stimulation) and allodynia (aggravation by usually nonpainful stimuli) with uniquely severe anguish and distress. The pain is constant and not completely relieved by rest, and it is aggravated by motion; activity; or temperature change (especially cold). Mirror image (advancement to the contralateral extremity) is as frequent as 25% of patients [23,51,79], especially in patients with a CNS-related cause, such as stroke, or shoulder-hand syndrome.

The best opportunity for early diagnosis is by careful observation of the patient's behavior and listening to the pain description. Patients with RSD-CRPS seem less able to cope with their circumstance and less able to trust their physicians, both during examination and when receiving reassurance. They fearfully withdraw from the examiner's touch and repeat strained, anxious questions, demanding an explanation for their distress. Situational stress may influence their episodes of severe pain, although patients seem totally unaware of these influences. Questionnaires answered by these patients deny psychologic distress causing or being caused by RSD-CRPS [80,81] despite data showing life stress as a significant factor [82–85]. This seems to be caused by a high incidence of alexithymia (the inability to verbalize one's emotions, thought to be caused by lack of awareness of mood) among patients with reflex dystrophy [86].

Although these patients deny emotional distress, they seem more dismayed, angry, and desperate about their dilemma than similar even more severely hand-injured patients [87], but often become annoyed when depression, anxiety, or psychiatric assessment is suggested, despite obvious clinical manifestations. They quickly feel rejected and resentful when the well-meaning but impatient surgeon points out their relative lack of physical findings. Even though these patients may appear anatomically capable, functional activity is usually impaired by pain, and the patient develops avoidance patterns and a sense of disassociation from the extremity. They frequently speak of their hand in the third person ("it") [Fig. 1], and as McKee observed, the involved hand is no longer included in characteristic conversational gesturing (N. McKee, personal communication, 2003). A study of patients even 3 to 9 years after onset demonstrated pain was still the predominant factor limiting function [85,88,89]. For the present, a careful history with meticulous characterization of the pain and observation of the patient's behavioral response remain the best tools for early recognition and diagnosis of RSD-CRPS. Any unexpected withdrawal response in a hand-injured patient, such as when sutures are removed, should alert the surgeon to provide immediate additional investigation and support.

Physical findings and stages

Physical findings

The first noticeable physical findings in RSD is the patient's avoidance of touch or functional use

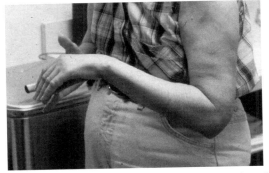

Fig. 1. Disassociation of RSD. This patient developed RSD after a Colles fracture and carried her hand like a foreign object.

caused by pain, with tremor or spasm present in 58% of cases, weakness or inability to move in 70%, and involuntary dystonic movement in 35% [24,89]. The first measurable changes, however, may be characterized as from either autonomic or low-grade inflammatory activity.

Edema is often the first noted abnormality. Mottled color change (redness or cyanosis) is often seen. Abnormal temperature is usually present, with warmness more common early and coolness later in the course of the disorder, and there may be either sweating or dryness. Joint swelling may be seen and a decreased active range of motion, more pronounced than is expected from the degree of swelling, with passive better than active range of motion until late changes occur. The pattern is of a vasomotor abnormality, with low-grade inflammatory change and disproportionate pain. Synovial tissue biopsy results reveal mild inflammatory change [90,91] and hyperplasia [92]. The degree of pain seems too severe, however, to be derived from mild synovial changes. Many authors [92–95] believe that RSD-CRPS represents exaggeration of a normal universal inflammatory response that does not diminish as it should in the normal course.

Stages of reflex sympathetic dystrophy and chronic regional pain syndrome
Betcher and Casten [93] classified the clinical features of RSD into three progressive stages [Figs. 2–4]. It is important to understand, however,

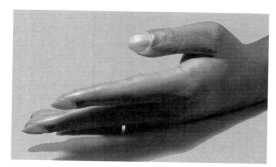

Fig. 3. Stage II RSD with shiny skin and loss of extension joint wrinkles 3 months after meningitis and septic shock.

that patients exhibit enormous variation in their presenting symptoms, duration, and mixture of characteristics in each stage. Many never progress beyond stage I, whereas others may rapidly progress to the dystrophic stage III within 3 to 6 months. These stages have no great clinical value, other than as a convenient description of the clinical change and its prognostic implications [Box 2].

Myofascial dysfunction and reflex sympathetic dystrophy
The most overlooked and underreported clinical finding in RSD-CRPS is proximal muscle trigger points that cause pain distally. Although most reports do not mention myofascial dysfunction trigger points in their clinical description of RSD-CRPS, several authors document their importance [89,96,97]. Indeed, in his original 1947 treatise

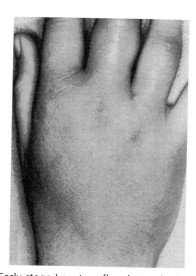

Fig. 2. Early stage I acute reflex dystrophy in a young man after minor trauma at work. He had intense pain, edema, and increased temperature. He responded to hand therapy and anti-inflammatory medication. (*From* Merritt WH. Reflex sympathetic dystrophy. In: McCarthy JG, editor. Plastic surgery, vol. 7. Philadelphia: WB Saunders; 1990. p. 4890; with permission.)

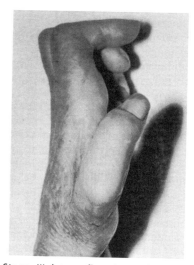

Fig. 4. Stage III late reflex dystrophy in a patient with causalgia from proximal electrical nerve injury. (*From* Merritt WH. Reflex sympathetic dystrophy. In: McCarthy JG, editor. Plastic surgery, vol. 7. Philadelphia: WB Saunders; 1990. p. 4892; with permission.)

Box 2: Stages of RDS

Stage I: acute

- Lasts approximately 3 months (variable)
- Constant burning or throbbing pain (intensity varies), atrophy, and hyperpathia
- Trigger points may develop
- Variable vasomotor changes, such as edema (aiding or nonprinting); color change (usually redness, sometimes cyanosis); temperature change (usually warming, sometimes coolness); increased sweating; sometimes dryness
- Decreased joint range of motion caused by pain
- Sometimes swollen fingernail ridging (occasional)
- Increased hair growth or pigmentation (occasional)

Stage II: subacute

- Lasts approximately 9 to 12 months (variable)
- Constant aggravating pain (intensity varies)
- Atrophy of skin and subcutaneous tissue
- Loss of fingertip pads (pencil pointing)
- Glossy, thin skin
- Decreased hair growth
- Cyanosis
- Brawny edema
- Joint ankylosis
- Palmar fasciitis and Dupuytren's nodules (occasional)
- Myofascial trigger points (usual)
- Subchondral patchy osteoporosis (usual)

Stage III: chronic

- Chronic intractable pain
- Pale, cool, dry extremity
- Thin, stretched skin
- Muscle atrophy
- Fixed flexion or extension contractures
- Diminished hair growth (usual)
- Patchy to generalized osteoporosis
- Patient is chronically depressed and may contemplate suicide

coining the term "reflex sympathetic dystrophy," Evans [20] observed multiple trigger points in 63% of his patients and the author noted a 67% incidence among his patients [1,98]. It behooves the clinician to know about myofascial dysfunction and its treatment. Like RSD, myofascial dysfunction is a clinical diagnosis without definitive laboratory criteria and is controversial. Myofascial dysfunction has the misfortune of being grouped among disorders of even less clear criteria, such as fibromyalgia, which causes some prejudice against the diagnosis. Referring myofascial trigger points, how-

ever, are more distinct clinical findings than in other less reputable muscle disorders, with specific palpable proximal trigger points arising in muscle or fascia, which elicit immediate referred pain or numbness at distant sites. The trigger point itself is a hyperirritable locus in a taut band of skeletal muscle and is usually found as a palpable lump. Pressure over this nodule causes pain in the distal extremity, which may vary from mild discomfort to intolerable pain that persists after the stimulation and, in rare instances, causes autonomic change, such as vasoconstriction, sweating, and color change. Generally, patients are unaware of their trigger points and surprised by their discovery. The relationship of the trigger point to their zone of referral is predictable, although they do not follow neurologic or segmental patterns and most commonly refer toward the region where the muscle inserts. Kellgren [99] noted in his own muscles that painful saline injections result in pain perceived at the region of insertion, rather than at the site of injection. These predictable referral zones were characterized by Trevell and Simons [100], who have offered the best criteria to identify the myofascial dysfunction trigger points and treatment suggestions.

As in RSD, the overwhelming symptom of myofascial dysfunction is unexplained pain, with lowered threshold, so that pain may be caused by such factors as minimal muscle activity, temperature change, or even emotional stress. Patients with myofascial dysfunction not associated with RSD differ, however, in that they have pain-free intervals, and relief occurs with rest, such as with splinting.

Treatment of myofascial dysfunction varies, but muscle stretch and vasocoolant spray or icing to inactivate the trigger points are popularized [100]. Heat [101]; injection of trigger points with local anesthetic [102], steroid [103], or saline [104]; ischemic compression by prolonged digital pressure [105]; massage [106]; ultrasound [103]; transcutaneous electrical neural stimulation (TENS); and a variety of pharmacologic treatments have been recommended [100]. Treatment success with myofascial dysfunction that is not associated with RSD-CRPS is high, especially when an eccentric exercise program is included to prevent recurrence. Because more than half of RSD-CRPS patients have myofascial trigger points that refer, the goal of therapy is to inactivate the hyperirritable trigger points, before such activities as strengthening exercises, work simulation, or even range-of-motion exercise are used in the painful referral zone. Unfortunately, patients with RSD usually have cold intolerance and rarely tolerate the use of vasocoolant spray or ice; other measures must be used, such as massage, ultrasound, pressure, TENS, and injection. It is important for any patient with myofascial trigger points to use a program of eccentric (stretch) strengthening exercise to avoid recurrence once the acute trigger points are controlled. This is compatible with the usual stress-loading program that is commonly used for RSD.

Clinical forms of reflex sympathetic dystrophy

Although current classification systems of RSD do not have much practical prognostic, etiologic, or therapeutic value, there are three clinical forms so distinct that they warrant separate discussion because of their specific clinical manifestations and therapeutic implications: (1) causalgia, (2) shoulder-hand syndrome, and (3) Sudeck's osteoporosis.

Causalgia and complex regional pain syndrome type II

Major causalgia (CRPS type II) is a distinct form of RSD caused by partial injury to a proximal major mixed nerve. Its onset is immediate and its course usually includes some degree of spontaneous improvement. Additionally, it has a superior response to sympathetic block and sympathectomy, compared with other forms of RSD-CRPS.

Causalgia has the most obvious peripheral irritation to the nervous system of all of the dystrophic syndromes. Nerve injuries are usually above the elbow and knee, and are most often caused by high-velocity missile wounds. In one series of war casualties, the incidence of causalgia was 58% with symptom onset within 6 hours in 75% of the patients. Sympathectomy improved all of the cases in this series [107]. The neurologic deficit and pain gradually improve to a variable degree in most patients, especially in the first 6 months [17,37,108], although numerous reports indicate that symptoms rarely ever completely disappear [1,39,40,98]. Sympathetic block usually provides temporary relief of causalgia and repeated blocks may produce sustained relief in some cases [109]. When only temporary relief consistently results, surgery is indicated, with sympathectomy remaining the treatment of choice [107]. Sunderland [17] and Seddon [110] point out that true causalgia is rarely seen in civilian practice, and suggest that the combat conditions of high emotional stress may be as important a feature as the high-velocity wound in the etiology of this disorder. The cause and onset of other types of RSD-CRPS are less well understood, and seem less likely to respond to sympathetic blocks or sympathectomy.

Shoulder-hand syndrome

When the pain of RSD originates in the shoulder, it should be separately identified because this may represent a proximal inciting cause. Although any RSD-CRPS of the finger, hand, or wrist may

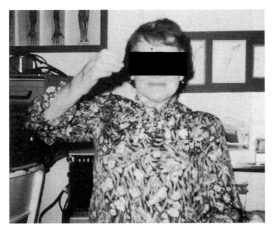

Fig. 5. Shoulder-hand syndrome developing subsequent to reflex dystrophy and Sudeck's osteoporosis of the hand after a Colles fracture. The patient responded to hand therapy and sympathetic blocks and 1 year later underwent successful capsulotomy of the metacarpophalangeal joints. (*From* Merritt WH. Reflex sympathetic dystrophy. In: McCarthy JG, editor. Plastic surgery, vol. 7. Philadelphia: WB Saunders; 1990. p. 4893; with permission.)

progress proximally to become shoulder-hand syndrome [**Fig. 5**], when the symptoms originate in the shoulder and progress distally to involve the hand, the clinician must be alert to the possibility of a visceral disease, such as ovarian carcinoma [61,111], pancreatic carcinoma [62], breast carcinoma [1,98], heart attack [112], gastric ulcer, Pancoast's tumor [113,114], and stroke [115]. When there is no obvious distal or proximal source for shoulder-hand syndrome, a thorough medical work-up is necessary [70].

Sudeck's osteoporosis

Sudeck's osteoporosis or atrophy is diagnosed because of the apparent skeletal involvement seen on radiographs [**Fig. 6**]. Although it resembles the osteoporosis of disuse [90], the onset of osteoporosis is much more rapid than can be explained by simple disuse, with findings as early as 4 to 6 weeks after onset of symptoms and changes that characteristically take as long as 10 years of disuse. Although treatment and results in Sudeck's osteoporosis are similar to those in other forms of RSD, this separate identification is warranted to consider calcitonin or bisphosphonate therapy, which may reverse the osteoblastic activity and the pain in Sudeck's osteoporosis [116,117].

Biologic mechanisms causing trophic changes

One of the most perplexing and controversial features of RSD-CRPS is the apparent physiologic

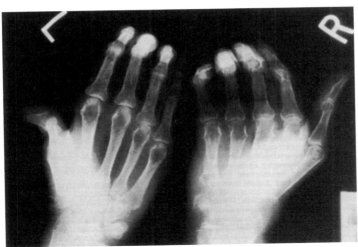

Fig. 6. Sudeck's patchy subchondral osteoporosis in the right hand caused by reflex dystrophy 18 months after a displaced radial fracture. The patient responded to systemic steroids, sympathetic blocks, and hand therapy to help her recover the use of the hand. (*From* Merritt WH. Reflex sympathetic dystrophy. In: McCarthy JG, editor. Plastic surgery, vol. 7. Philadelphia: WB Saunders; 1990. p. 4894; with permission.)

and anatomic change that may occur without any apparent peripheral cause. These dystrophic changes can become dramatic, with permanent stiffness, atrophy, osteoporosis, tapered fingertips, and tight shiny skin. Furthermore, the changes may progress in the involved extremity; may appear in the contralateral extremity; or may appear in a new site weeks, months, and even years after the original onset [51]. The mechanisms for these changes remain unclear. Disuse is a widely accepted explanation, but anyone witnessing the often rapid alteration in these patients cannot accept such a simple explanation. There is increasing evidence and belief that complex internal neurogenic pain-neurotransmitter systems and intrinsic physiologic pain inhibition mechanisms may someday provide an explanation for these changes associated with RSD, and afford therapeutic possibilities.

Neurogenic inflammation: the role of substance P and other neuropeptides

When noxious external stimulation, such as cuts or burns, activates peripheral unmyelinated afferent pain fibers, a characteristic pain and inflammatory response is expected. Proinflammatory cells like lymphocytes and mast cells accumulate in the affected tissue, releasing cytokines and histamine, and activate inflammatory mediators, such as prostaglandins, which are responsible for sensitizing C nociceptor afferent nerve endings. Interestingly, in RSD-CRPS, these cell types were never found in significant quantities [91,118], leading some to propose that the inflammation in RSD is caused by neuropeptides. Whereas a noxious stimulus causing cellular inflammation is mediated to the CNS

through nociceptive pain afferents, simultaneous conduction occurs in the same fibers away from the CNS in response to the stimulus. This backflow, known as "axon reflux," results in the release of vasoactive neuropeptide substances, such as substance P, calcitonin gene-related peptide, bradykinin, serotonin, somatostatin, neurokinin, and others. Some investigators regard RSD as a variety of chronic neuropeptide-induced neuropathic pain [1,10,119–121], others believe it is an exaggerated and sustained normal inflammatory response [95], and still others hold the traditional view that an altered sympathetic nervous system is responsible for these changes [15]. A comprehensive explanation for these mechanisms remains lacking.

Today, more than 20 neuropeptide neurotransmitter substances are being characterized [122], many of which are known to be inflammatory mediators [123]. The most likely source of inflammation in RSD-CRPS may be the afferent pain receptors themselves. These unmyelinated bidirectional afferent pain receptors not only respond to produce pain centrally but are also capable of releasing inflammatory mediators peripherally in response to either peripheral (trauma) or central stimulation. Note that the highest concentrations of these nerve endings are in the hands, feet, and face, the most common locations for RSD. For example, afferent nociceptor neurons are known to synthesize and release the undecapeptide neurotransmitter substance P in the CNS, where it is believed to mediate pain transmission [122], but up to 90% of this neuropeptide is actually transmitted from the cell body to the peripheral terminals of these afferent fibers, from which it can be released to contribute to inflammation [123,124]. In experimental substance P injection [125,126], or by stimulation of peripheral nerves at an intensity known to release substance P [127,128], inflammatory response has been caused, including vasodilatation, increased vascular permeability, pavementing of leukocytes in venules, stimulation of phagocytosis, degranulation of mast cells, and a host of other characteristic inflammatory changes. Substance P even has inflammatory immunologic properties that are largely stimulatory, such as stimulation of T lymphocytes [129], increased production of immunoglobulin A [130], and release of lysosomal enzymes with generation of thromboxane [131]. Furthermore, this neurotransmitter has been shown to enhance proliferation of fibroblasts [132], possibly causing fibroplasia and ankylosis and can evoke release of prostaglandin [133]. Among the neurotransmitters, substance P is attractive to implicate in RSD because it seems to generate such a profound generalized inflammatory response while being a primary pain transmitter. It is the most studied (the first neurotransmitter identified and purified) [123], but efforts to produce and use substance P antagonists have shown neither high affinity nor selectivity [124]. They seem only to inhibit specific parts of the inflammatory response induced by substance P.

Other neurotransmitter substances known to be released from unmyelinated afferent pain endings also elicit various inflammatory responses. Two that coexist with substance P are calcitonin gene-related peptide and neurokinin A. Calcitonin gene-related peptide is a potent vasodilator that has been used therapeutically to reverse vasoconstriction in Raynaud's disease [134], and neurokinin A increases vascular permeability and causes vasodilatation.

To clarify the role of neurogenic inflammation, a provocative study compared RSD-CRPS patients with control subjects in response to electrically induced neuropeptide stimulation, measuring vasodilatation and protein extravasation (edema) [135]. Both demonstrated evidence of increased neuropeptide release, but the control subjects had no protein extravasation, whereas the RSD-CRPS patients had steadily increased extravasation (edema). Leis and coworkers [136] compared intradermal substance P injection in the affected and unaffected limbs of RSD-CRPS patients and compared this with control subjects. The substance P–induced protein extravasation (edema) was significantly increased in the RSD-CRPS patients from the controls, but the response was equal in the affected and unaffected limbs of the RSD-CRPS patients, leading the authors to conclude that RSD-CRPS patients have impaired inactivation of substance P because both arms responded. This implies that the

endorphin pain control system is limited or inactivated in these patients.

The extent to which this complicated neurotransmitter system may function independently of external stimuli may vary, but the reality that RSD-CRPS can occur spontaneously or after a stroke makes a CNS explanation attractive. This must involve a complex regulatory system with the endorphin pain control system involved, and dysregulation of this neuropeptide system could result in the changes known as RSD-CRPS. Indeed, analysis of blood samples obtained from 61 patients with RSD showed significantly increased systemic levels of bradykinin and calcitonin gene-related peptide compared with 21 control subjects [137]. Unfortunately, it proves difficult to measure substance P in humans, and this evidence for its presence remains indirect [138].

Role of the sympathetic nervous system

Abnormal sympathetic activity is hypothesized to be the predominant etiologic factor in most reports on RSD-CRPS [6,23]. The major proof for this conclusion, however, remains the clinical response to sympathetic block, which is sufficiently variable that it is no longer a requirement for diagnosis [1,2, 10,33,133,139–141]. Concluding etiologic cause by the response to treatment is a treacherous approach, especially with such varied response among different patients, and even in the same patient on different occasions [1,10,142,143]. Yet, current concepts hold that pain relieved by regional block of the sympathetic ganglia identifies patients with "sympathetically maintained pain." Many authors now contest this concept [14,142, 144,145]. Experimental findings do not show hyperactivity of the sympathetic nervous system [146–148], and in the early stages of RSD there seems to be sympathetic hypofunction, with increased arterial flow, rather than sympathetic overactivity and vasoconstriction [148]. Proponents for sympathetically maintained pain point out evidence that the afferent pain nociceptors may become hypersensitized to normal sympathetic norepinephrine release [15]. There is a growing number of investigators, however, who question the role of the sympathetic nervous system in any way other than a modulatory fashion [1,98,133,136,144,149–153]. Unfortunately, most reported series of sympathetic blocks are not placebo controlled, and RSD-CRPS patients are known to be heavy placebo responders [149,151,152]. Indeed, placebo-controlled studies showed sympathetic block to be no more effective than the placebo [149,151,153].

Many of RSD-CRPS clinical findings do seem to involve sympathetic manifestations, with abnormalities of temperature, skin color and appearance, hair growth, sweat pattern, and edema, but it is just as possible that these are mediated by neurogenic secretion from the afferent nociceptive fibers as from the sympathetic efferents, but surely both of these systems must be implicated ultimately to understand the disorder. If proinflammatory neuropeptide secretion from the afferent sensory nerve terminals is largely responsible for inflammatory and autonomic changes (by lowering the sympathetic response threshold), it becomes understandable how anti-inflammatory drugs (eg, steroids and dimethyl sulfoxide), drugs that produce pharmacologic sympathetic block, and local anesthetic sympathetic nerve blocks may reduce the peripheral neurotransmission in some cases in which the sympathetic modification is great. These measures may be ineffective, however, in other patients in whom the sympathetic modification is minimal. When the primary reflex or stimulus for neurotransmitter release is at a higher cortical level, CNS modulators (eg, TENS, biofeedback therapy, antiepileptic medication, antidepressive drugs, acupuncture, dorsal root stimulation, and hypnosis) may prove to be of greater benefit. These latter methods probably rely on the endogenous (enkephalin-endorphin) CNS pain control neurotransmitter system rather than peripheral modification of afferent response. Endorphin inhibition of substance P from the spinal cord, spinal trigeminal nucleus, and primary sensory neurons in culture has been well documented experimentally and may account for the success of these central treatment techniques in RSD and the frequency of placebo effect [122].

The debate whether this disorder is primarily mediated from the sympathetic versus the afferent nociceptive system becomes moot if one recognizes that this is likely to vary, depending on the degree and level of CNS neuropeptide dysregulation, accounting for marked individual variation in manifestations and response.

Role of the opioid pain control system

Much research verifies an intrinsic pain-inhibiting system (enkephalins and endorphins), represented at descending levels in the midbrain, medulla, and spinal cord. Although the role of this modulating system in RSD is not described, in a disorder with unexplained pain as its dominant feature this must surely be important. Endorphins have a direct inhibitory effect on the CNS production and release of pain-producing neuropeptides, such as substance P [122].

RSD has a 30% or greater placebo block response rate [143,153]. Study of patients treated with placebo suggests the significant roll of endorphins in producing pain relief [153]. There is general consensus, however, that the patient's confidence and expectation of relief are essential for activating this pain inhibition system [154]. The critical importance of a positive, confident, compassionate, and consistent approach to patients with RSD may have a rational scientific basis and a humanitarian one. This seems especially rational with use of central treatment methods, such as acupuncture, biofeedback, TENS, dorsal column stimulation, stress loading, antiepileptic medication, and physical therapy. These patients may need faith in these treatment methods for the treatment to prove beneficial.

If, indeed, central endogenous pain control is required for coping with RSD, the hopeless attitude found among those who have had the disorder more than 6 months and difficulties with interpersonal relationships, which are frequently complicated and antagonistic, certainly could complicate successful treatment. This may be one reason late treatment proves so difficult.

Psychologic findings

The first question to answer is whether patients with RSD-CRPS are significantly different psychologically from other patients with hand injuries. Hardy and Merritt [87] compared psychologic test results in patients with RSD with those in control subjects who had hand injury but not RSD. This study showed significant differences in the psychologic profile of patients with RSD in 4 of the 10 tests performed. Patients with RSD tested significantly higher in anxiety, depression, interpersonal sensitivity, and somatization. One test, body cathexis, approached significance ($P = .58$), with dystrophy patients testing lower than controls. Intelligence, concepts of personal control, and obsessive compulsive features were not significantly different. A patient with RSD might be characterized as someone more anxious and depressed than other hand-injured patients and with more frequent complaints of somatic distress and less ability to relate interpersonally. The study suggested these patients are more dissatisfied with their bodies.

It has been suggested that patients with RSD have greater pain because of a lower threshold. Hardy answered this by means of visual linear analog scale testing [155] and the ischemic ratio pain test [156] and did not show a difference in pain threshold or overall pain complaints in the two groups; however, review of precipitating causes in this series did show less serious injuries in the reflex dystrophy group than in the control group, despite equivalent pain. None in this series had causalgia, so it seems that the non–nerve-injured patients with RSD do have a significantly different psychologic make-up than other hand-injured patients. Now there is widespread acceptance of Hardy's observations;

however, most investigators believe these psychologic differences are a result rather than a cause of RSD [6], but it may be otherwise.

Psychiatric evaluation of 34 of the author's patients with RSD-CRPS revealed most were from dysfunctional backgrounds having endured difficulties, such as parental alcoholism, death of parents, rape, and other childhood abuse. All but four of these patients fulfilled the clinical criteria for a diagnosis of alexithymia. The psychiatrist doing the study was blinded insofar as each patient's diagnosis, and the evaluation was clinical. One of the patients in the series had causalgia and one had RSD associated with carcinoma, both of which were included in the four that did not have alexithymia. Although only the psychiatrist doing the study has reported the prevalence of alexithymia in patients with RSD-CRPS, others have recognized the increased incidence of chronic pain syndromes among alexithymic patients and it is reported that alexithymia may contribute to chronic pain by means of sympathetic arousal [157].

Alexithymia means "a lack of words for mood or emotion." Formulated by Nemiah and Sifneos [158], this construct is discussed predominantly in the psychosomatic literature to depict a personality profile marked by inability to verbalize one's feelings and inability to discriminate between feelings and physical sensation. Studies of alexithymic patients suggest that disassociation from traumatic events during childhood may play a role in its etiology [159]. As a coping mechanism in a dysfunctional environment children may grow up emotionally undeveloped, without awareness of their feelings and with a continuum of unfulfilled dependency needs, a quick sense of rejection, and often unconsciously suppressed anger. Emotional stress in such individuals who are "blind to their emotions" goes unrecognized and may be transmitted at the midbrain level as physical stress, possibly stimulating neuropeptide response in the CNS. Unfortunately, there has been no study of RSD-CRPS patients by use of the Toronto Alexithymic Scale, which provides an established testing mechanism for diagnosis. Treatment of alexithymia is largely by general psychiatric support because this disorder represents a fundamental developmental problem, not usually altered by conventional psychotherapy.

Any patient complaining of disproportionate pain after a minor injury or operation who seems anxious and depressed should immediately be treated by compassionate intensive hand therapy and support. This is especially true in patients who give endless, detailed, concrete descriptions of their physical manifestations and who seem oblivious to their anger, depression, or other emotions and do not gesture with the involved hand. The worst approach is to minimize the patient's unconscious plea for support by appearing nonchalant and belittling the symptoms. These patients already have unfulfilled dependency needs and feel easily rejected. Although unaware of their own emotions, they are highly sensitive to the negative countertransference that can occur when dealing with someone who complains of great distress and has minimal objective findings.

Psychophysiologic etiology

Any etiologic theory about RSD-CRPS must reconcile a vast array of differing inciting causes, a wide variation of clinical manifestations, inconsistent results of very different treatment techniques, and contradictory research results. If predisposing personality characteristics and severe psychic stress (eg, combat) lead toward RSD, then afferent unmyelinated pain endings may release neuropeptides that cause persistent pain and inflammation in response to either physical or emotional trauma.

Expectation of relief may be able to activate a descending system of opioids that can inhibit the neuropeptides causing pain and inflammation. Exactly how these may become etiologic factors is open to speculation, but an attractive unifying hypothesis is that a varying CNS bias may lead to dysregulation of the neuropeptide system with inappropriate reflexive response to psychic or physical trauma.

Relationships between personality characteristics, psychologic stress, and somatic illness are accepted in a few other illnesses, such as peptic ulcer disease and shingles. Some physiologic manifestations of stress occur through the autonomic nervous system [160], and study of normal subjects reveals consistent but different individualized patterns of sympathetic response for each person. It is distinctly possible that personality characteristics (eg, alexithymia), unusual conditions of stress at the time of injury (eg, military combat), the nature of neural insult (eg, high-velocity nerve wounding or midbrain stroke), or the emotional state of the patient (eg, anxiety or depression) may bias the CNS toward dysregulation and imbalance of the complex mediators of pain and neurogenic inflammation. Electrical stereotactic brainstem stimulation in conscious patients suggests some fundamental alteration at the midbrain level that distinguishes RSD-CRPS patients from those with somatic chronic peripheral pain [161]. This suggests that mesencephalic reticulothalamocortical circuits are hypersensitive to innocent afferent input, causing inappropriate pain neuropeptide release at this cortical level. In these patients the pain of RDS-CRPS seems a distinct entity from somatic pain, arising from alteration of the CNS at the midbrain level, which once established persists, despite removal or absence of the original peripheral stimulus. Functional MRI study shows widespread prefrontal hypersensitivity, increased anterior cingulate activity, and decreased activity in the contralateral thalamus [162]. Interestingly, unsuccessful sympathetic blocks did not change the cortical response on MRI, but successful sympathetic blocks and successful placebo blocks both did alter the cortical responses [162]. Many authors now suspect that CNS mechanisms are more important than the peripheral sympathetic nervous system in the cause of this disorder [136,163–169].

If such central mechanisms are largely responsible, those with alexithymia could be expected to be at greater risk of central misrepresentation from emotional stress and minor injury. In a controlled study, Gertzen and coworkers [85] confirmed Hardy and Merritt's [87] earlier findings that RSD-CRPS patients have significantly greater depression and anxiety than control subjects. In addition, Gertzen and coworkers [85] found that 80% of these patients had a recent stressful "life event" compared with 20% of the controls, suggesting that stress was a major etiologic factor in this series. Others also suggest major stressful life events are a precipitating factor [82]. Interestingly, there have been reports of spontaneous resolution of RSD-CRPS after cerebral contusion head injury [170]; the successful use of electroconvulsive therapy [171] and hypnotherapy [172] also suggests implication of the CNS.

Other factors that could bias the CNS toward neuropeptide dysregulation include circumstances surrounding an injury, along with the psychologic make-up of the patient and his or her characteristic response to stress. Causalgia (CRPS type II) occurs more frequently under stressful battle conditions than in civilian settings [110,173], and antagonistic relationships with previous physicians and with employers in work-related injury do seem to prevail in patients with RSD-CRPS. If stressful circumstances in patients with predisposed personalities can produce these alterations in the CNS, then regardless of the treatment used, it behooves physicians and therapists to encourage expression of the fear and anger these circumstances have caused in hopes of reducing this central hypersensitivity. Such a biased CNS midbrain could initiate pain-causing descending excitation, ultimately releasing neuropeptide inflammatory mediators that might cause the inflammatory and sympathetic responses seen in RSD-CRPS. Alternatively, it is conceivable that the confident, reassured, and optimistic patient may be able to counter this process with

the descending endogenous enkephalin-endorphin system, which is known to inhibit pain and substance P at the spinal cord level. Indeed, studies by Leis and coworkers [136] of the response in RSD-CRPS patients injected with substance P demonstrated less inactivation in RSD-CRPS patients than in control subjects, even on the asymptomatic side, suggesting such a mechanism.

A centrally mediated system causing midbrain neuropeptide dysregulation could explain the wide variation in precipitating causes and responses of patients, with some having predominantly a neurogenic insult leading to the disorder, such as stroke and gunshot major nerve injury, and others having a central bias that makes them highly susceptible with minor injury or no injury at all. This could also account for the remarkably high incidence of placebo effect in this disorder, mediated by the CNS.

Diagnostic techniques

No one laboratory study is specific for RSD-CRPS, and it remains a clinical diagnosis, even though numerous objective measurements are useful to support the diagnosis. Because RSD is often associated with a variety of other disorders, such as a diabetes, herpes infection, carcinoma, heart disease, thyroid disease, arthritis, and stroke, abnormal laboratory studies should not exclude the diagnosis. Typical patients with RSD have normal sedimentation rate, C-reactive protein level, leukocyte count, and concentrations of other acute-phase reactants, despite the appearance of inflammation [92]. Neurogenic inflammation usually causes minimal, if any, laboratory study change.

Radiography and bone scan

Radiologic studies have provided a definitive objective test for RSD-CRPS when positive, with classic Sudeck's atrophy radiologic findings that are considered diagnostic on plain film [57,90]. Unfortunately, considerable demineralization must occur for osteopenia to become visible on standard radiographic views [174], which places the patient in a later stage with worse prognosis by the time the diagnosis can be made on routine radiographs. Radionuclide scintigraphic studies using three-phase technetium-labeled diphosphonate bone scanning provide an important diagnostic tool, abnormal scans being reported variably from 50% [175,176] to 80% [177]. Although increased uptake is not present in all patients, it is a useful test when positive, because it is seen well before standard radiographic change. Doury [64], however, points out that children, and in rare cases adults, may actually show decreased uptake. Investigators who use bone scan as their diagnostic prerequisite classify such decreased uptake as "pseudo dystrophy" [178]. With current methods, a normal bone scan does not rule out the diagnosis [3,6, 179,180]. An abnormal scan has high specificity but poor sensitivity [181]; however, it remains a useful adjunctive diagnostic technique because changes occur early. When abnormal bone scan is present, the rapidity of bone resorption in RSD is far greater than that seen with disuse osteoporosis, and reflects marked regional hyperemia, with evidence of microvascular hyperpermeability [92]. Although bone scan remains a useful diagnostic tool in RSD, it should not be held as a prerequisite for diagnosis and does not afford prognostic information, although it may provide rationale for calcitonin or bisphosphonate therapy.

MRI

Changes on MRI of the involved extremity are seen early in RSD-CRPS but are too nonspecific to be diagnostic and vary at different stages of the disease [64,92].

Thermography

Temperature measurement by infrared thermography is appealing for RSD because it is noninvasive and safe [182], and is regarded by some to be the favored test in diagnosis of RSD [8]. Studies show such a spectrum of temperature variability in RSD-CRPS, however, that its value is limited [79, 183–186]. Thermography seems most useful to help the clinician communicate with the patient about the illness and to monitor progress.

Other diagnostic tests

Galvanic skin conduction in the palms is reported to be abnormal in RSD. Quantitative sweat response (the quantitative sudomotor axon reflex test) has been popularized by Low and coworkers [187] with reported abnormalities of sweat response to thermography testing in patients with RSD.

Capillary blood velocity determination with microscopic epi-illumination of digital skin, combined with laser Doppler flux, offers a sensitive assessment of skin blood flow [188]. Koman and coworkers [6] point out the importance of using stress, such as cold stress, to afford reproducible dynamic response patterns. These methods are not universally available, however, and their precise role in the diagnosis and treatment of RSD is yet to be determined. Electromyographic and nerve conduction studies show no specific abnormality associated with RSD [91].

Response to sympathetic block has been regarded by many as the best traditional criterion for diagnosis of patients with RSD. Recent recognition that this response is variable, however, and is absent in as many as 30% or more, has led to the redesignation of CRPS, with subclassification for those who respond to blocks as having sympathetically mediated pain. The role of the sympathetic nervous system remains controversial; however, a positive sympathetic block response does provide a valuable indicator of therapy options.

Functional assessment

It is imperative to clarify precisely which changes are most responsible for inhibiting function in patients with RSD, usually best accomplished as a functional assessment by hand therapists. This helps the patient focus on measures to gain control of specific problems and provides objective parameters for positive therapeutic reinforcement. For example, if cold causes increased pain and decreased function, temperature biofeedback therapy and methods of cold avoidance should be taught, whereas in a different patient, edema control may be a more important functional variable.

Although sophisticated diagnostic instrumentation and tests of autonomic function exist, from a practical point of view, most patients need simple functional assessment by a physician and hand therapist, with simple reproducible measurements to monitor progress, such as volume displacement measurement of edema; resting temperature measurements comparing fingers on the affected hand with those of the unaffected extremity; sweat assessment; color and appearance observation; range of motion; strength; fine manipulation; sensory testing with two-point discrimination; moving two-point discrimination; and Semmes-Weinstein monofilament testing and temperature cold recovery time when it is not too painful (length of time for temperature to return to baseline after cold exposure). Pain assessment is by use of a visual analog scale and a pain diagram drawn by the patient. These simple tests afford an easily reproducible method to monitor success of the therapeutic effort and offer the patient important feedback.

Treatment techniques

There is a wide spectrum of treatment methods with inconsistent results for RSD-CRPS, ranging from psychotherapy to sympathectomy. Although all techniques are directed at interruption of the reflex pain cycle, the existence of so many different methods is testimony that none is universally successful [9]. Although there is no consensus regarding the best treatment, there is general belief that the earlier treatment is instituted, the better the prognosis. One must be honest with patients that predicting the course and result of treatment in this disorder is like predicting the weather: there may be some idea of what to expect, but do not be surprised if the prediction is incorrect. To that extent, the clinician must be willing to individualize treatment with as many modifications and changes as are needed to find a regimen that offers benefit.

The following treatment methods vary greatly and are not at all inclusive but are those most frequently used. In general, start with the least invasive and morbid techniques and gradually try different methods until a regimen succeeds, always attempting to maintain a positive, constructive, albeit honest outlook. The physician's and hand therapist's interest and concern may, in fact, be the most important therapeutic tool in this puzzling disorder.

Surgical treatment

Except for certain specific exceptions, avoid efforts to seek surgical solutions for RSD. Sunderland [17] summarized surgical treatment results as follows:

> Operations have been performed for pain at nearly every possible site in the pathway from the peripheral receptors to the sensory cortex. At every level, the story is the same - some encouraging results, but a disheartening tendency for the pain to recur...many procedures for the relief of pain have had their crowded hour of general enthusiastic adoption, only to fade gradually into oblivion.

Sympathectomy

Most surgical techniques, such as periarterial sympathectomy [107], posterior rhizotomy (dorsal root section) [173], cordotomy (spinothalamic transection), neurolysis, and neurectomy [189,190], have proved of little value for RSD-CRPS. Sympathectomy remains useful in well-selected patients, however, especially in cases with proximal nerve injury, such as causalgia. Sympathectomy is generally less useful in the slowly developing dystrophy caused by minor trauma or CNS origin, such as stroke [107].

The patient most likely to benefit from sympathectomy is one who obtains repeated, dramatic, temporary relief from sympathetic blocks but for whom the relief never lasts longer than the duration of the anesthetic and in whom there is no placebo effect with use of saline for the block. Patients who do not respond to sympathetic blocks are not likely to respond to sympathectomy, and some other treatment should be attempted [13,20, 189]. Causalgia is the one form of RSD most likely to benefit from sympathectomy [191].

Surgical control of peripheral irritants

Many patients with RSD have an associated identifiable peripheral nerve irritant (dystrophic focus) that seems disproportionately painful and might be considered for elective surgical correction, such as painful neuromas, intraneural fibrosis, previous carpal tunnel release, and so forth. The patient must be protected from the surgeon's lust to find a simple surgical solution. The wary surgeon gains control of the inappropriate symptom complex before elective surgery when the patient's symptoms have narrowed to an appropriate level. This may be accomplished through pharmacologic treatment, a goal-oriented hand therapy program, autonomic blocks, and other measures [192]. The author has reviewed too many litigation cases in which surgeons arduously and heroically attempted operation after operation, even amputation, to try to resolve their patients' desperate complaints, usually resulting in temporary relief later obviated by recurrent symptoms.

An important exception that warrants emergency surgery is acute carpal tunnel syndrome with RSD-CRPS symptoms following Colles fractures or similar trauma. The timing and progressive nature of this problem indicates need for immediate surgery to avoid a severe chronic pain syndrome [193].

Once the patient with RSD-CRPS has adequate pain control, elective surgery can be considered, but in these circumstances the surgeon must be aware of significant risk for exacerbation of symptoms, and a long-acting or continuous axillary block anesthetic should be administered to avoid redevelopment of a pain reflex cycle [1]. Study of patients with and without blocks clearly verifies this approach [194].

Implanted electrical stimulation

Use of implantable neurostimulation systems for treatment of chronic pain has gained increasing popularity at pain management centers. When painful peripheral nerves are treated, improvement by peripheral nerve block is a prerequisite, along with temporary success by transcutaneous nerve stimulation [195]. Caution should be exercised in this area, however, because most reports of success do not separate patients with RSD-CRPS from other pain patients. Cooney [195] suggests that implanted electrical stimulation should be confined to patients whose pain is "somatically" derived and not from "sympathetic overstimulation/RSD." In the author's limited experience, a few patients had initial promising results after implant placement but later redeveloped symptoms. The ability to control the stimulation level themselves may lead some patients to cope better with their chronic problem, however, and it remains a worthwhile attempt for those who do not respond to more conservative efforts.

Stellate ganglion and other nerve blocks

Percutaneous stellate ganglion sympathetic nerve block remains the most widely accepted form of RSD-CRPS treatment in the United States. Blocks are not uniformly successful and are no longer required for diagnosis, although widely used to classify sympathetically maintained pain (CRPS type I or II) [1,6]. Sympathetic block seems best suited for patients whose manifestations seem predominantly sympathetic, such as abnormal skin color, temperature, and sweat. The most favorable scenario is a patient treated within 6 months after onset of symptoms, [50,196,197], as is true for all other methods of RSD-CRPS treatment.

The nerve-injured causalgia patients (CRPS type II) are most likely to benefit from percutaneous sympathetic block (at least for the duration of the anesthetic). This is also the group of patients most likely to benefit from sympathectomy [1,189, 198]. In patients who do not have causalgia, sympathetic block fails in more than one third of patients [50,197,198]. Ochoa [149,151] is convinced that sympathetic blocks afford either no relief or relief only attainable because of the placebo response. When the patient obtains relief the block should be regarded as a successful treatment, however, regardless of whether it is caused by the placebo effect or the pharmacologic agent used. The patient really does not care.

If neuropeptide dysfunction is an important mechanism in patients with RSD-CRPS, it can be understood how sympathetic modification of the afferent pain endings could be beneficial in some patients, such as causalgia with predominantly peripheral insult, and not in others whose stimulus may be at a higher established central level. Reflex pain firmly established at the central level is more likely to respond to methods that activate the endogenous opioid internal pain control system, which is known to interfere with pain neurotransmitter production and secretion (eg, substance P) [151]. This endogenous mechanism might explain why "placebo blocks" are frequently successful in as many as 30% of patients [149,151,199,200].

Brachial plexus blocks are useful to determine whether a patient's stiffness is caused by pain or fibrosis by assessing the passive range of motion while they are anesthetized and paralyzed. Patients sometimes obtain improvement with brachial plexus blocks and not with stellate ganglion blocks [201]. Repeated local long-acting nerve blocks are sometimes successful in breaking the pain cycle in selected patients whose symptoms are confined to a specific neurologic region, such as that supplied by the superficial radial nerve, or an isolated digit, such as an amputation stump with painful digital neuroma.

Intravenous regional pharmacologic infusion

Infusion of intravenous guanethidine sympathetic block into an extremity isolated by arterial tourniquet (Bier block) has been a popular treatment technique, especially in England, although it was never approved for this purpose in the United States [202–205]. Although guanethidine blocks usually last only 15 to 20 minutes, the duration of response is longer than stellate ganglion blocks because there is a 5-day half-life for displacing norepinephrine in the postganglionic system [203,206].

Other pharmacologic agents used with regional infusion for RSD-CRPS include reserpine [207,208], phentolamine [209], bretylium tosylate [210], and steroids [22]. Currently, reserpine and phentolamine are not approved for parenteral use in the United States, and only bretylium tosylate and steroids remain available. Parenteral bretylium tosylate is approved for cardiac ventricular arrhythmias and its activity is similar to guanethidine, inhibiting norepinephrine release and uptake. There are reports of its successful use in patients with RSD-CRPS, usually used in conjunction with steroids [211–213].

Recent randomized, double-blind controlled comparison of intravenous guanethidine, reserpine, and saline showed no difference at 24 hours [44]. Similar studies using phentolamine showed no advantage over placebo [149,151]. As yet, there has been no controlled study of bretylium tosylate. Whether the benefit of intravenous sympathetic block is predominantly a placebo response or the result of modulation of the afferent pain system by sympathetic control remains controversial, but the many reports of its successful use, especially early in the patient's course, maintain its worth as a treatment option.

Acupuncture

Acupuncture with electrodes or transdermal needles has been used for patients with RSD-CRPS with varying results [214]. It is interesting that the most successful series, reported by Chan and Chow [215], was in Chinese patients in Hong Kong with excellent results in 70% and improvement in 90%

of patients, but they pointed out that these were Chinese patients with confidence in acupuncture, whose expectation of relief may have played a role in activating the release of endorphin pain inhibitors in the CNS. In the West, this technique has usually been used as an adjunctive measure without as much success, possibly because patients have less faith in the method and less probability of activating the endogenous pain control system.

Biofeedback therapy

Temperature biofeedback is a useful adjunctive treatment for patients with RSD-CRPS whose clinical manifestations include pronounced temperature change. In those patients capable of biofeedback training, control of the temperature difference correlated with control or better tolerance of their pain [216]. Why voluntary control of this autonomic function provides pain control remains a provocative question. Although usually used as an adjunctive measure by hand therapists, there are reports of biofeedback as a successful primary treatment [44,127,217,218], and other self-hypnosis techniques [172]. It is best suited for patients with pronounced temperature change treated early in the course of their disorder.

Transcutaneous nerve stimulation

Successful use of TENS has been reported in RSD-CRPS [7,219–223]. Its mechanism is hypothesized to be by activation of the endogenous opioid analgesic system to release endorphins [223] that may inhibit pain at the level of the spinothalamic tract [224,225]. Animal and human studies suggest such a mechanism [104]. TENS may be particularly useful when there are minimal inflammatory or autonomic changes and pain is the predominant manifestation. It is generally used as adjunctive therapy to assist with pain control. Like all other methods, TENS is reported most effective when initiated early.

Pharmacologic medical treatment

As in all other aspects of RSD-CRPS, controversy exists in regard to which medications are effective. Pharmacologic choices vary according to clinician's concept of etiophysiologic mechanisms and to some extent by the clinical manifestations. The United States Food and Drug Administration has to date approved no single pharmacologic agent as safe and effective for RSD-CRPS. There is no one drug of choice.

Review of the huge spectrum of reported pharmacologic treatment regimens is beyond the scope of this article. Examples are mentioned in the treatment classifications for differing etiologic concepts, however, according to whether one believes a particular patient's problem is predominantly from an exaggerated inflammatory response, overactivity or an increased sensitivity of the sympathetic nervous system, a predominantly CNS-mediated reflex, or a principally peripheral vascular disorder. Clearly, these mechanisms are not independent of one another and opinions differ about which is most etiologically important. Medications should be directed to the manifestations that seem to prevail in individual patients.

Sympatholytics

Unfortunately, most of the older nonspecific oral alpha and beta sympathetic blockers result in such prohibitive side effects that they are not tolerated. Clonidine is among the most useful of the sympatholytics. It is a α_2-adrenergic agonist that is active in the dorsal horn and brainstem to suppress CNS activity and peripheral sympathetic tone [226]. The transdermal patch form is more useful to reduce side effects and may be a very effective adjunctive treatment along with hand therapy and other measures. Clonidine may also be given orally in doses of 0.1 to 0.4 mg daily and may be particularly useful for weaning narcotic-addicted patients by blocking their withdrawal effects [227].

Phenoxybenzamine is a combined α_1- and α_2-antagonist and has been reported as a successful oral sympathetic blocker for RSD-CRPS treatment, but its nonselective features can cause widespread side effects [228].

Calcium channel blockers, such as nifedipine, are not true sympathetic blockers but function to decrease sympathetic smooth muscle tone and improve blood flow, warming digits by preventing calcium release and reducing vasoconstriction. These are beneficial in selected patients with RSD because of "cool" extremities or Raynaud's disease [229,230]. Verapamil, diltiazem, amlodipine, and nifedipine are the principal calcium antagonists available; however, verapamil has predominantly cardiac effect and is not useful for RSD-CRPS.

Anti-inflammatory medications

Corticosteroids have long proved beneficial in some patients with RSD-CRPS, either with a short-term, high-dose method [91] or with long-term use [231]. Control studies with placebo confirm steroid benefit [148]. Kozin [23], however, observed that steroid response is not as good in patients who have predominantly pain, without inflammatory or autonomic manifestations.

Nonsteroidal anti-inflammatory drugs, such as ibuprofen, are of questionable value in the treatment of RSD-CRPS without convincing studies either for or against their use. Much of their benefit is thought to be caused by inhibition of prostaglandins, which are proinflammatory mediators [232].

Recent interest in the etiologic hypothesis that RSD-CRPS is caused by an exaggerated neuropeptide-induced inflammatory tissue response caused by free radicals has led to the use of free radical scavengers, such as intravenous mannitol and dimethyl sulfoxide, for acute RSD [94,133].

Central-acting pharmacologic agents

Antiepileptic drugs are among the most interesting and useful pharmacologic medications for RSD and other neuropathic pain syndromes. It is puzzling that phenobarbital, one of the oldest and most widely used anticonvulsants, is known to sometimes cause RSD [64], whereas the anticonvulsant gabapentin is one of the most successful newer drugs for pain control of RSD-CRPS [218]. The central changes by which antiepilepsy drugs can either cause or control RSD certainly poses a provocative question. In the high dosages used for epilepsy, gabapentin can cause sedation, confusion, diplopia, vertigo, and ataxia. Fortunately, those who benefit from treatment of neuropathic pain usually do so at lower dosages, usually started at 100 mg three times a day. Gabapentin is structurally related to γ-aminobutyric acid, a neurotransmitter that plays a role in pain transmission and modulation. Its precise mechanism of action is not understood but a randomized, double-blind, placebo-controlled multicenter study showed significant benefit in neuropathic pain syndromes [233]. Gabapentin alters γ-aminobutyric acid synthesis and release in blood serotonin levels [234]. Gabapentin is eliminated by renal excretion, so it must be used carefully in patients with renal insufficiency, especially if the creatinine clearance is less than 60 mL/min [235,236].

Clonazepam is a benzodiazepine that facilitates binding of the inhibitory neurotransmitter γ-aminobutyric acid to its specific channel receptors and has been used successfully to treat allodynia in patients with chronic pain syndromes. Baclofen is a strong γ-aminobutyric acid receptor agonist and seems particularly useful for lancinating pain and ongoing muscle spasms and cramps. It seems especially useful for treatment of the dystonia that often occurs in patients with RSD [227,237]. Tramadol is a CNS-active analgesic, neither nonsteroidal nor true opioid, which inhibits reuptake of serotonin and norepinephrine [238,239]. When tolerated, it seems a much better choice than opioids for RSD pain.

Antidepressants, anxiety, narcotic, and sleep medications

In RSD-CRPS, sleep disturbance is typical in a pattern usually characteristic of depression (awakening in the early morning hours). Although these alexithymic-prone patients usually deny any awareness of depression, they generally need medication for sleep, and when tolerated, tricyclic antidepressants, such as amitriptyline, are useful. Amitriptyline, however, must be used with care in the elderly and in patients with heart disease, narrow-angle glaucoma, prostatism, or seizure disorders [227]. On psychiatric testing, patients with RSD are significantly depressed and anxious, and because it is difficult clinically to distinguish between depression and anxiety, psychiatric evaluation is indicated to determine if patients need antidepressant or anxiety medications [240]. Diazepam has been previously recommended for RSD-CRPS [109] but it is a poor choice because although it is a useful antianxiety medication, it is ineffective for depression and patients with RSD-CRPS may develop antianalgesia response and physical dependence after long use [241].

Opioid narcotic use is currently popular in pain management centers in the United States because available long-acting opioids permit normal daily activity in many patients with chronic pain. The RSD patient should not be grouped with those who have chronic back and other types of somatic pain, however, and caution is recommended for use in RSD-CRPS patients [227]. If one accepts the concept of an internal opioid pain mechanism in humans, use of exogenous opioids could conceivably inhibit production of the internal endorphin system and interfere with any treatment programs believed to activate this endorphin internal pain control system (eg, TENS, acupuncture, stress-loading hand therapy, implanted electrical stimulation, and so forth).

I believe narcotic treatment for RSD is a better short-term treatment for the physician than the patient, and the more time-consuming and troublesome techniques to help patients slowly cope with their pain are a better approach in all but absolute treatment failures. One should exhaust other treatment techniques before resorting to chronic narcotic use. Certainly, short-acting opioid preparations are contraindicated for long-term use in patients with this disorder, such as propoxyphene, oxycodone, meperidine, and pentazocine, because they can cause addiction and CNS toxic effects [242].

Calcitonin and bisphosphonates

Calcitonin is a hormone in a separate category that regulates bone metabolism. Its success for treating

RSD was totally unexpected, with unforeseeable benefits, other than antiosteoclast properties. It has been the most frequently used treatment method in France and some other European countries for more than 20 years [243–246], using high doses of recombinant human calcitonin. As with other treatments, better results are reported when patients are treated soon after onset [243] and it seems best suited for patients with positive three-phase bone scan [1,98].

The success of calcitonin led to considerations for bisphosphonate use [247] because of their known action as potent osteoclast blocking agents and their believed action to inhibit neuropeptide release from afferent nerve endings [117]. Pamidronate disodium is typically used to relieve pain from Paget's disease, multiple myeloma, and osteolytic painful metastases and has been the most successful intravenous bisphosphonate preparation for RSD-CRPS [117,248–250]. Alendronate sodium also showed efficacy but had a 40% recurrence rate at 1 year [251]. This method of treatment also seems most suitable in patients with abnormalities on bone scan [252].

Hand therapy

Hand therapy is the foundation of treatment for most patients with RSD-CRPS, whereas TENS, pharmacologic treatment, nerve blocks, and even surgery serve as adjunctive measures. It is imperative to establish baseline measurement criteria to monitor progress, best accomplished in the hand therapy arena, whatever treatment method is chosen.

These patients typically do not believe they are slowly improving until shown proof through objective measurements, such as reduced edema, increased grip strength, improved range of motion, temperature control, and so forth. This proof may afford an important positive outlook. "Rest and motion" [243] are management principles that emphasize the need for partial rest in a splinted functional position and frequent physical activity and motion to the fullest pain-free extent. Heat is valuable to relax muscle spasm and improve joint motion; however, heat with dependency in a whirlpool should be avoided in patients with edema because this aggravates swelling [27] and tends to depersonalize management.

Muscle trigger points of myofascial dysfunction must be treated, but the usual methods of ice, massage, and cold spray are often intolerable in patients with RSD-CRPS. Warm massage, stretch exercises, and injection of persistent trigger points are usually preferable.

Techniques, such as ultrasound over the stellate ganglion [253] or the involved peripheral nerves [254], biofeedback [255], desensitization [192], and stress loading [256], involve intense personal support by the therapist. No single modality or method succeeds in all patients, and individualization and flexibility are essential. The importance of psychologic support and encouragement cannot be overemphasized and may be essential to treatment success. It seems valuable to have the same therapist work with a particular patient if good rapport is established.

Psychotherapy

RSD-CRPS is not a psychiatric disorder [6,99], just as peptic ulcer disease is not a psychiatric disorder; however, neither of these disorders is separate from CNS and psychogenic effect. Most cases of RSD are not surgical, but certainly the patients do not regard their disorder as emotional and do not easily accept psychotherapy or even psychiatric evaluation. Consultation is most easily accomplished by introducing the psychiatrist in the hand therapy arena, as a supportive person to help with the emotional impact of losing hand function. Most patients are comfortable with this explanation and cooperative with the psychiatrist, who can explore etiologic patterns, assist with the patient's current conflicts, and identify when there is need for psychotropic medication for depression.

There are a few isolated reports of successful treatment of RSD-CRPS by psychotherapy alone, and all of these stress the importance of helping patients feel responsible and in control [40,79,217,257, 258]. The importance of consistent psychologic support, sympathy, reassurance, and stubborn encouragement for these patients cannot be overemphasized. In general, the support from a psychiatrist or psychologist is beneficial, but the primary caregiver must also continue to give support.

Ten practical principles in the treatment of reflex sympathetic dystrophy

Any arrogance about diagnosis or treatment of RSD-CRPS must be held suspect because of the lack of distinctive criteria for diagnosis or a unifying etiologic hypothesis, and because of such a remarkable array of inciting causes (sometimes no apparent cause at all) and treatment techniques (none of which are universally successful). Until there is better understanding of this disorder, the following 10 principles are offered as a practical treatment approach [Box 3]. These principles are offered as a method for possible help and to minimize harm, recognizing that the fundamental mechanisms underlying this disorder

Box 3: Ten practical principles in the treatment of RSD

1. **The best treatment is prevention.** Take seriously any preoperative or postoperative patient whose pain complaints seem disproportionate and who asks extensive, anxious, detailed questions, requiring additional attention and reassurance from the physician. Similarly, the postoperative patient who is quiet but seems to withdraw and disassociate from the physician because of pain also needs additional therapeutic support. This support is usually best provided by hand therapy, in which objective parameters are measured and nonpainful mobilization activities are encouraged. If the patient improves, one can never prove that this would have evolved into RSD. Many clinicians and therapists, however, believe additional support and early intervention may prevent the disorder in some patients [259]. The worst therapeutic approach is to belittle or minimize the painful patient's complaint because of the lack of objective findings. If the studies by Hardy and Merritt [87] and Gurtzen and coworkers [85] are correct, these are sensitized patients who are already significantly anxious and depressed, have poor self-image, feel easily rejected, and somatize their anger. Minimizing their complaints may add fuel to stress-related features that may play a role in this disorder. In today's managed care environment, providing this important, early, intense support based on the intuition of the clinician proves increasingly difficult.

2. **The earlier the treatment, the better the prognosis**. With few exceptions, most authors believe that RSD-CRPS becomes increasingly recalcitrant to therapeutic efforts after 6 months.

3. **Individualize treatment methods to the particular patient's manifestations.** Patients can be characterized by objective measured parameters as having symptoms that are predominantly sympathetic, inflammatory, or central manifestations (when objective peripheral response is minimal but pain is great). Clinicians should use sympathetic blocks, for example, if sympathetic symptoms predominate, such as changes in temperature, color, and sweat. Temperature biofeedback treatment could be attempted when there is major temperature change. If inflammatory symptoms predominate, such as stiffness, joint discomfort, swelling, and pain with joint motion, anti-inflammatory agents, such as a short-term burst of steroids, should be used. Central stimulation (eg, TENS), antiepileptic medication

(eg, gabapentin), hypnosis, acupuncture, and stress loading should be used when central pain predominates. If early Sudeck's bone atrophy or a marked change on bone scan is present, calcitonin or bisphosphonate can be considered. All treatment techniques should include regular hand therapy support with monitoring of objective parameters.

4. **Start with the least invasive and morbid treatment techniques.** By use of objective monitoring, gradually alter or try new treatments starting with those least likely to cause harm until one of these regimens shows objective improvement. Maintain a positive outlook and reassure the patient that many different treatment methods can be explored until one demonstrates improvement. Do not expect much subjective pain improvement until objective measured improvement to the patient can be demonstrated, which may instill hope and confidence needed for pain control. These patients rarely think they are better until they are shown to be by measurement, and the physician must maintain a stubborn optimism with compassionate honesty about the goal to help patients cope with their pain rather than to eliminate the pain.

5. **Minimize stressful situations**. RSD-CRPS patients seem particularly prone to conflict, usually feel victimized and poorly understood, and often express distress that no one understands or believes their degree of suffering. It is easy to become impatient with their constant complaints, but it is crucial to listen patiently and help modify any stress-producing situations to minimize rather than aggravate their problem.

6. **Encourage litigation settlement as soon as possible.** Unrealistic unconscious expectations of dramatic cure, wealth from litigation settlement, or revenge against an employer or spouse create additional progressive disappointment, resentment, and depression unless these expectations are recognized and gently eliminated whenever possible. In some patients, these expectations may arise from unfulfilled childhood dependency needs and are immature and unrealistic but are also unconscious. The patient must be encouraged to avoid measures that additionally complicate and increase stress. It helps to listen to the patient vent his or her frustrations and anger, which requires the patience of a saint (hand therapists generally have greater sainthood potential than hand surgeons). Unfortunately, litigation increases stress and encourages victimization, implying that the worse the problem, the better

the settlement. Although a healthier therapeutic environment exists after settlement, the problem of RSD usually persists and still may sometimes result in suicide.

7. **Control the disproportionate pain and other marked symptoms of RSD before elective surgery.** Do not expect surgery to cure disproportionate pain [1,194,260]. There is a popular misguided belief that most RSD is altogether from a single peripheral cause, possibly because a precipitating irritant is frequently identified. One should avoid a surgical search for such a cause, at least until the disproportionate pain is controlled, except in certain specific acute situations. Surgery typically results in temporary relief [173], followed by exacerbation or worsening and requests for additional surgery, and the surgeon is often held responsible for the worsening symptoms. Amputation is not likely to rid the patient of the pain, although it certainly will of the extremity [261]. When surgery is done on a patient with RSD who has developed control of the pain or any patient with a past history of RSD, long-acting blocks should be used during surgery [194] to avoid exacerbating RSD symptoms, even if the patient has a general or local anesthetic. Use of perioperative calcitonin prophylaxis has also been reported to prevent recurrence of RSD-CRPS [262]. There are two situations in which surgery is clearly indicated for RSD, one of which is emergent: when RSD is associated with acute traumatic carpal tunnel syndrome after injury, such as Colles fracture, emergent surgical release of the carpal tunnel is indicated to avoid progressive dystrophic change [193]; another surgical indication is when sympathetic blocks consistently relieve pain only to the time limit of the block, at which point sympathectomy can then be recommended.

8. **Regard the patient with RSD as an impaired individual with a chronic illness.** Brand and Yancey [263] pointed out the need to treat chronic pain patients with the same compassion offered patients with rheumatoid arthritis or diabetes. A positive, optimistic outlook designed to instill confidence and expectation of improvement should be provided, but do not imply a greater understanding or ability than is actually present. Although one must admit to patients the ignorance of the basic underlying problem and that one cannot confidently promise to solve it, one must try to remain optimistic and supportive. One can help patients cope by showing compassion and continued support, much the same as treating patients with connective tissue disease and other chronic disorders. Some patients may "need their pain" even while they seek relief. These patients complicate their own management with noncompliant behavior and intolerance to drugs and other treatment regimens; retaining a positive outlook and diluting the responsibility by a team approach with the hand therapist and psychologic counseling are helpful when managing these difficult patients.

9. **Never discharge the patient with RSD.** Patients with RSD who improve are at significant risk for redevelopment of the syndrome, often at a new location [194]. The complex psychophysiologic features of this disorder may relate to unfulfilled dependency needs in some patients, and an important therapeutic feature may be the opportunity to return annually to express their current status to their caregivers. Those who do not need to return will not, but others seem to appreciate the opportunity to express how they have coped with their difficulties, and one suspects it may afford benefit to prevent recurrence. The author made the mistake of discharging a "cured" patient only to have her return a year later with severe mirror image disease.

10. **Do not call these patients "turkeys."** The compassion needed to manage patients with RSD successfully is incompatible with such a rude designation, and furthermore shows lack of respect for and knowledge of the Meleagris Gallopavo, the noble American wild turkey.

and the optimal treatment method still remain unknown.

Summary

Can one prevent RSD? Certainly not in every situation because some highly predisposed patients apparently develop the disorder spontaneously. Empirical observation has convinced many that on recognition of the earliest signs (eg, disproportionate pain, swelling, vasomotor instability, and so forth), immediate therapeutic intervention may obviate development in some patients. One cannot expect consistently to prevent such a poorly understood disorder; however, there are six measures that may hopefully reduce the possibility of RSD.

1. **Communication.** As early as 1942, Miller suggested that a significant preventive factor is communication with the patient, expressing

reassurance of support and assistance for relief of his or her anxiety and pain [264].

2. **Early active motion**. Early active motion and function within the patient's pain threshold should be encouraged. Newer methods of management, such as relative motion splinting that permits immediate active motion after long extensor repair or sagittal band rupture [265], or secure plate fracture fixation and early active motion [266], do much to discourage the self-victimization that accompanies immobilization and seems related to RSD.

3. **Avoid external fixation**. Whenever possible, prolonged use of external fixation should be avoided [146]. One report noted development of RSD in 9.8% of patients after external fixation of distal radius wrist fractures and a 5.5% incidence after external minifixation in the hand. An even higher incidence was suggested in patients with distraction external fixation. If RSD-CRPS symptoms arise, abandon external fixation in favor of immobilization.

4. **Remove painful casts**. Remove any cast or splint that the patient believes is too tight or is causing pain. In general, RSD is more common in patients who are immobilized, and perception by the patient that a tight cast is causing their symptoms is frequent, even though the clinician may find no evidence on physical inspection. Nonetheless, the cast should be removed and replaced as often as necessary to rid the patient of burning, incessant pain. If unrelenting pain continues, it is appropriate to abandon immobilization completely (other than perhaps a soft dressing), but only after a physical examination to be certain that there is no other explanation for the pain (eg, acute carpal tunnel syndrome, infection, or ischemia) and thorough communication with the patient about the need to control the pain have taken place. Whenever the patient has subjective relief, the immobilization can be gently replaced. The patient is likely to have better function despite a nonunion or tendon rupture than he or she would ever have with the disaster of late RSD.

5. **Avoid painful therapy**. Avoid measures that increase inflammation. For example, avoid painful, forced passive range-of-motion therapy or dynamic splints until acute inflammation subsides. Pain is the indication to limit passive forced motion, which should remain within a relatively pain-free range.

6. **Block patients with a history of RSD**. Patients with a history of RSD are at greater risk for recurrence [194]. When surgery is necessary in such a patient, a long-acting block of the operative area should be performed before any incision is made, even under a general anesthetic. Keep the CNS unaware of the procedure as long as possible to avoid recurrence of the reflex or cycle of pain. Recurrent or migratory RSD is reported to occur in 15% to 75% of RSD-CRPS patients [36,45,46,51–54].

The study of RSD-CRPS brings into sharp focus the poor understanding of the mechanisms involved in the interrelationship of CNS physiology and hand function and reminds one of the large amount of cerebral cortex dedicated to hand activity. Once this challenge is unraveled, Pulvertaft's [4] belief that the hand is indeed the "mirror of man's emotion" may be verified.

References

[1] Merritt WH. Reflex sympathetic dystrophy. In: Achauer BM, editor. Plastic surgery indications, operations and outcomes, vol. 4. Chicago: Mosby; 2000. p. 2381.

[2] Amadio PC, Mackinnon SE, Merritt WH, et al. Reflex sympathetic dystrophy syndrome: consensus report of the ad hoc committee of the American Association for Hand Surgery on the definition of reflex sympathetic dystrophy syndrome. J Plast Reconstr Surg 1991;87:371–5.

[3] Manning D. Reflex sympathetic dystrophy, sympathetically maintained pain, and complex regional pain syndrome: diagnoses of inclusion, exclusion or confusion? J Hand Ther 2000;13:260–8.

[4] Pulvertaft RG. Psychological aspects of hand injuries. Hand 1975;7:93.

[5] Tahmoush AJ. Causalgia: redefinition as a clinical pain syndrome. Pain 1981;10:187.

[6] Koman LA, Poehling GG, Smith TL. Complex regional pain syndrome: reflex sympathetic dystrophy and causalgia. In: Green DP, Hotchkiss RN, Pederson WC, editors. Green's operative hand surgery. 4th edition. New York: Churchill-Livingstone; 1999.

[7] Gellman H. Reflex sympathetic dystrophy: alternative modalities for pain management. Instr Course Lect 2000;49:549–57.

[8] Hooshmand H. Chronic pain: reflex sympathetic dystrophy. Prevention and management. Boca Raton (FL): CRC Press; 1993.

[9] Lankford LL. Reflex sympathetic dystrophy. In: Green DP, editor. Operative hand surgery, vol. 1. New York: Churchill-Livingstone; 1982. p. 539.

[10] Merritt WH. Complications of hand surgery and trauma. In: Greenfield LJ, editor. Complications in surgery and trauma. Philadelphia: JB Lippincott; 1984. p. 852.

[11] Poplawski ZJ, Wylie AM, Murray JS. Posttraumatic dystrophy of the extremities: a clinical

review and trial of treatment. J Bone Joint Surg Am 1983;65:642–55.

[12] Thompson JE. The diagnosis and management of post-traumatic pain syndromes (causalgia). Aust N Z J Surg 1979;49:299.

[13] Boas RA. Complex regional pain syndromes: symptoms, signs, differential diagnosis. In: Jänig W, Stanton-Hicks M, editors. Reflex sympathetic dystrophy: a reappraisal. Seattle: IAST Press; 1996. p. 72–9.

[14] Stanton-Hicks M, Jänig W, Hassenbusch S, et al. Reflex sympathetic dystrophy: changing concepts in taxonomy. Pain 1995;63:127–33.

[15] Campbell JN, Raja SN, Seilig DK, et al. Diagnosis and management of sympathetically maintained pain. Prog Pain Res Manage 1994; 1:85–100.

[16] Bruehl S, Harden R, Galer B, et al. External validation of IASP diagnostic criteria for complex regional pain syndrome and proposed research diagnostic criteria. Pain 1999;81:147–54.

[17] Sunderland S. Nerve and nerve injuries. Edinburgh: Churchill-Livingstone; 1972.

[18] Bonicalvi V, Canavero S. Comments on Kingery pain. 73:123–39 [letter], 1997. Pain 1999;79: 317–8.

[19] Mitchell SW. Causalgia. Injuries of nerves and their consequences. Philadelphia: Lea Brothers & Company; 1872. p. 292.

[20] Evans J. Sympathetic dystrophy: report of 57 cases. Intern Med 1947;26:417.

[21] Plewes LW. Sudeck's atrophy in the hand. J Bone Joint Surg 1956;38:195.

[22] Hartley J. Reflex hyperemic deossification (Sudeck's atrophy). J Mount Sinai Hosp 1955; 22:268.

[23] Kozin F. Reflex sympathetic dystrophy syndrome. Bull Rheum Dis 1986;36:1.

[24] Veldman PH, Reynen HM, Artz IE, et al. Signs and symptoms of reflex sympathetic dystrophy: prospective study of 829 patients. Lancet 1993; 342:1012–6.

[25] Doury PC. Reflex sympathetic dystrophy (algodystrophy). Int Med Special 1985;6:67.

[26] McCarty DJ. Arthritis and allied conditions. 9th edition. Philadelphia: Lea & Febiger; 1979.

[27] Khoury R, Kennedy SF, MacNamara TE. Facial causalgia: report of case. J Oral Surg 1980;38:782.

[28] Biggs JT, Miranda FJ. Dental causalgia: a chronic oral pain syndrome. Quintessence Int 1983; 14:595.

[29] Massler M. Dental causalgia. Quintessence Int 1981;12:341.

[30] Arden RL, Bahu SJ, Zuazu MA, et al. Reflex sympathetic dystrophy of the face: current treatment recommendations. Laryngoscope 1998;108: 437–42.

[31] Jaeger B, Singer E, Kroening R. Reflex sympathetic dystrophy of the face: a report of two cases and review of the literature. Arch Neurol 1986;43:693.

[32] Drucker W, Hubay C, Holden W, et al. Patho-genesis of post-traumatic sympathetic dystrophy. Am J Surg 1959;97:454.

[33] Pollock LJ, Davis L. Peripheral nerve injuries. New York: Paul B. Hobber; 1933.

[34] Parrillo SJ. Reflex sympathetic dystrophy in children. Pediatr Emerg Care 1998;14:217–20.

[35] Greipp ME. Follow-up study of 14 young adults with complex regional pain syndrome Type I. J Neurosci Nurs 2000;32:83–8.

[36] Sherry DD, Wallace CA, Kelley C, et al. Short- and long-term outcomes of children with complex regional pain syndrome type I treated with exercise therapy. Clin J Pain 1999;15: 218–23.

[37] Mitchell JK. Remote consequences of injuries of nerves and their treatment. Philadelphia: Lea; 1895.

[38] Horowitz SH. Brachial plexus injuries with causalgia resulting in trans-axillary rib resection. Arch Surg 1985;120:1189.

[39] Rowlingson JC. The sympathetic dystrophies. Int Anesthesiol Clin 1983;21:117.

[40] Shumaker Jr HB, Seigel IJ, Upjohn RH. Causalgia. II. The signs and symptoms with particular reference to vasomotor disturbance. Surg Gynecol Obstet 1948;86:452.

[41] Nath RK, Mackinnon SE, Stelnicki E. Reflex sympathetic dystrophy: the controversy continues. Clin Plast Surg 1996;23(3):435–46.

[42] Ulmer JL, Mayfield FN. Causalgia: a study of 75 cases. Surg Gynecol Obstet 1946;83:789.

[43] Procacci P, Francini F, Zoppi M, et al. Cutaneous pain threshold changes after sympathetic block in reflex dystrophies. Pain 1975;1:167.

[44] Blanchard J, Ramamurthy S, Walsh N, et al. Intravenous regional sympatholysis: a double-blind comparison of guanethidine, reserpine, and normal saline. J Pain Symptom Manage 1990; 5:357–61.

[45] Greipp ME. Reflex sympathetic dystrophy syndrome: a retrospective pain study. J Adv Surg 1990;15:1452.

[46] Greipp ME, Thomas AF. New thoughts on reflex sympathetic dystrophy syndrome. J Neurosci Nurs 1990;22:313–6.

[47] Tanelian DL. Reflex sympathetic dystrophy: a re-evaluation of the literature. Pain Forum 1996;5: 247–56.

[48] Zar JH. Biostatistical analysis. 2nd edition. Englewood Cliffs (NJ): Prentice Hall; 1984.

[49] Subbarao J, Stillwell GK. Reflex sympathetic dystrophy syndrome of the upper extremity: analysis of total outcome management of 125 cases. Arch Phys Med Rehabil 1981;62:549.

[50] Wang JK, Johnson KA, Ilstrup DM. Sympathetic blocks for reflex sympathetic dystrophy. Pain 1985;23:13.

[51] Maleki J, LeBel A, Bennett G, et al. Patterns of spread in complex regional pain syndrome, type I (reflex sympathetic dystrophy). Pain 2000; 88:259–66.

[52] Greipp ME. A follow-up study of 14 young

adults with complex regional pain syndrome type I. J Neurosci Nurs 2000;32:83–8.

[53] Greipp ME, Thomas AF, Renkun C. Children and young adults with reflex sympathetic dystrophy syndrome. Clin J Pain 1988;4:217–21.

[54] Tong HC, Nelson VS. Recurrent and migratory reflex sympathetic dystrophy in children. Pediatr Rehabil 2000;4:87–9.

[55] Macdonald RI, Lichtman DM, Hanlon JJ, et al. Complications of surgical release for carpal tunnel syndrome. J Hand Surg 1978;3:70.

[56] Lichtman DM, Florio RL, Mack GE. Carpal tunnel release under local anesthesia: evaluation of the outpatient procedure. J Hand Surg 1979;4:544.

[57] Atkins RM, Duckworth T, Kanis JA. Algodystrophy following Colles' fracture. J Hand Surg [Br] 1989;14:161–4.

[58] Atkins RM, Duckworth T, Kavis JA. Features of algodystrophy after Colles' fracture. J Bone Joint Surg 1990;72:105–10.

[59] Atkins RM, Tindale W, Bickerstaff D, et al. Quantitative bone scintigraphy in reflex sympathetic dystrophy. Br J Rheumatol 1993;32:41–5.

[60] Markoff M, Farole A. Reflex sympathetic dystrophy syndrome: case report with review of the literature. Oral Surg 1986;661:23.

[61] Medsgar Jr TA, Dixon JA, Garwood VF. Palmar fasciitis and polyarthritis associated with ovarian carcinoma. Ann Intern Med 1982;96:424.

[62] Michaels RM, Sorber JA. Reflex sympathetic dystrophy as a probable paraneoplastic syndrome: case report and literature review. Arthritis Rheum 1984;27:1183.

[63] Burch GE, Giles TD. Cardiac causalgia. Arch Intern Med 1970;125:809.

[64] Doury PC. Algodystrophy: a spectrum of disease, historical perspectives, criteria of diagnosis, and principles of treatment. Hand Clin 1997; 13:327–37.

[65] Doury PC. L'algodystophie de la grossesse ou du post-partum. Semin Hop 1996;72:117–24.

[66] Doury PC. L'algodystrophie du rachis. Rev Rhum Ed Fr 1989;56:697–701.

[67] Doury PC, Dirheimer Y, Pattin S. Algodystrophy: diagnosis and therapy of a frequent disease of the locomotor apparatus. Berlin: Springer Verlag; 1981.

[68] Morettin LB, Wilson M. Severe reflex algodystrophy (Sudeck's atrophy) as a complication of myelography: report of two cases. AJR Am J Roentgenol 1970;110:156.

[69] Querol I, Cisneros T. Reflex sympathetic dystrophy syndrome following herpes zoster. Cutis 2001;68:179–82.

[70] Johnson EW, Pannozzo AN. Management of shoulder/hand syndrome. JAMA 1966;195:108.

[71] McLelland J, Ellis SJ. Causalgia as a complication of meningococcal meningitis. BMJ 1986; 292:1710.

[72] Desantis A, Ceccarelli G, Cesana BM, et al. Shoulder/hand syndrome in neurosurgical patients treated with barbiturates. J Neurosurg Sci 2000;44:69–75.

[73] Taylor LP, Posner JV. Phenobarbital rheumatism in patients with brain tumor. Ann Neurol 1989;25:92–4.

[74] Horton P, Gerster J. Reflex sympathetic dystrophy syndrome and barbiturates: a study of 25 cases treated with barbiturates compared with 124 cases treated without barbiturates. Clin Rheumatol 1984;3:493–9.

[75] Vergne P, Bertin P, Bonnet C, et al. Drug-induced rheumatic disorders: incidence, prevention and management. Drug Saf 2000;23: 279–93.

[76] Das A, Puvanendran K. Syringomyelia and complex regional pain syndrome as complications of multiple sclerosis. Arch Neurol 1999; 56:1021–4.

[77] de Carvalho M, Nogueira A, Pinto A, et al. Reflex sympathetic dystrophy associated with amyotrophic lateral sclerosis. J Neurol Sci 1999; 169:80–3.

[78] Ku A, Lachmann E, Tunkel R, et al. Upper limb sympathetic dystrophy associated with occult malignancy. Arch Phys Med Rehabil 1996;77: 726–8.

[79] Shumaker Jr HB, Seigel IJ, Upjohn RH. Causalgia. II. The signs and symptoms with particular reference to vasomotor disturbance. Surg Gynecol Obstet 1948;86:452.

[80] van der Lan L, Spaendonck K, Horstink M, et al. The symptom checklist-90. Revised questionnaire: no psychological profiles in complex regional pain syndrome-dystonia. J Pain Symptom Manage 1999;17:357–62.

[81] DeGood DE, Cundiff GW, Adams LE, et al. A psychosocial and behavioral comparison of reflex sympathetic dystrophy, low back pain and headache patients. Pain 1993;54: 317–22.

[82] van Houdenhove B. Algoneurodystrophy: a psychiatrist's point of view. Clin Rheumatol 1986;5:399–406.

[83] van Houdenhove B, Vasquez G. Is there a relationship between reflex sympathetic dystrophy and helplessness? Case reports and a hypothesis. Gen Hosp Psychiatry 1993;15: 325–9.

[84] van Houdenhove B, Vasquez G, Onghena P, et al. Etiopathogenesis of reflex sympathetic dystrophy: a review and biopsychosocial hypothesis. Clin J Pain 1992;8:300–6.

[85] Gertzen JH, de Bruijn HP, de Bruijn Kofman AT, et al. Reflex sympathetic dystrophy: early treatment and psychological aspects. Arch Phys Med Rehabil 1994;75:442–6.

[86] Theogaraj J, Merritt WH. Psychological evaluation of patients with RSD. Presented at the first annual meeting of the American Society for Peripheral Nerve. Charlottesville, VA, May 5–7, 1990.

[87] Hardy MA, Merritt WH. Psychological evalua-

tion pain assessment in patients with RSD. J Hand Ther 1988;1:155–64.

[88] Gertzen JH. Reflex sympathetic dystrophy: outcome and measurement. Acta Orthop Scand Suppl 1998;279:69:1–3.

[89] Galer BS, Henderson J, Perander J, et al. Course of symptom and quality of life measurement in complex regional pain syndrome: a pilot study. J Pain Symptom Manage 2000;20: 286–92.

[90] Genant HK, Kozin F, Bekerman C, et al. The reflex sympathetic dystrophy syndrome. Radiology 1975;117:21–32.

[91] Kozin F, McCarty DJ, Sims J, et al. The reflex sympathetic dystrophy syndrome, I. Clinical and histological studies: evidence for bilaterality, response to corticosteroids and articular involvement. Am J Med 1976;60:321.

[92] Masson C, Audran M, Pascaretti C, et al. Further vascular, bone, and autonomic investigations in algodystrophy. Acta Orthop Belg 1998;64: 77–87.

[93] Betcher AM, Casten D. Reflex sympathetic dystrophy: criteria for diagnosis and treatment. Anesthesiology 1955;16:994.

[94] Goris RJ, Dongen LM, Winters HA. Are toxic oxygen radicals involved in the pathogenesis of reflex sympathetic dystrophy? Free Radic Res 1987;3:13–8.

[95] Jäng W. The puzzle of reflex sympathetic dystrophy: mechanisms, hypothetic, open questions. In: Jänig W, Stanton-Hicks M, editors. Reflex sympathetic dystrophy: a reappraisal. Progress in pain research and management. Seattle (WA): IASP Press; 1996. p. 1–24.

[96] Rashig S, Galer BS. Proximal myofascial dysfunction in complex regional pain syndrome: a retrospective prevalence study. Clin J Pain 1999; 15:151–3.

[97] Steinbrocker O. Shoulder-hand syndrome: present perspective. Arch Phys Med Rehabil 1968; 49:388.

[98] Merritt WH. Reflex sympathetic dystrophy. In: McCarthy JG, editor. Plastic surgery, vol. 7. Philadelphia: WB Saunders; 1990. p. 4884–921.

[99] Kellgren JH. Observations on referred pain arising from muscle. Clin Sci 1938;3:175.

[100] Trevell JG, Simons D. Myofascial pain and dysfunction: the trigger point manual. Baltimore: Williams & Wilkins; 1983.

[101] Modell W, Trevell J. The treatment of painful disorders of skeletal muscle. N Y State J Med 1948;48:2050.

[102] Berges PU. Myofascial pain syndrome. Postgrad Med 1973;53:161.

[103] Zohn DA, Mennell J. Musculoskeletal pain: principles of physical diagnosis and physical treatment. Boston: Little, Brown; 1976.

[104] Frost FA, Jessen B, Siggard-Anderson J. A controlled, double blind comparison of mepivacaine injection versus saline injection for myofascial pain. Lancet 1980;1:499.

[105] Prudden B. Pain erasure: the Bonnie Prudden way. New York: M. Evans; 1980.

[106] Williams HL, Elkins EC. Myalgia of the head. Arch Phys Ther 1942;23:14.

[107] Jebara VA, Saade B. Causalgia, a wartime experience: report of 20 treated cases. J Trauma 1987; 27:519.

[108] Echlin F, Owens Jr FM, Wells WL. Observations on major and minor causalgia. Arch Neurol Psychol 1949;62:183.

[109] Kleinert H, Cole N, Wayne L, et al. Posttraumatic sympathetic dystrophy. Orthop Clin North Am 1973;4:917.

[110] Seddon H. Surgical disorders of the peripheral nerve. Edinburgh: Churchill-Livingstone; 1972.

[111] Taggart AJ, Iveson MI, Wright V. Shoulder/hand syndrome and symmetrical arthralgia in patients with tubo-ovarian carcinoma. Ann Rheum Dis 1984;43:391–3.

[112] Edeiken J. Shoulder-hand syndrome following myocardial infarction, with special reference to prognosis. Circulation 1957;41:14.

[113] Lankford LL. Reflex sympathetic dystrophy. In: Green DP, editor. Operative hand surgery, vol. 3. New York: Churchill-Livingstone; 1993. p. 627–60.

[114] Kubalek I, Fain O, Paries J, et al. Treatment of reflex sympathetic dystrophy with pamidronate: 29 cases. Rheumatology 2001;40: 1394–7.

[115] Calder JS, Holten I, McAllister RMR. Evidence for immune system involvement in reflex sympathetic dystrophy. J Hand Surg [Br] 1998; 23:147–50.

[116] Nuti R, Vattimo A, Martini G, et al. Carbocalcitonin treatment in Sudeck's atrophy. Clin Orthop Rel Res 1987;215–7.

[117] Derbekyan V, Novales-Dias J, Lisbona R. Pancoast tumor as a cause of reflex sympathetic dystrophy. J Nucl Med 1993;34:1992–4.

[118] Davis S, Petrillo C, Eichberg R, et al. Shoulder-hand syndrome in hemiplegic population: 5-year retrospective study. Arch Phys Med Rehabil 1977;58:353.

[119] Gracely RH, Lynch SA, Bennett GJ. Painful neuropathy: altered central processing maintained dynamically by peripheral input. Pain 1992;51:175–94.

[120] Jänig W. Experimental approach to reflex sympathetic dystrophy and related syndromes [editorial]. Pain 1991;46:241–5.

[121] Mailis A, Furlan A. Sympathectomy for neuropathic pain. Cochrane Database Syst Rev 2003; 2:CD-002918.

[122] Leeman SE, Gamse R, Lackner D, et al. Effect of capsaicin pretreatment on capsule evoked release of immunoreactive somatostatin and substance P from primary sensory neurons. Naunyn Schmiedebergs Arch Pharmacol 1981; 316:38.

[123] Levine JD, Goetzl E, Basbaum AI. Contrast of the nervous system to pathophysiology of

rheumatoid and other polyarthritides. Rheum Dis Clin North Am 1987;13:369.

[124] Foreman JC, Jordan CC, Piotrowski W. Inner action of neurotensin with the substance P receptor mediating histamine release from rat mast cells and the flare in human skin. Br J Pharmacol 1982;77:531.

[125] Pak J, Martin GM, Magness JL, et al. Reflex sympathetic dystrophy: review of 140 cases. Minn Med 1970;53:507.

[126] Lembeck F, Gamse R, Juan H. Substance P and sensory nerve endings. In: Von Euler US, Pernow B, editors. Substance P, 37th Noble Symposium, Stockholm, 1976. New York: Raven Press; 1977. p. 169.

[127] Bill A, Stjernschantz J, Mandahla A, et al. Substance P: release on trigeminal stimulation; effects in the eye. Acta Physiol Scand 1979; 101:371.

[128] Jansco N, Jansco-Gabor A, Szolesanyi J. Direct evidence for direct neurogenic inflammation and its prevention by denervation and by pretreatment with capsaicin. Br Pharmacol Chemother 1967;31:138.

[129] Payan D, Goetzl E. Modulation of lymphocyte function by sensory neuropeptides. J Immunol 1985;135:783s.

[130] Stanisz AM, Defus D, Bienenstock J. Differential effects of vasoactive intestinal peptides, substance P, and somatostatin on immunoglobulin synthesis and proliferation of lymphocytes from Peyer's patches, mesenteric lymph nodes, and spleen. J Immunol 1986;136:152.

[131] Hartung HP, Toyka KV. Activation of macrophages by substance P: induction of oxidative burst and thromboxane release. J Pharmacol 1983;89:301.

[132] Nilsson J, von Euler AM, Dalsgaard CJ. Stimulation of connective tissue cell growth by substance P and substance K. Nature 1985;315:61.

[133] van der Laan L, Goris RJ. Reflex sympathetic dystrophy: an exaggerated regional inflammatory response? Hand Clin 1997;13:373–85.

[134] Merritt WH. Comprehensive management of Raynaud's syndrome. Clin Plast Surg 1997;24: 133–59.

[135] Weber M, Birklein F, Neundorfer B, et al. Facilitated neurogenic inflammation in complex regional pain syndrome. Pain 2001;91: 251–7.

[136] Leis S, Weber M, Isselmann A, et al. Substance-P-induced protein extravasation is bilaterally increased in complex regional pain syndrome. Exp Neurol 2003;183:197–204.

[137] Blair SJ. Role of neuropeptides in pathogenesis of RSD. Programs and abstracts RSD. Brussels; 1996. p. 18.

[138] Birklein F, Weber M, Ernst M, et al. Experimental tissue acidosis leads to increased pain in complex regional pain syndrome (CRPS). Pain 2000;87:227–34.

[139] Spebar MJ, Rosenthal D, Collins Jr GJ, et al. Changing trends in causalgia. Am J Surg 1981; 142:744.

[140] Jäng W. The puzzle of reflex sympathetic dystrophy: mechanisms, hypothetic, open questions. In: Jänig W, Stanton-Hicks M, editors. Reflex sympathetic dystrophy: a reappraisal. Progress in pain research and management. Seattle (WA): IASP Press; 1996. p. 1–24.

[141] Kline SC, Holder LE. Segmental reflex sympathetic dystrophy: clinical and scintigraphic criteria. J Hand Surg [Am] 1993;18:853–9.

[142] Farcot JM, Gautherie M, Foucher G. Regional intravenous sympathetic nerve blocks. Hand Clin 1997;13:499–517.

[143] Ochoa JL, Verdugo RJ. Reflex sympathetic dystrophy: a common clinical avenue for somatoform expression. Neurol Clin 1995;13:351–63.

[144] Schott GD. An unsympathetic view of pain. Lancet 1995;345:634–6.

[145] Cooke ED, Ward C. Vicious circles in reflex sympathetic dystrophy: a hypothesis. Discussion paper. J R Soc Med 1990;83:96–9.

[146] Baron R, Blumberg H, Jänig W. Clinical characteristics of patients with complex regional pain syndrome in Germany, with special emphasis on vasomotor function. In: Jänig W, Stanton-Hicks M, editors. Reflex sympathetic dystrophy, a reappraisal. Progress in pain research and management. Seattle (WA): IASP Press; 1996. p. 25–48.

[147] Schuind F, Burny F. Can algodystrophy be prevented after hand surgery? Hand Clin 1997; 13:455–76.

[148] Christensen K, Jensen EM, Noer I. The reflex dystrophy syndrome: response to treatment with systemic corticosteroids. Acta Chir Hand 1982;148:653.

[149] Ochoa JL. Reflex sympathetic dystrophy: a tragic error in medical science. Hippocrates Lantern 1995;3:1–6.

[150] Roberts WJ. An hypothesis on the physiological basis for causalgia and unrelated pain. Pain 1986;24:297–311.

[151] Ochoa JL. Reflex? Sympathetic? Dystrophy? Triple questioned again. Mayo Clin Proc 1995; 70: 1124–6.

[152] Kingery WS. A critical review of controlled clinical trials for peripheral neuropathic pain in complex regional pain syndromes. Pain 1997; 73:123–39.

[153] Gracely RH, Dubner R, Wolskee PJ, et al. Placebo and naloxone can alter post-surgical pain by separate mechanisms. Nature 1983; 306:264.

[154] Fields HL, Levine JD. Placebo analgesia: a role for endorphins? Trends Neurosci 1984;1:271.

[155] Revill SI, Robinson JO, Rosen M, et al. The reliability of a linear analog scale for evaluating pain. Anesthesia 1976;31:1191.

[156] Sternbach RA. Recent advances in psychologic pain therapy. Adv Pain Res Ther 1984;7:251.

[157] Friedlander L, Lumley M, Farchione T, et al.

Testing the alexithymia hypothesis: physiological and subjective responses during relaxation and stress. J Nerv Ment Dis 1997;185:233–9.

[158] Nemiah JC, Sifneos PE. Affect and fantasy in patients with psychosomatic disorders. Psychosom Med 1970;2:26–34.

[159] Kooiman CG, Spinhoven P, Trijsburg RW, et al. Perceived parental attitude: alexithymia and defense style in psychiatric outpatients. Psychother Psychosom 1998;67:81–7.

[160] Branch C. Aspects of anxiety. Philadelphia: JB Lippincott; 1965.

[161] Tasker RR, Organ LW, Hawrylyshyn P. Deafferentation and causalgia. In: Bonica JJ, editor. Pain. New York: Raven Press; 1980.

[162] Apkarian AV, Thomas PS, Krauss BR, et al. Prefrontal cortical hyperactivity in patients with sympathetically mediated chronic pain. Neurosci Lett 2001;311:193–7.

[163] Wasner G, Schattschneider J, Binder A, et al. Complex regional pain syndrome: diagnostic, mechanisms, CNS involvement and therapy. Spinal Cord 2003;41:61–75.

[164] McCabe CS, Haigh RC, Halligan PW, et al. Referred sensation in patients with complex regional pain syndrome type I. Rheumatology (Oxford) 2003;42:1067–73.

[165] Galer BS, Butler S, Jensen M. Case reports and hypothesis: a neglect-like syndrome may be responsible for the motor disturbance in reflex sympathetic dystrophy (complex regional pain syndrome -1). J Pain Symptom Manage 1995; 10:385–92.

[166] Rommel O, Gehling M, Dertwinkel R, et al. Hemisensory impairment in patients with complex regional pain syndrome. Pain 1999;80: 95–101.

[167] Riedl B, Beckmann T, Neundörfer B, et al. Autonomic failure after stroke: is it indicative for pathophysiology of complex regional pain syndrome? Acta Neurol Scand 2001;103:27–34.

[168] Ribbers GM, Mulder T, Geurts AC, et al. Reflex sympathetic dystrophy of the left hand and motor impairments of the unaffected right hand: impaired central motor processing? Arch Phys Med Rehabil 2002;83:81–5.

[169] Sieweke N, Birklein F, Riedl B, et al. Patterns of hyperalgesia in complex regional pain syndrome. Pain 1999;80:171–7.

[170] Shibata M, Nakao K, Galer B, et al. A case of reflex sympathetic dystrophy (complex regional pain syndrome type I) resolved by cerebral contusion. Pain 1999;79:313–5.

[171] King JH, Nuss S. Reflex sympathetic dystrophy treated by electroconvulsive therapy: intractable pain, depression and bilateral electrode ECT. Pain 1993;55:393–6.

[172] Gainer MJ. Hypnotherapy for reflex sympathetic dystrophy. Am J Clin Hypn 1992;34:227–32.

[173] Sunderland S. Pain mechanisms in causalgia. J Neurol Neurosurg Psychiatry 1976;39:471.

[174] Arriagada M, Arinoviche R. X-ray bone densi-

tometry in the diagnosis and follow-up of reflex sympathetic dystrophy syndrome. J Rheumatol 1994;21:498–500.

[175] Kozin F, Genant H, Bekerman C, et al. The reflex sympathetic dystrophy syndrome II: Roentgenographic and scintigraphic bilaterality and of periarticular accentuation. Am J Med 1976;60:332–8.

[176] Allen G, Galer B, Schwartz I. Epidemiology of complex regional pain syndrome: a retrospective chart review of 134 patients. Pain 1999;80: 539–44.

[177] Sandroni P, Benrud-Larson L, McClelland R, et al. Complex regional pain syndrome type I: incidence and prevalence in Olmsted County, a population-based study. Pain 2003;103:199–207.

[178] Driessens E. Infrequent presentations of reflex sympathetic dystrophy and pseudodystrophy. Hand Clin 1997;13:413–22.

[179] Zyluk A. The usefulness of quantitative evaluation of three-phase scintigraphy in the diagnosis of post-traumatic reflex sympathetic dystrophy. J Hand Surg [Br] 1999;24:16–21.

[180] Pawl R. Controversies surrounding reflex sympathetic dystrophy: a review article. Curr Rev Pain 2000;4:259–67.

[181] Werner R, Davidoff G, Jackson D, et al. Factors affecting the sensitivity and specificity of the three-phase technetium bone scan in the diagnosis of reflex sympathetic dystrophy syndrome in the upper extremity. J Hand Surg [Am] 1989;14:520–3.

[182] Hendler N, Uematesu S, Long D. Thermographic validation of physical complaints in psychogenic pain patients. Psychosomatics 1982; 23:283.

[183] Holden WD. Sympathetic dystrophy. Arch Surg 1948;57:373.

[184] Mayfield FH, Divine JW. Causalgia. Surg Gynecol Obstet 1945;80:631.

[185] Cronin KD, Kirsner RLG. Diagnosis of reflex sympathetic dysfunction: use of skin potential response. Anesthesia 1982;37:848.

[186] Tahmoush AJ, Malley J, Jennings JR. Skin conductance, temperature, and blood flow in causalgia. Neurology 1983;33:1483.

[187] Low PA, Caskey PE, Tuck RR, et al. Quantitative sudomotor axon reflex test in normal and neuropathic subjects. Ann Neurol 1983;14:573–80.

[188] Fagrell B, Froneck A, Intaglietta M. A microscope television system for dynamic studies of blood flow velocity in human skin capillaries. Am J Physiol 1977;233:H318–21.

[189] Abram SE. Pain of sympathetic origin. In: Raj P, editor. Practical management of pain. New York: Yearbook Medical; 1986. p. 451.

[190] Greenberg RP, Price DD, Becker DP. Complications of persistent postoperative pain. In: Greenfield LJ, editor. Complications in surgery and trauma. Philadelphia: JP Lippincott; 1983. p. 709.

[191] Bonica JJ. Causalgia and other reflex sympa-

thetic dystrophies. Adv Pain Res Ther 1979;3:141–66.

[192] Hardy MA, Moran CA, Merritt WH. Desensitization of the traumatized hand. VA Med J 1982;109:134.

[193] Jupiter JB, Seiler JG, Zienowicz R. Sympathetic maintained pain (causalgia) associated with demonstrable peripheral nerve lesions. J Bone Joint Surg Am 1994;76:1376–84.

[194] Reuben SS, Rosenthal EA, Steinberg RB. Surgery on the affected upper extremity of patients with a history of complex regional pain syndrome: a retrospective study of 100 patients. J Hand Surg [Am] 2000;25:1147–51.

[195] Cooney WP. Electrical stimulation and the treatment of complex regional pain syndromes of the upper extremity. Hand Clin 1997;13:519–26.

[196] Kasdan ML, Johnson AL. Reflex sympathetic dystrophy. Occup Med 1998;13:521–31.

[197] Chelimsky TC, Low PA, Naessens JM, et al. Value of autonomic testing in reflex sympathetic dystrophy. Mayo Clin Proc 1995;70:1029–40.

[198] Shumaker Jr HB. A personal overview of causalgia and other reflex dystrophies. Ann Surg 1985;201:278.

[199] Beecher HK. Measurement of subjective responses. New York: Oxford University Press; 1959.

[200] Bonica JJ. Pain. Philadelphia: Lea & Febiger; 1953.

[201] Durrani Z, Winnie AP. Diagnostic and therapeutic brachial plexus blocks for RSD, unresponsive to stellate ganglion block. Anesth Analg 1992;74:77.

[202] Hannington-Kiff JG. Intravenous regional sympathetic block with guanethidine. Lancet 1974;1:1019–20.

[203] Bonelli A, Conoscente F, Moveilia PG, et al. Regional intravenous guanethidine versus stellate block in reflex sympathetic dystrophies: a randomized trial. Pain 1983;16:297–307.

[204] Field J, Monk C, Atkins RM. Objective improvements in algodystrophy following regional intravenous guanethidine. J Hand Surg [Br] 1993;18:339.

[205] Hannington-Kiff JG. Pharmacologic target blocks in hand surgery and rehabilitation. J Hand Surg [Br] 1984;9:29–36.

[206] Woosley RL, Niews AS. Drug therapy: guanethidine. N Engl J Med 1976;295:1053.

[207] Benzon H, Chomka CM, Brunner EA. Treatment of reflex sympathetic dystrophy with regional intravenous reserpine. Anesth Analg 1980;59:500–2.

[208] Gorsky BH. Intravenous perfusion with reserpine for Raynaud's phenomenon. Reg Anaesth 1977;2:5.

[209] Arnér S. Intravenous phentolamine tests: diagnostic and prognostic use in reflex sympathetic dystrophy. Pain 1991;46:17–22.

[210] Hord AH, Rooks MD, Stephans BO, et al. Intravenous regional bretylium and lidocaine for treatment of reflex sympathetic dystrophy: a randomized, double-blind study. Anesth Analg 1992;74:818.

[211] Duncan KH, Lewis RC, Racz G, et al. Treatment of upper extremity reflex sympathetic dystrophy with joint stiffness using sympatheticolytic Bier blocks and manipulation. Orthopedics 1988;11:883–6.

[212] Ford SR, Forest Jr WH, Eltherington L. The treatment of reflex sympathetic dystrophy with intravenous regional bretylium. Anesthesiology 1988;68:137–40.

[213] Hanowell LH, Kanefield JK, Soriano III SG. A recommendation for reduced lidocaine dosage during intravenous regional bretylium treatment of reflex sympathetic dystrophy [letter]. Anesthesiology 1989;71:811–2.

[214] Hill S, Lin M, Shandler Jr P. Reflex sympathetic dystrophy and electroacupuncture. Tex Med 1991;87:76–81.

[215] Chan CS, Chow SP. Electroacupuncture in the treatment of posttraumatic sympathetic dystrophy (Sudeck's atrophy). Br J Anaesth 1981;53:899.

[216] Hardy MA, Merritt WH. A model to study sympathetic dystrophy: psychological testing and biofeedback results. Presented at the annual meeting of the Plastic Surgery Research Council. Hershey (PA), May 1982.

[217] Alioto JT. Behavioral treatment of reflex sympathetic dystrophy. Psychosomatics 1981;22:539–40.

[218] Grunert BK, Divine CA, Sanger JR, et al. Thermal self-regulation for pain control and reflex sympathetic dystrophy syndrome. J Hand Surg [Am] 1990;15:615–8.

[219] Kesler R, Saulsbury F, Miller L, et al. Reflex sympathetic dystrophy in children: treatment with transcutaneous nerve stimulation. An Pediatr (Barc) 1988;82:728–32.

[220] Richlin DM, Carron H, Rowlingson JC, et al. Reflex sympathetic dystrophy: successful treatment by transcutaneous nerve stimulation. J Pediatr 1978;93:84.

[221] Meyer GA, Fields HL. Causalgia treated by selective large fiber stimulation of peripheral nerve. Brain 1972;95:163.

[222] Stilz RJ, Carron H, Saunders DB. Case history #96. Reflex sympathetic dystrophy in a 6-year-old: successful treatment by transcutaneous nerve stimulation. Anesth Analg 1977;56:438.

[223] Wall PD, Sweet WH. Temporary abolition of pain in man. Science 1977;155:108.

[224] Law JD. Spinal cord stimulation for intractable pain due to reflex sympathetic dystrophy. CNI Review 1993;17–22.

[225] Peets JM, Pomeranz B. Acupuncture-like transcutaneous electrical nerve stimulation analgesia is influenced by spinal cord endorphins, but no serotonin: an intrathecal pharmacological study. Adv Pain Res Ther 1985;9:519.

[226] Portenoy RK. Neuropathic pain. In: Portenoy RK, Kanner RN, editors. Pain management:

theory and practice. Philadelphia: Davis; 1996. p. 83–125.

[227] Mackin GA. Medical and pharmacologic management of upper extremity neuropathic pain syndromes. J Hand Ther 1997;10:96–109.

[228] Ghostine SWY, Comair YG, Turner DM, et al. Phenoxybenzamine in the treatment of causalgia. J Neurosurg 1984;60:263.

[229] Jensen NH. Accurate diagnosis and drug selection in chronic pain patients. Postgrad Med J 1991;67:2–8.

[230] Prough DS, McLeskey CH, Poehling GG, et al. Efficacy of oral nifedipine in treatment of reflex sympathetic dystrophy. Anesthesiology 1985;62: 796–9.

[231] Glick EN, Helal B. Postraumatic neurodystrophy: treatment by corticosteroids. Hand 1976; 8:45.

[232] Vane JR. Inhibition of prostaglandin synthesis as a mechanism of action for the aspirin-like drugs. Nature 1971;231:232–5.

[233] Backonja M, Beydoun A, Edwards KR, et al. Gabapentin for the symptomatic treatment of painful neuropathy in patients with diabetes mellitus: a randomized, controlled trial. JAMA 1998;280:1831–6.

[234] Taylor CP, Gee NS, Su PV, et al. A summary of mechanistic hypotheses of gabapentin pharmacology. Epilepsy Res 1998;29:233–49.

[235] Dyck PJ, Litchy WJ, Lehman KA, et al. Variables influencing neuropathic endpoints: the Rochester diabetic neuropathic study of healthy subjects. Neurology 1995;45:1115–21.

[236] Vollmer KO, Von Hodenberg A, Kolle EU. Pharmakinetics and metabolism of gabapentin in rat, dog and man. Arzneimittelforschung 1986;36:830–9.

[237] van Hilten BJ, van de Beek W-JT, Hoff JI, et al. Intrathecal baclofen for the treatment of dystonia in patients with reflex sympathetic dystrophy. N Engl J Med 2000;343:625–30.

[238] Drissen B, Ryman W. Interaction of the central analgesic, tramadol, with the uptake and release of 5-hydroxytryptamine in the rat brain in vitro. Br J Pharmacol 1992;105:147–51.

[239] Rauck RL, Rouff GE, McMillan JI. Comparison of tramadol and acetaminophen with codeine for long-term pain management in elderly patients. Curr Ther Res 1994;55:1417–31.

[240] Roth M, Mountjoy CQ. The distinction between anxiety states and depressive disorders. In: Paykel ES, editor. Handbook of affective disorders. New York: Oxford University Press; 1982. p. 70.

[241] Neumann M. Nonsurgical management of pain secondary to peripheral nerve injuries. Orthop Clin North Am 1988;19:165.

[242] Pappagallo M, Campbell JN. The pharmacologic management of chronic back pain. In: Frymoyer JW, editor. The adult spine. principles and practice. 2nd edition. Philadelphia: Lippincott-Raven; 1997. p. 275–85.

[243] Arlet J, Maziéres B. Medical treatment of reflex sympathetic dystrophy. Hand Clin 1997;13: 477–83.

[244] Eisinger J, Acquaviva P, D'Omezon Y, et al. Traitement des algodystrophies par la calcitonie: resultats préliminaires. Marseille Médical 1973;110:373–6.

[245] De Bastiani G, Nogarin L. Perusim: tratamento della syndromi algodistrofiche con la calcitonina. Minerva Med 1978;69:1485–95.

[246] Munzenberg KL. Therapie des Sudeck syndrom mit calcitonin. Dtsch Med Wochenschr 1978; 103:26–9.

[247] Devogelaer JP, Dall, Aremellina S, et al. Dramatic improvement of intractable reflex sympathetic dystrophy syndrome by IV infusion of the second-generation bisphosphonate [abstract]. J Bone Miner Res 1988;3:213.

[248] Rehman MT, Clayson AD, Marsh D, et al. Treatment of reflex sympathetic dystrophy with intravenous pamidronate [abstract]. Bone 1992; 13:116.

[249] Maillefert JF, Chatard C, Owen S, et al. Treatment of refractory reflex sympathetic dystrophy with pamidronate [letter]. Ann Rheum Dis 1995;54:687.

[250] Cortet B, Flipo RM, Coquerelle P, et al. Treatment of severe, recalcitrant reflex sympathetic dystrophy: assessment of efficacy and safety of the second-generation bisphosphonate pamidronate. Clin Rheumatol 1997;16:51–6.

[251] Adami S, Fossaluzza V, Gatti D, et al. Bisphosphonate therapy of reflex sympathetic dystrophy syndrome. Rheum Dis 1997;56:201–4.

[252] Varenna M, Zucchi F, Ghiringhelli D, et al. Intravenous clodronate in the treatment of reflex sympathetic dystrophy syndrome: a randomized, double-blind, placebo-controlled study. J Rheumatol 2000;27:1477–83.

[253] Goodman CR. Treatment of shoulder-hand syndrome: combined with ultrasonic applications of stellate ganglion and physical medicine. N Y State J Med 1971;71:559.

[254] Portwood MM, Lieberman JS, Taylor RG. Ultrasound treatment of reflex sympathetic dystrophy. Arch Phys Med Rehabil 1987;68:116.

[255] Blacker HM. Volitional sympathetic control. Anesth Analg 1980;59:785–8.

[256] Watson HK, Carlson L. Treatment of reflex sympathetic dystrophy of the hand with an active stress loading program. J Hand Surg [Am] 1987; 12:779.

[257] Litz T, Payne RL. Causalgia: report of recovery following relief of emotional stress. Arch Neurol Psych 1945;53:222.

[258] Verdugo RJ, Ochoa JL. Abnormal movements in complex regional pain syndrome: assessment of their nature. Muscle Nerve 2000;23: 198–205.

[259] Phelps RG, Wilentz S. Reflex sympathetic dystrophy. Int J Dermatol 2000;39:481–6.

[260] Veldman PH, Goris RJ. Surgery on extremities

with reflex sympathetic dystrophy. Unfallchirurg 1995;98:45–8.

[261] Deilissen PW, Classen AT, Veldman PH, et al. Amputation for reflex sympathetic dystrophy. J Bone Joint Surg Br 1995;77:270–3.

[262] Marx C, Wiedersheim P, Michel B, et al. Preventing recurrence of reflex sympathetic dystrophy in patients requiring an operative intervention at the site of dystrophy after surgery. Clin Rheumatol 2001;20:114–8.

[263] Brand P, Yancey P. Pain: the gift nobody wants. New York: Harper Collins; 1993.

[264] Bruehl S, Carlson CR. Predisposing psychological factors in the development of reflex sympathetic dystrophy: a review of the empirical evidence. Clin J Pain 1992;8:287–99.

[265] Merritt WH, Howell J, Tune R, et al. Achieving immediate active motion by using relative motion splinting after long extensor tendon repair and sagittal band ruptures with tendon subluxation. Operative techniques in plastic and reconstructive surgery, vol. 7. Philadelphia: WB Saunders; 2000.

[266] Freeland AE, Jabaley ME, Huges JL. Stable fixation of the hand and wrist. New York: Springer-Verlag; 1986.

CLINICS IN PLASTIC SURGERY

Clin Plastic Surg 32 (2005) 605–616

Bridging the Neural Gap

Renata V. Weber, MD, Susan E. Mackinnon, MD*

- Nerve repair: when to repair primarily
- Bridging the gap: current techniques
- Nerve transfer: alternative to conduits
- Neurorrhaphy: end-to-end versus end-to-side
- Allografts: overcoming immunosuppression?
- Bioengineering conduits: the future?
- Summary
- References

Although the future of nerve surgery holds exciting possibilities, the current reality is that the results of nerve repair have not significantly improved over the past several decades. The initial principles set forth by Sir Sidney Sunderland during World War II still hold true. A major limitation to overall success in peripheral nerve surgery is time for regeneration. This principle remains true regardless of the technique used for the repair. Without prompt motor nerve input, denervated muscle becomes resistant to nerve regeneration. Although one can help speed up the regenerative process to some extent, success is hindered by additional issues, such as number of coaptation sites, supply of donor nerves, and the limitations of nerve substitutes. At every coaptation site, a percentage of nerve fibers are lost. Excessive tension is harmful to a repair site, and, in the case of a large gap, a nerve graft is often used to fill in the deficit. Autogenous nerve grafts are in limited supply, with sural nerve grafts being the primary source. Alternatives to the standard treatment include vein grafts, synthetic nerve conduits, nerve transfers, and nerve transplantation. Schwann cell–lined nerve conduits and tissue-engineered substitutions are still in their infancy and have some limited clinical application.

Nerve repair: when to repair primarily

Prompt primary neurorrhaphy is the procedure of choice whenever possible. Because a percentage of fibers are lost at each repair site, the fewer neurorrhaphies are present the greater is the percentage of proximal nerve axons that will reach the target organ. Of those fibers that do cross the repair, some investigators believe that as many as 50% of regenerating sensory or motor axons may never reach the correct end organ [1]. With the introduction of transgenic mice with fluorescent axons, the riddles of the type and percentage of nerve fibers lost and how the nerve inherently "knows" to find its preinjured target organ may be solved.

Excessive tension across a nerve repair is known to increase the scarring at the coaptation site and impair regeneration. In an uninjured nerve, a 15% strain of the nerve causes a reduction in microvascular flow; for an hour after relaxation, a delay

Division of Plastic and Reconstructive Surgery, Washington University School of Medicine, Campus Box 8238, 660 South Euclid Avenue, St. Louis, MO 63110, USA
* Corresponding author.
E-mail address: mackinnons@wustl.edu (S.E. Mackinnon).

doi:10.1016/j.cps.2005.05.003

of peak velocity to 66% of initial value persists [2]. Mild tension, by contrast, is actually believed to be beneficial to the repair by stimulating neurotropic growth factors. In a recent rodent study of sciatic nerve gap repaired primarily [3], there was no difference in ultimate nerve repair at 4 weeks among various groups ranging from no gap to a 6-mm gap; however, at a 9-mm gap, the repair under tension did not have the same robust nerve regeneration as the groups with shorter gaps or no gap. This difference was evident by both functional recovery and histologic examination of the distal nerve segment. The study indicates that, above a threshold tension, nerve repair precipitously drops. In this study, the nerve gap of 6 to 9 mm corresponded to a tension between 0.39 Newtons and 0.56 Newtons.

In clinical practice, the authors do not measure the tension across a neurorrhaphy but rather rely on experience and clinical judgment. The two ends of a nerve are mobilized to bring them in reasonable approximation. Strain on the nerve decreases the microcirculation, and excessive tension will cause the repair to break down. Based on experimental models, Trumble and McCallister [4] recommend limiting elongation of unscarred peripheral nerves to 10%, after which the microvascular blood flow to the nerve is decreased by half. When determining percentage of elongation, one determines the total length of exposed nerve. Each half is accessed separately, and up to one tenth of the length for each side can be stretched without risk for ischemia [5]. The greater the mobilization of the nerve, the greater the amount of elongation that may be safely performed. In addition, tricks such as positioning the arm in adduction or placing the wrist and fingers in flexion will significantly decrease the tension across the repair, depending on the location of the injury, and may increase the total length of available nerve. However, the authors recommend avoiding postural manipulation to force primary repair. Not only will gapping occur when the joint near the repair is moved, but this technique may create significant stiffness from prolonged immobilization [6].

In a recent experimental study, the authors found that redundancy and configuration of the nerve graft did not inhibit axonal regeneration [7]. A 2.5-cm isograft was used to repair the rat sciatic nerve in four different fashions, including a 2.5-cm graft tacked into a sinusoidal and an omega-shaped configuration to bridge a 0.5-cm gap. After 6 weeks, histomorphometric analysis revealed no significant differences in regeneration between the four groups, suggesting that regeneration through the isograft is independent of the graft geometry and redundancy.

Excessive tension will inhibit nerve regeneration. However, a small amount of tension to achieve primary repair is acceptable. At the other extreme, redundant nerve graft reconstruction, such as for the nonanatomic rerouting of a nerve graft, will not inhibit nerve regeneration.

Another technique for overcoming a short nerve graft is to expand the nerve using low-pressure tissue expanders placed under the skin. In early experimental studies, there does not appear to be any change in latency or velocity after or during expansion [8]. The delayed repair after 2 weeks of nerve expansion shows functional recovery as good as that of primary repair [9], although some decrease in function was noted in another investigation in which as much as 30% of a rat sciatic nerve was elongated [10]. Clinically, this technique is limited because of the delay required for the expansion to occur. The conductive property of the nerve is affected, more in the distal segment than in the proximal segment. The expansion of a normal nerve or proximal segment of a transected nerve is better tolerated than distal segment expansion, suggesting that the presence of an axon may have a beneficial effect in minimizing the deforming mechanical insult. Slow nerve expansion appears to have a limited but possible role in the management of the unique short nerve gap [10].

Although they are technically feasible, tissue expansion techniques have not found a major clinical role in nerve reconstruction. The combination of time-consuming process and relative technical complexity makes the process less desirable as a first option for neural gap repair.

When the nerve is ready for repair, the authors prefer a circumferential epineural repair using 9-0 nylon sutures. Any repair that withstands gentle range of motion is considered a "tension-free" repair, although it may still be under some mild yet acceptable tension. Giddins and colleagues [11] showed in a cadaveric study comparing suture size with the strength of an acute repair of the median nerve that 9-0 nylon withstood the greatest distractive forces. Ten-0 snapped at a lower tension, and 8-0 sutures pulled out of the nerve tissue. However, in clinical practice, 10-0 and 8-0 sutures are often used, based on the size of the nerve, the thickness of the epineurium, and the amount of inflammation. From a practical point of view, if the nerve ends cannot be approximated with a single 6-0 nylon and repaired with an 8-0 nylon or smaller suture, then an alternative to primary repair should be considered.

Epineural repair is the traditional method of repair once the severed ends are freshened surgically. Alignment is achieved by external markers, such as a vessel on the surface, and by matching the fascicular patterns. In theory, a grouped fascicular repair is more accurate, and some investigators believe that if the individual fascicles are misaligned, the axon may never find its other half [12]. The proponents of the perineural repair stress that this misalignment may be avoided by repairing larger fascicular groups individually [13,14]. Initial studies showed that the techniques were equally effective [15]. The disadvantage of a perineural repair is that the extensive dissection and the permanent intraneural stitches may lead to increase fibrosis [16]. In practice, it is often difficult accurately to align the fascicles, because trauma, edema, and scarring can distort the normal topography. The authors' preferred method for repair is an epineural repair using the native vessels as a guide. The smallest number of epineural sutures that approximates and keeps the repair intact through a full range of motion is used.

At the time of surgery, the range of movement that the repair will accept is noted, and postoperative protective range of motion is initiated in the early postoperative period.

After neurorrhaphy, the authors immobilize the area for 1 to 2 weeks but start gentle protected range of motion at 2 to 3 days. Nerve repair of the rodent sciatic nerve has shown that healing nerves achieved 63% of the strength of the control by 8 weeks [17]. In a monkey study of median and ulnar nerve, the repairs had regained 77% of the bursting strength of the normal median and ulnar nerves by 4 weeks [18]. No consensus exists on the length of time necessary for immobilization. One recent clinical study suggests that early range of motion may not be as detrimental to the long-term results as was previously believed. Patients with isolated digital nerve injuries were compared with patients with combined flexor tendon and digital nerve injuries. The patients with isolated nerve injuries were immobilized for 21 days, whereas patients with the combined tendon and nerve injuries were started on protected motion at approximately 4 days postoperatively. At follow-up, all patients regardless of the postoperative protocol had less sensibility in the repaired nerve when compared with an uninjured nerve in the same hand. No significant difference was found in final two-point discrimination and Semmes-Weinstein testing between the two repaired groups, challenging the long-held belief that nerve repairs should be completely immobilized after surgery [19].

Bridging the gap: current techniques

A nerve gap is the distance between two ends of a severed nerve. It includes not only the loss of nerve tissue from the injury or necessary debridement of the nerve ends but also the distance the nerve has retracted [20]. Because of the elastic property of a nerve, transecting an intact nerve will cause the nerve ends to retract. A primary repair is universally held to be ideal, and multiple animal studies support the idea that a single nerve repair results in a better outcome than a nerve repair with two neurorrhaphy sites [21]. An exception to this is a repair performed in the face of extreme tension and contamination; it is better to have two neurorrhaphy sites under favorable conditions than a single neurorrhaphy under unfavorable ones [6,22]. If primary repair by mobilization and elongation cannot be achieved, the most common technique for repairing defects in peripheral nerves is autologous nerve grafts. The nerve grafts serve as a guide for the axon as it regrows toward the distal stump. The sural nerve is by far the most commonly used donor nerve, although other suitable donor nerves include the lateral and medial antibrachial cutaneous nerve [23,24] and the terminal portion of the anterior interosseus nerve that innervates the pronator quadratus [25]. In complete median or ulnar nerve injuries, expendable denervated portions of these nerves, such as the nerve to the third web space or the dorsal cutaneous branch of the ulnar nerve, may be used as graft material to reconstruct more critical portions of the same injured nerve [26].

One current practice that accounts for the success of nerve grafts is the use of small, thin grafts that are cabled when necessary. Historically, full-thickness nerve trunks were used as grafts [27]. Those early grafts were placed under more tension than is used today. For the graft to be successful, it must survive long enough for the nerve to regenerate through it. Small, thin grafts revascularize more easily than larger nerves, a factor that contributes to the success of functional outcome. No agreement exists on the maximum length that may be bridged by a nerve graft; however, in some situations, 20-cm and longer nerve grafts have been used with various degrees of success [28,29]. Free vascularized nerve grafts were introduced in 1976 by Taylor and Ham [30] to deal with these longer gaps. For smaller defects, a vascularized graft and conventional graft do not appear to differ in clinical outcome; however, Doi and colleagues [31] recommend using free vascularized nerve grafts when the gap distance is greater than 6 cm with associated soft tissue loss over the repaired area. Current use of free vascularized sural nerve grafts is for reconstruction of upper extremity gaps greater than 20 cm in length [32,33]. Pedicled vascularized ulnar nerve [34,35] has been described for a contralateral C7 nerve root transfer to the median nerve in extreme cases, and, recently, a vascularized great auricular nerve [36] was used to bridge a 4-cm gap in the facial nerve.

Thin-caliber nerve grafts will revascularize by the process of inosculation. Large-caliber nerve grafts need to be vascularized, or the central portions will undergo ischemic necrosis.

Although nerve grafts are the standard of care for the management of nerve gaps, their major disadvantage is the limited number of donor nerves available. This problem has led to the development of new techniques for bridging the nerve gap. For distances of less than 3 cm, either a nerve conduit or an autologous vein graft serves equally well as a nerve graft [37]. The initial recommendation was to limit the use of autogenous vein grafts in a nerve gap less than or equal to 3 cm in nonessential peripheral sensory nerves [38]. Since that time, surgeons have used conduits of various types for both sensory and motor nerves. Biologic conduits made from bone, vein, artery, collagen [39], and muscle have been used [40], as well as synthetic conduits made from silicone and polyglycolic acid [41,42]. Nondegradable nerve guides have fallen out of favor because they have the disadvantage of leaving foreign material that potentially may cause chronic reactions with excessive scarring.

Veins, especially grafts longer than 3 cm, are believed to collapse because of their thin walls and absence of pressure from within. The surrounding scar tissue can cause compression, preventing the nerves from completing the regrowth via the graft. To improve regeneration through the conduit, one study showed that a vein conduit turned inside out had superior results to a nerve graft [43]. Vein grafts were filled with several types of biodegradable matrix to keep the lumen from scarring. It was the introduction of Schwann cells to the conduit that pushed the limit of nerve regeneration through a 6-cm gap [44]. In experimental studies with Schwann cell–lined bioengineered conduits, gaps as large as 8 cm can be bridged [45]. Placing pieces of morselized neural tissue within the conduit will improve regeneration [46].

Biodegradable nerve guides thus promise to be a successful alternative to nerve grafts. These nerve tubes degrade with minimal foreign body reaction [47]. Tissue engineers are creating Schwann cell–lined biodegradable tubes in various media. It must be emphasized that not all nerve conduits will allow regeneration, even when they are biodegradable [48]. Experimental and clinical studies of each "new" conduit are necessary, because it is not appropriate to extrapolate that all biodegradable conduits work equally well. Currently, there is only one double-blinded prospective clinical study evaluating the use of a biodegradable polyglycolic acid conduit [49].

Nerve gaps as large as 3 cm in small-diameter nerves may be successfully reconstructed with a fluid-filled (not blood-filled) biodegradable nerve conduit. With larger-diameter nerves, the nerve gap must be equal to or less than 1 cm. In either case, the authors recommend using morselized nerve harvested from a short section of the proximal nerve stump to line the conduit and support nerve regeneration (Hess et al, submitted for publication).

Nerve transfer: alternative to conduits

A nerve transfer is an alternative method of repairing a large nerve gap. The procedure has a higher learning curve than a standard nerve repair. A nerve gap easily repaired with a graft or neural tube should be considered the gold standard. Nerve transfers should be reserved for situations such as the following:

A brachial plexus injury where no nerve or only very proximal nerve is available for grafting

A high proximal injury that requires a long distance for regeneration

To avoid scarred areas in locations with potential for injury to critical structures

In the case of major limb trauma with segmental loss of nerve tissue that would require several grafts

As an alternative to nerve grafting when time from injury to reconstruction is prolonged

Partial nerve injuries with a defined functional loss

Spinal-cord root avulsion injuries

Nerve injuries where the level of injury is uncertain, such as idiopathic neuritides or radiation trauma, and nerve injuries with multiple levels of injury

The more commonly used motor nerve transfers are modeled after their analogous tendon transfers, so similar principles hold true for both. Only an expendable nerve fascicle is used. Nerves with redundant fascicles or branches make excellent donor nerves. Unlike a tendon transfer, a nerve transfer does not rely on amplitude and excursion of the tendon muscle unit, nor is it limited to the one tendon–one function and the straight-line-of-pull principles. The type of muscle fiber unit and the insertion of the tendon will influence the ultimate effectiveness of that muscle's contraction in its new position [50,51]. The major advantages of a nerve transfer over a tendon transfer are that (1) nerve transfers can restore sensibility in addition to motor function; (2) a nerve that innervates multiple muscle groups may be restored with a single nerve transfer; and (3) the insertion and attachments of the muscle or muscles in question are not disrupted, so the original muscle function and tension are maintained. Although a synergistic nerve transfer is ideal, antagonistic nerve transfers may be used successfully in some cases, such as that of branches of median nerve used to restore radial nerve function [52].

A significant advantage of nerve transfers over long nerve grafts is that they make it possible to convert a proximal high-level nerve injury to a low-level nerve injury. This property is especially important in high median nerve and ulnar nerve injuries. The donor nerves close to the injured nerve and the motor end-plate are selected, and nerve grafts are rarely needed in addition to a nerve transfer. An internal neurolysis allows for separation of donor and recipient fascicles from the main nerve, so that an end-to-end repair is performed. Nerve transfers for motor and sensory nerves have similar criteria that are listed in Boxes 1 and 2 [52,53].

When choosing donor nerves for transfer, one prefers a nerve that innervates a synergistic muscle group, because it facilitates postoperative re-education. Although a nerve supplying a nonsynergistic or even antagonistic muscle group may be used, more retraining may be necessary to learn to contract the newly reinnervated muscle. The authors' preferred method for the neurorrhaphy is an end-to-end repair. In rare instances, they perform a nerve transfer with an end-to-side neurorrhaphy [26]. Their experimental studies show that, whereas sensory nerves will spontaneously sprout from an epineural or perineural window, a motor nerve requires a partial neurectomy to facilitate end-to-side regeneration [54].

Nerve transfers are possible in part because of the redundancy in proximal mixed nerve fibers. Knowledge of the internal topography facilitates the separation of fascicle groups even in the proximal extremity. Although it was once believed that nerve fibers to a distinct fascicular group remained separate proximally and merged distally, close to the

Box 2: Criteria for sensory nerve transfer

Donor sensory nerve near the target sensory nerve
Expendable donor sensory nerve (noncritical sensory distribution)
Donor sensory nerve with a large number of pure sensory axons
Denervated distal end of donor nerve spliced end-to-side to adjacent normal sensory nerve
Sensory re-education improves functional recovery

target organ, we now know that these fibers run adjacent to one another even in the proximal limb, albeit following extensive interfascicular plexus pathways [Fig. 1] [55]. Motor fibers for a specific distal function are grouped together and thus may be electrically identified intraoperatively when being selected for possible nerve transfer. Motor nerves preferentially regenerate in a motor environment [56]. Nonetheless, the most commonly used grafts are all sensory nerves. Brushart and colleagues [57] developed the concept of preferential motor reinnervation in rodent models and

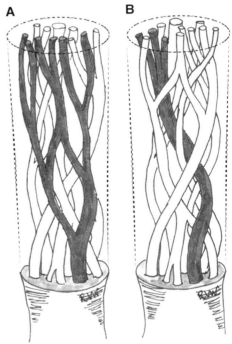

Fig.1. Nerve topography. (*A*) Nerve fibers destined for a particular fascicular group were thought to remain separate until the distal limb. (*B*) Recent anatomic studies demonstrate that fibers of a distinct fascicular group are located adjacent to one another even in the proximal limb. At the proximal level, there is significant plexus interconnection.

Box 1: Criteria for motor nerve transfer

Donor nerve near motor end plates of target muscle (smallest distance = shortest time to reinnervation)
Expendable or redundant donor motor nerve
Donor nerve with pure motor nerve fibers
Donor motor nerve with a large number of motor axons
Donor nerve innervates a muscle that is synergistic to the target muscle (preferred but not required to facilitate re-education)
Motor re-education improves functional recovery

Table 1: **List of common nerve transfers**

Injured nerve	Donor nerves	Recipient nerves	Function restored
Musculo-cutaneous	FCU fascicle of ulnar n. FCR fascicle of median n.	Brachialis br. Biceps bachii br.	Elbow flexion
Suprascapular	Spinal accessory n.	Suprascapular n.	Shoulder abduction, external rotation
Accessory	Medial pectoral br.	Spinal accessory n.	Shoulder elevation and abduction
Axillary	Triceps br. of radial n.	Deltoid br.	Shoulder abduction
Radial	FCR, FDS ± PL br. of median n.	Posterior interosseus n. ECRB br.	Wrist, finger extension
Median	FCU fascicle of ulnar n.	Anterior interosseus n.	Thumb opposition, finger flexion
Ulnar	Distal anterior interosseus n. of median n.	Ulnar motor br.	Hand intrinsics
Median (sensory)	Ulnar sensory n.	n. to first web space	Sensation to key pinch area
Ulnar (sensory)	Dorsal sensory n. of radial n. n. to third web space of median n.	n. to fourth and fifth digits	Sensation to fourth and fifth digits
Ulnar (sensory)	Lateral antebrachial cutaneous n..	Dorsal ulnar n.	Sensation to ulnar border of hand

Abbreviations: br., branch; ECRB, Extensor carpi radialis brevis; FCR, Flexor carpi radialis; FCU, Flexor carpi ulnaris; FDS, Flexor digitorum superficialis; n., nerve; PL, Palmaris longus.

subsequently demonstrated similar findings in nonhuman primates; this property is likely to be conserved in human peripheral nerves [58].

The authors have recently shown that the phenotype of the nerve graft significantly affects nerve regeneration [59]. A single motor nerve graft was as successful as two or three motor cable grafts in enhancing nerve regeneration. In fact, there existed a dose-recognized inhibitory effect of sensory nerve grafts on regeneration of mixed tibial nerve [60].

The future may see the use of motor nerve allografts or expendable motor nerve autografts for the reconstruction of motor nerve injuries. At present, the more commonly used nerve transfers the authors perform are presented in Table 1 and Fig. 2.

Neurorrhaphy: end-to-end versus end-to-side

As we gain greater knowledge of the internal topography of the nerves of both upper and lower limbs, the number of possible combinations of transfers continues to increase. The major debate at the forefront of this area of inquiry is whether an end-to-side neurorrhaphy is equivalent to an end-to-end neurorrhaphy. In the last 2 decades, there has been an explosion of research evaluating end-to-end versus end-to-side repairs, but it is generally accepted that end-to-side will provide only limited sensory recovery [61]. An end-to-side transfer will allow motor reinnervation through collateral sprouting only when there has been a direct nerve

injury at the repair site, such as a partial neurectomy. Such end-to-side transfers are commonly performed in hemihypoglossal nerve transfers to the facial nerve for reanimation with clinical success. A perineural window will create a localized mild injury on the donor nerve, which is transient [62–64]. Other investigators found no adverse effect at all [65,66]. The authors believe that, without some direct injury, minimal motor nerve sprouting occurs without any appreciable functional recovery [54]. Some have suggested that these axons represent spontaneous collateral sprouts from the intact donor nerve, whereas others believe that the nerves populating the end-to-side limb are simply composed of daughter axons of regenerating units seeking a sensory or motor target as a result of trauma to the donor nerve [67]. In two separate studies, end-to-side neurorrhaphies between rat transected tibial and intact peroneal nerves were evaluated. The experimental groups included both an epineurotomy and a perineurotomy group. No functional recovery was documented in any gastrocnemius muscles reinnervated with an end-to-side neurorrhaphy, and muscle weight in these groups remained significantly lower than those in gastrocnemius muscles reinnervated by an end-to-end neurorrhaphy. Retrograde labeling techniques indicate that sensory reinnervation but no motor reinnervation occurred. The number of sensory fibers increased as the degree of injury to the donor nerve increased from epineural to perineural injury in the end-to-side limb. These findings support previous

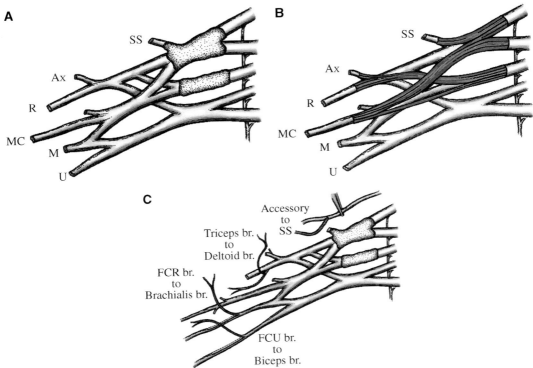

Fig. 2. Nerve transfer. A proximal brachial plexus injury (*A*) has been classically treated with excision and primary grafting of the nerve defect (*B*). (*C*) Nerve transfers are increasingly used in place of multiple nerve grafts. The suprascapular nerve is often neurotized end-to-side into the spinal accessory to restore shoulder rotation. The long head of the triceps branches may be used to reinnervate the deltoid branch of the axillary nerve in isolated traction injuries. The authors' preferred approach to restoration of elbow flexion uses both redundant fascicles from the median and ulnar nerves neurotized directly to the biceps brachii and brachialis branches. Accessory, spinal accessory nerve; Ax, axillary nerve; Biceps br., biceps brachii branch of musculocutaneous nerve; Brachialis br., brachialis branch of musculocutaneous nerve; Deltoid br., deltoid branch of axillary nerve; FCR br., flexor carpi radialis redundant fascicles of the median nerve; FCU br., flexor carpi ulnaris redundant fascicles of the ulnar nerve; M, median nerve; MC, musculocutaneous nerve; R, radial nerve; SS, suprascapular nerve; Triceps br., triceps branch of the radial nerve; U, ulnar nerve.

reports that progressive injury to the conjunctival layers of peripheral nerves proportionally increased axonal population along the end-to-side limb [68]. Interestingly, only limited sensory recovery occurred with an end-to-side repair.

Allografts: overcoming immunosuppression?

With a paucity of donor nerves, substitutes for nerve grafts have been at the forefront of investigations. Nerve allografts are currently enjoying a resurgence. Increased knowledge about cold preservation, immunosuppression, and axonal regeneration makes it clear that techniques minimizing the graft antigenicity, in combination with induction of tolerance, can lead to results similar to nerve autograft. Nerve allografts act as a temporary scaffold across which host axons regenerate. Eventually, the allograft tissue is completely replaced with host

material [69]. Once regeneration of the nerve occurs through the graft, the allograft is no longer needed, and immunosuppression may be discontinued. The new nerve will remyelinate itself by repopulating the missing segment with autologous Schwann cells. Because long-term immunosuppression is not needed in peripheral nerve allografts, such negative effects may be limited. Although systemic immunosuppression with cyclosporin A or FK506 has been shown to prevent acute rejection of the allograft, significant side effects and permanent tolerance to a foreign antigen may occur. Initial studies and clinical trial with FK506 appear to enhance the rate of nerve regeneration [70]. Although this effect is beneficial, the risks of total immunosuppression generally outweigh the benefits, so its clinical use is limited. The senior author has a unique expertise and has successfully restored motor and sensory nerve function in two out of two patients treated with FK506 and in five out of six patients treated with cyclosporin [71]. The authors' clinical experience with nerve allografts and FK506 indicates that functional recovery is similar or better than when a long nerve autograft is used without FK506 [68].

Recent targets of the immunosuppression cascade have shifted focus to the costimulatory pathway, such as the CD40/CD40 ligand [72] and the B7/CD28 ligand [73] interactions and the RIB 5/2 ligand [74], a nondepleting anti-CD4 monoclonal antibody. Attempts to combine modalities to maximize regenerative potential have met with variable results, although in some cases a synergistic effect has been noted. Nerve allografts treated with a combination of cold preservation and subimmunosuppressive, less toxic doses of FK506 demonstrated an equal degree of nerve regeneration when compared with nerve allografts treated with higher immunosuppressive doses of FK506 [75]. The combination of FK506 with cold preservation took advantage of the neuroenhancing properties of FK506 to produce significantly better regeneration than that noted in autografts. Combining the administration of monoclonal antibodies with intercellular adhesion molecule–1 and lymphocyte function–associated antigen–1 [76] or cold preservation of nerve allografts [77] with systemic cyclosporin reduces the dose required of the systemic immunosuppression to allow nerve regeneration through the allograft. An additional strategy employed in animal models to confer donor-specific tolerance to peripheral nerve allografts is pretreating the host with ultraviolet-B–irradiated splenocytes derived from the transplant donor, which are administered through the portal venous circulation. Although this method does induce a prolonged period of donor-specific immune unresponsiveness to nerve allografts in the rat, it is fairly invasive and more effective when combined with other immunosuppressive regimens. It has not been as effective as a singular treatment in larger animal models [78].

Cold preservation alone has an immunosuppressive effect on nerve allografts [79]. Although Schwann cells remain viable in experimental rat models for as long as 3 weeks, the cellular adhesion molecule expression is downgraded by 7 weeks [80,81]. Recent data show that short allografts cold preserved for 7 weeks lose their immunogenicity and facilitate axonal regeneration equivalent to that of autografts [82]. Earlier data show that Schwann cells can be expanded in culture and transplanted into peripheral nerve allografts without causing significant disruption of neural architecture or tumor formation [83]. Recent work in a subhuman primate long-graft (6-cm) model showed that 8-week cold preserved allografts were acellular and did not facilitate nerve regeneration. By contrast, when 8-week cold preserved allografts were cannulated and autologous Schwann cells injected along the graft, regeneration was equal to that of a nerve autograft [84].

Bioengineering conduits: the future?

At the opposite end of the spectrum, advances in bioengineering have allowed for the creation of composite neural tubes lined with Schwann cells and neurotrophic agents to facilitate the regenerative process. Trophic (growth-promoting) factors studied include nerve growth factor, brain-derived neurotrophic factor, fibroblastic growth factors, ciliary neurotrophic factor, and interleukin-6 [85,86]. Although many of these growth factors and cytokines are released into the surrounding tissues after a nerve injury, the mechanism by which they stimulate axonal regeneration is not yet clear. In theory, a gap at the nerve repair site should allow regenerating axons correctly to identify the target end organ; investigations have shown that optimal nerve regeneration requires tightly coapted nerves with no gap and accurate alignment [87]. Finally, the capacity of certain axon membrane glycoproteins preferentially to attract either motor or sensory axons has been investigated as a method of guiding nerve regeneration [88].

The ultimate bioengineered nerve conduit will be able to enhance regeneration, block invasion of scar tissue, and autodegrade when it is no longer needed. Schwann cells inside a conduit are known to improve nerve regeneration, and early clinical trials of Schwann cell–lined neural tubes are in progress. Growth factors have been studied to determine the usefulness and timing of the doses. Insulin-derived growth factor [89] does not promote nerve regeneration through a nerve guide, whereas nerve growth factor [90] and fibroblastic growth factor [91] show enhanced nerve regeneration across the guide. One external modality to enhance nerve regeneration is the use of pulsed electromagnetic fields. Although the rate of regeneration is not increased, the number of motor neurons as well as their ability to reach the target organ is significantly improved [92]. This effect appears to be driven by an up-regulation of brain-derived neurotrophic factor [93]. At present, there is no benign modality of increasing the rate at which a nerve regenerates; however, it has been experimentally possible to alter the rate at which the motor end plates resorb. Leupeptin, a calpain inhibitor, blocks the calpain protease-mediated absorption of the motor end plates and may offer an important advancement in nerve repair and nerve recovery at the peripheral and spinal cord levels [94].

Summary

The gold standard for bridging a nerve gap remains a nerve autograft. Since the first implementation of a nerve allograft in 1870 by Philipeaux and Vulpian, significant contributions to suturing technique, neural topography, and the biology of nerve regeneration have transformed the way we approach nerve gaps. Although primary neurorrhaphy and autografts are the most common methods of repair, several newer options are at our disposal. Nerve transfers have revolutionized our approach to nerve gaps, from devastating brachial plexus injuries to highly selected upper and lower motor and sensory nerve injuries. Nerve allografts, bioengineered nerve conduits, and therapies to augment the regenerative properties of the peripheral nerve are the current objects of investigation in academic laboratories and industry. Breaking these barriers of nerve regeneration limitation will push peripheral nerve surgery to the next level. Nerve allografts have the advantage of being closest to an autologous nerve. When the morbidity associated with even temporary immunosuppression becomes negligible, allografts may have a prominent role in grafting in cases of larger nerve volume loss. Industry-driven tissue engineering is already being implemented in bioengineered nerve conduits. The future of bioengineered grafts may entail a combination of tissue typing, trophic factors, and perhaps the use of embryonic stem cells to create effective nerve substitutes.

References

[1] Trumble TE, Archibald S, Allan CH. Bioengineering for nerve repair in the future. Journal of the American Society for Surgery of the Hand 2004; 4(3):134–42.

[2] Driscoll PJ, Glasby MA, Lawson GM. An in vivo study of peripheral nerves in continuity: biomechanical and physiological responses to elongation. J Orthop Res 2002;20(2):370–5.

[3] Sunderland IR, Brenner MJ, Singham J, et al. Effect of tension on nerve regeneration in rat sciatic nerve transection model. Ann Plast Surg 2004;53(4):382–7.

[4] Trumble TE, McCallister WV. Repair of peripheral nerve defects in the upper extremity. Hand Clin 2000;16(1):37–52.

[5] Allan CH, Trumble TE. Biomechanics of peripheral nerve repair. Oper Tech Orthop 2004;14: 184–9.

[6] Millesi H. Microsurgery of the peripheral nerves. Hand 1973;5:157–60.

[7] Kawamura DH, Hadlock TA, Fox IK, et al. Regeneration through nerve isografts is independent of nerve geometry. J Reconstr Microsurg 2005; 21(4):243–9.

[8] Hall GD, Van Way CW, Kung FT, et al. Peripheral nerve elongation with tissue expansion techniques. J Trauma 1993;34(3):401–5.

[9] Ohkaya S, Hirata H, Uchida A. Repair of nerve gap with the elongation of Wallerian degenerated nerve by tissue expansion. Microsurgery 2000; 20(3):126–30.

[10] Skoulis TG, Lovice D, von Fricken K, et al. Nerve expansion. The optimal answer for the short nerve gap. Behavioral analysis. Clin Orthop 1995; 314:84–94.

[11] Giddins GE, Wade PJ, Amis AA. Primary nerve repair: strength of repair with different gauges of nylon suture material. J Hand Surg [Br] 1989; 14(3):301–2.

[12] Millesi H. The current state of peripheral nerve surgery in the upper limb. Ann Chir Main 1984; 3:18–34.

[13] Bora Jr FW. Peripheral nerve repair in cats. The fascicular stitch. J Bone Joint Surg Am 1967; 49:659–66.

[14] Grabb WC, Bement SL, Koepke GH, et al. Comparison of methods of peripheral nerve suturing in monkeys. Plast Reconstr Surg 1970;46: 31–8.

[15] Cabaud HE, Rodkey WG, McCarroll Jr HR, et al. Epineurial and perineurial fascicular nerve repairs: a critical comparison. J Hand Surg [Am] 1976;1(2):131–7.

[16] Zhao Q, Dahlin LB, Kanje M, et al. Specificity of muscle reinnervation following repair of the transected sciatic nerve. A comparative study of different repair techniques in the rat. J Hand Surg [Br] 1992;17(3):257–61.

[17] Temple CL, Ross DC, Dunning CE, et al. Tensile strength of healing peripheral nerves. J Reconstr Microsurg 2003;19(7):483–8.

[18] Higgs PE, Weeks PM. The rate of bursting strength gain in repaired nerves. Ann Plast Surg 1979;3(4):338–40.

[19] Yu RS, Catalano III LW, Barron OA, et al. Limited, protected postsurgical motion does not affect the results of digital nerve repair. J Hand Surg [Am] 2004;29(2):302–6.

[20] Millesi H. The nerve gap. Theory and clinical practice. Hand Clin 1986;2(4):651–63.

[21] Myckatyn TM, MacKinnon SE. A review of research endeavors to optimize peripheral nerve reconstruction. Neurol Res 2004;26:124–38.

[22] Seddon HJ, editor. Surgical disorders of peripheral nerves. Edinburgh (UK): Churchill Livingstone; 1975.

[23] Dvali L, Mackinnon S. Nerve repair, grafting, and nerve transfers. Clin Plast Surg 2003; 30(2): 203–21.

[24] Myckatyn TM, Mackinnon SE. Surgical techniques of nerve grafting (standard/vascularized/allograft). Oper Tech Orthop 2004;14:171–8.

[25] Novak CB, Mackinnon SE. Distal anterior interosseous nerve transfer to the deep motor branch

of the ulnar nerve for reconstruction of high ulnar nerve injuries. J Reconstr Microsurg 2002; 18(6):459–64.

[26] Humphreys DB, Mackinnon SE. Nerve transfers. Operative techniques. Plast Reconstr Surg 2002; 9:89–99.

[27] Brunnell S. Nerve grafts. Am J Surg 1939;44:64.

[28] Lenoble E, Sokolow C, Ebelin M, et al. Results of the primary repair of 28 isolated median nerve injuries in the wrist. Ann Chir Main 1989; 8:347–51.

[29] Millesi H. Indication, technique and results of nerve grafting. Handchirurgie Suppl 1977;2:1–24.

[30] Taylor GI, Ham FJ. The free vascularized nerve graft. A further experimental and clinical application of microvascular techniques. Plast Reconstr Surg 1976;57(4):413–26.

[31] Doi K, Tamaru K, Sakai K, et al. A comparison of vascularized and conventional sural nerve grafts. J Hand Surg [Am] 1992;17(4):670–6.

[32] Doi K, Kuwata N, Kawakami F, et al. The free vascularized sural nerve graft. Microsurgery 1984; 5(4):175–84.

[33] Hasegawa T, Nakamura S, Manabe T, et al. Vascularized nerve grafts for the treatment of large nerve gap after severe trauma to an upper extremity. Arch Orthop Trauma Surg 2004; 124(3):209–13.

[34] Gu YD, Chen DS, Zhang GM, et al. Long-term functional results of contralateral C7 transfer. J Reconstr Microsurg 1998;14(1):57–9.

[35] Waikakul S, Orapin S, Vanadurongwan V. Clinical results of contralateral C7 root neurotization to the median nerve in brachial plexus injuries with total root avulsions. J Hand Surg [Br] 1999;24(5):556–60.

[36] Koshima I, Nanba Y, Tsutsui T, et al. New one-stage nerve pedicle grafting technique using the great auricular nerve for reconstruction of facial nerve defects. J Reconstr Microsurg 2004;20(5): 357–61.

[37] Chiu DT, Janecka I, Krizek TJ, et al. Autogenous vein graft as a conduit for nerve regeneration. Surgery 1982;91(2):226–33.

[38] Chiu DT, Strauch B. A prospective clinical evaluation of autogenous vein grafts used as a nerve conduit for distal sensory nerve defects of 3 cm or less. Plast Reconstr Surg 1990;86(5): 928–34.

[39] Kim DH, Connoly SE, Zhao S, et al. Comparison of macropore, semipermeable and nonpermeable collagen conduits in nerve repair. J Reconstr Microsurg 1993;9:415–20.

[40] Chen LE, Seaber AV, Urbaniak JR, et al. Denatured muscle as a nerve conduit: a functional, morphologic, and electrophysiologic evaluation. J Reconstr Microsurg 1994;10:137–44.

[41] Keeley RD, Nguyen KD, Stephanides MJ, et al. The artificial nerve graft: a comparison of blended elastomerhydrogel with polyglycolic acid conduits. J Reconstr Microsurg 1991;7:93–100.

[42] Meek MF, Coert JH. Clinical use of nerve con-

duits in peripheral-nerve repair: review of the literature. J Reconstr Microsurg 2002;18:97–109.

[43] Wang KK, Costas PD, Bryan DJ, et al. Inside-out vein graft repair compared with nerve grafting for nerve regeneration in rats. Microsurgery 1995;16(2):65–70.

[44] Strauch B, Rodriguez DM, Diaz J, et al. Autologous Schwann cells drive regeneration through a 6-cm autogenous venous nerve conduit. J Reconstr Microsurg 2001;17(8):589–95.

[45] Zhang F, Blain B, Beck J, et al. Autogenous venous graft with one-stage prepared Schwann cells as a conduit for repair of long segmented nerve defects. J Reconstr Microsurg 2002;18: 295–300.

[46] Saito I, Oka Y, Odaka M. Promoting nerve regeneration through long gaps using a small nerve tissue graft. Surg Neurol 2003;59(3):148–54.

[47] Ijkema-Paassen J, Jansen K, Gramsbergen A, et al. Transection of peripheral nerves, bridging strategies and effect evaluation. Biomaterials 2004; 25(9):1583–92.

[48] Belkas J, Munro CA, Shoichet MS, et al. Peripheral nerve regeneration through a synthetic hydrogel nerve tube. Restor Neurol Neurosci 2005;23(1):19–29.

[49] Weber RA, Breidenbach WC, Brown RE, et al. A randomized prospective study of polyglycolic acid conduits for digital nerve reconstruction in humans. Plast Reconstr Surg 2000;106(5): 1036–45.

[50] Guelinckx PJ, Faulkner JA. Parallel-fibered muscles transplanted with neurovascular repair into bipennate muscle sites in rabbits. Plast Reconstr Surg 1992;89:290–8.

[51] Guelinckx PJ, Carlson BM, Faulkner JA. Morphologic characteristics of muscles grafted in rabbits with neurovascular repair. J Reconstr Microsurg 1992;8:481–9.

[52] Weber RV, Mackinnon S. Nerve transfers in the upper extremity. Journal of the American Society for Surgery of the Hand 2004;4(3):200–13.

[53] Mackinnon SE, Novak CB. Nerve transfers: new options for reconstruction following nerve injury. Hand Clin 1999;15:643–66.

[54] Goheen-Robillard B, Myckatyn TM, Mackinnon SE, et al. End-to-side neurorrhaphy and lateral axonal sprouting in a long graft rat model. Laryngoscope 2002;112(5):899–905.

[55] Brandt KE, Mackinnon SE. Microsurgical repair of peripheral nerves and nerve grafts. In: Aston SJ, Beasley RW, Thorne CHM, editors. Grabb and Smith's plastic surgery. 5th edition. New York: Lippincott-Raven; 1997. p. 79–90.

[56] Brushart TM. Motor axons preferentially reinnervate motor pathways. J Neurosci 1993;13: 2730–8.

[57] Brushart TM, Gerber J, Kessens P, et al. Contributions of pathway and neuron to preferential motor reinnervation. J Neurosci 1998;18:8674–81.

[58] Madison RD, Archibald SJ, Lacin R, et al. Factors contributing to preferential motor reinnerva-

tion in the primate peripheral nervous system. J Neurosci 1999;19:11007–16.

[59] Nichols CM, Brenner MJ, Fox IK, et al. Effects of motor versus sensory nerve grafts on peripheral nerve regeneration. Exp Neurol 2004;190(2): 347–55.

[60] Hess JR, Myckatyn TM, Hunter DA, et al. The effects of fascicle quantity and composition in the fiber regeneration across a mixed peripheral nerve gap. [in press].

[61] Tarasidis G, Watanabe O, Mackinnon SE, et al. End-to-side neurorrhaphy: a long-term study of neural regeneration in a rat model. Otolaryngol Head Neck Surg 1998;119(4):337–41.

[62] Sanapanich K, Morrison WA, Messina A. Physiologic and morphologic aspects of nerve regeneration after end-to-end or end-to-side coaptation in a rat model of brachial plexus injury. J Hand Surg [Am] 2002;27(1):133–42.

[63] Zhang Z, Soucacos PN, Bo J, et al. Reinnervation after end-to-side nerve coaptation in a rat model. Am J Orthop 2001;30(5):400–6.

[64] Cederna PS, Kalliainen LK, Urbanchek MG, et al. "Donor" muscle structure and function after end-to-side neurorrhaphy. Plast Reconstr Surg 2001; 107(3):789–96.

[65] Yan JG, Matloub HS, Sanger JR, et al. A modified end-to-side method for peripheral nerve repair: large epineurial window helicoid technique versus small epineurial window standard end-to-side technique. J Hand Surg [Am] 2002; 27(3):484–92.

[66] Tham SK, Morrison WA. Motor collateral sprouting through an end-to-side nerve repair. J Hand Surg [Am] 1998;23(5):844–51.

[67] Rovak JM, Cederna PS, Kuzon Jr WM. Terminolateral neurorrhaphy: a review of the literature. J Reconstr Microsurg 2001;17(8):615–24.

[68] Bertelli JA, dos Santos AR, Calixto JB. Is axonal sprouting able to traverse the conjunctival layers of the peripheral nerve? A behavioral, motor, and sensory study of end-to-side nerve anastomosis. J Reconstr Microsurg 1996;12(8):559–63.

[69] Atchabahian A, Doolabh VB, Mackinnon SE, et al. Indefinite survival of peripheral nerve allografts after temporary Cyclosporine A immunosuppression. Restor Neurol Neurosci 1998; 13(3–4):129–39.

[70] Jost SC, Doolabh VB, Mackinnon SE, et al. Acceleration of peripheral nerve regeneration following FK506 administration. Restor Neurol Neurosci 2000;17(1):39–44.

[71] Mackinnon SE, Doolabh VB, Novak CB, et al. Clinical outcome following nerve allograft transplantation. Plast Reconstr Surg 2001;107(6): 1419–29.

[72] Niimi M, Pearson TC, Larsen CP, et al. The role of the CD40 pathway in alloantigen-induced hyporesponsiveness in vivo. J Immunol 1998; 161(10):5331–7.

[73] Larsen CP, Elwood ET, Alexander DZ, et al. Long-term acceptance of skin and cardiac allografts after blocking CD40 and CD28 pathways. Nature 1996;381(6581):434–8.

[74] Doolabh VB, Tung TH, Wayne Flye M, et al. Effect of nondepleting anti-CD4 monoclonal antibody (Rib 5/2) plus donor antigen pretreatment in peripheral nerve allotransplantation. Microsurgery 2002;22(8):329–34.

[75] Grand AG, Myckatyn TM, Mackinnon SE, et al. Axonal regeneration after cold preservation of nerve allografts and immunosuppression with tacrolimus in mice. J Neurosurg 2002;96:924–32.

[76] Fox DJ, Doolabh VB, Mackinnon SE, et al. Decreased Cyclosporin A requirement with anti-ICAM-1 and anti-LFA-1 in a peripheral nerve allotransplantation model. Restor Neurol Neurosci 1999;15(4):319–26.

[77] Strasberg SR, Hertl MC, Mackinnon SE, et al. Peripheral nerve allograft preservation improves regeneration and decreases systemic cyclosporin A requirements. Exp Neurol 1996;139(2): 306–16.

[78] Genden EM, Mackinnon SE, Yu S, et al. Pretreatment with portal venous ultraviolet B–irradiated donor alloantigen promotes donor-specific tolerance to rat nerve allografts. Laryngoscope 2001; 111(3):439–47.

[79] Evans PJ, Mackinnon SE, Levi AD, et al. Cold preserved nerve allografts: changes in basement membrane, viability, immunogenicity, and regeneration. Muscle Nerve 1998;21:1507–22.

[80] Evans PJ, Mackinnon SE, Best TJ, et al. Regeneration across preserved peripheral nerve grafts. Muscle Nerve 1995;18:1128–38.

[81] Atchabahian A, Mackinnon SE, Hunter DA. Cold preservation of nerve grafts decreases expression of ICAM-1 and class II MHC antigens. J Reconstr Microsurg 1999;15:307–11.

[82] Fox IK, Jaramillo A, Hunter DA, et al. Prolonged cold-preservation of nerve allografts. Muscle Nerve 2005;31(1):59–69.

[83] Ogden MA, Feng FY, Myckatyn TM, et al. Safe injection of cultured Schwann cells into peripheral nerve allografts. Microsurgery 2000;20(7): 314–23.

[84] Fox IK, Nichols CM, Brenner MJ, et al. Schwann cell injected cold preserved nerve allografts for reconstruction of the long nerve gap: preliminary results. In: American Society for Peripheral Nerve Annual Meeting 2005 program book. Fajardo (Puerto Rico); 2005. p. 51.

[85] McCallister WV, Tang P, Smith J, et al. Axonal regeneration stimulated by the combination of nerve growth factor and ciliary neurotrophic factor in an end-to-side model. J Hand Surg [Am] 2001;26(3):478–88.

[86] Bothwell M. Functional interactions of neurotrophins and neurotrophin receptors. Ann Rev Neurosci 1995;18:223–53.

[87] Brushart TM, Mathur V, Sood R, et al. Joseph H. Boyes Award. Dispersion of regenerating axons across enclosed neural gaps. J Hand Surg [Am] 1995;20(4):557–64.

[88] Martini R, Schachner M, Brushart TM. The L2/HNK-1 carbohydrate is preferentially expressed by previously motor axon–associated Schwann cells in reinnervated peripheral nerves. J Neurosci 1994;14(11):7180–91.

[89] Fansa H, Schneider W, Wolf G, et al. Influence of insulin-like growth factor-I (IGF-I) on nerve autografts and tissue-engineered nerve grafts. Muscle Nerve 2002;26(1):87–93.

[90] Santos X, Rodrigo J, Hontanilla B, et al. Local administration of neurotrophic growth factor in subcutaneous silicon chambers enhances the regeneration of the sensory component of the rat sciatic nerve. Microsurgery 1999;19(6):275–80.

[91] Wang S, Cai Q, Hou J, et al. Acceleration effect of basic fibroblast growth factor on the regeneration of peripheral nerve through a 15-mm gap. J Biomed Mater Res 2003;66A(3):522–31.

[92] Brushart TM, Hoffman PN, Royall RM, et al. Electrical stimulation promotes motoneuron regeneration without increasing its speed or conditioning the neuron. J Neurosci 2002;22(15):6631–8.

[93] Al-Majed AA, Neumann CM, Brushart TM, et al. Brief electrical stimulation promotes the speed and accuracy of motor axonal regeneration. J Neurosci 2000;20(7):2602–8.

[94] Badalamente MA, Hurst LC, Stracher A. Neuromuscular recovery after peripheral nerve repair: effects of an orally-administered peptide in a primate model. J Reconstr Microsurg 1995;11(6):429–37.

CLINICS IN
PLASTIC
SURGERY

Clin Plastic Surg 32 (2005) 617–634

Cortical Plasticity Following Upper Extremity Injury and Reconstruction

Dimitri J. Anastakis, MD[a],*, Robert Chen, MD[b],
Karen D. Davis, PhD[c], David Mikulis, MD[d]

Abbreviations

COG, center of gravity
EMG, electromyography
FFMT, free functioning muscle transfer
fMRI, functional MRI
ICF, intracortical facilitation
IPJ, interphalangeal joint
M1, primary motor cortex
MEG, magnetoencephalography
MEP, motor evoked potential
MMax, maximum compound muscle action potential evoked by peripheral nerve stimulation
MRI, magnetic resonance image

MT, motor thresholds
PET, positron emission tomography
S1, primary sensory cortex
SICI, short-interval intracortical inhibition
SMC, sensorimotor cortex
TMS, transcranial magnetic stimulation

An increasing body of research exists describing cortical plasticity following upper extremity injury and reconstruction. Plastic surgeons, because of the motor and sensory reconstruction they perform, need to understand cortical plasticity following upper extremity injury, reconstruction, and rehabilitation. In 2000, Lundborg [1] reviewed the sig-

[a] Divisions of Plastic and Orthopaedic Surgery, University of Toronto, University Health Network, 399 Bathurst Street, 4 FP-140, Toronto, Ontario M5T 2S8, Canada
[b] Division of Neurology, University of Toronto, University Health Network, 399 Bathurst Street, Toronto, Ontario M5T 2S8, Canada
[c] Division of Neurosurgery, University of Toronto, University Health Network, 399 Bathurst Street, Toronto, Ontario M5T 2S8, Canada
[d] Department of Medical Imaging, University of Toronto, University Health Network, 399 Bathurst Street, Toronto, Ontario M5T 2S8, Canada
* Corresponding author.
E-mail address: dimitri.anastakis@uhn.on.ca (D.J. Anastakis).

doi:10.1016/j.cps.2005.05.008

nificance of sensory changes in the hand and associated cortical plasticity. However, this comprehensive overview did not address cortical plasticity following motor function loss, reconstruction, and rehabilitation.

This article provides an overview of the methods used to study cortical plasticity and the current knowledge of cortical plasticity as it relates to motor reconstruction and rehabilitation. Cortical plasticity following peripheral nerve injury and repair, toe transfer for thumb reconstruction, and free-functioning muscle transfer for upper limb paralysis reconstruction will be highlighted.

The notion that the adult brain is static in terms of its functional organization has been replaced with a model based on pliability and responsiveness to environmental changes. In this model, the central nervous system changes as it learns and relearns or in response to an injury. These changes occur at biochemical, electrophysiologic, and structural levels. Today's view of the adult central nervous system is that of an adaptive and responsive system.

The word *plastic* originates from the Greek word *plastikos*, which means to mold or form. In modern English, the word plastic refers to the capability of being molded or modeled. In general terms, brain plasticity is the brain's capability to adapt to varying conditions. These conditions may be motor or sensory in nature and can occur throughout the neuraxis. *Synaptic plasticity* refers to the ability of synapses to change in response to changes in motor or sensory function. Synaptic changes include biochemical alteration in sensitivity or excitability, number, and cortical and subcortical representation [2–5].

A large region of the sensorimotor cortex is dedicated to sensorimotor functions of the hand and upper extremity [Fig. 1]. As a result, hand and upper extremity injuries have a profound effect on the brain. Even with the current state of knowledge, we lack a comprehensive understanding of what happens to the human sensorimotor cortex following upper extremity injury, reconstruction, and rehabilitation.

Plasticity occurs in the sensorimotor cortices (ie, primary motor [M1] and primary sensory [S1]) in response to a variety of experiences, from learning a new piano piece to losing a hand in an accident. Research in primates and humans has confirmed that the sensorimotor cortex has the capacity for adaptive change following numerous experiences, including motor skills learning. Changes in cortical representations occur in association with motor skill acquisition [6–9] and the practice of basic movements [10]. Karni and colleagues (1995) [7] demonstrated evidence of M1 plasticity during motor skill learning in normal subjects using rapid sequences of finger movements. The authors found a slowly evolving long-term, experience-dependent reorganization of M1, which may represent the acquisition and retention of motor skills. The influence of training is characterized by expansion of motor and sensory repre-

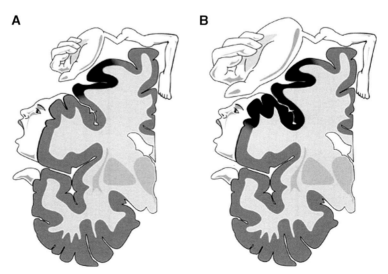

A **B**

Fig. 1. The homunculus. (*A*) A large region of the sensorimotor cortex is dedicated to the hand. Note the disproportionate amount of representation given to the thumb. (*B*) Expansion of motor representation occurs during acquisition of a new motor skill.

sentations most strongly connected to the learned skill. Magnetoencephalographic (MEG) and transcranial magnetic stimulation (TMS) studies have identified similar results in highly trained musicians [11] and blind individuals who have used Braille for a long time [12]. The acquisition of a new motor skill, be it playing a musical instrument or using a new thumb following toe transfer, is associated with cortical plasticity in motor representation, namely expansion of motor and sensory representations during the acquisition of the new skill [see Fig. 1].

Experimental techniques for studying cortical plasticity

Cortical plasticity in humans is studied using non-invasive techniques, such as TMS [13,14], electroencephalography, MEG, functional MRI (fMRI), and positron emission tomography (PET) [15,16]. A comparison of PET, MEG, fMRI, and TMS is provided in Table 1. The authors' group has investigated motor system reorganization using two methods: TMS and fMRI. TMS can measure different inhibitory and excitatory circuits in the motor cortex not assessable by other means, whereas fMRI has high spatial resolution for assessment of motor and sensory representations. Together, these two complementary methods measure different aspects of cortical plasticity.

Functional magnetic resonance imaging

Signal intensity from fMRI images is influenced by the relative proportion of oxyhemoglobin to deoxyhemoglobin in the blood and is therefore blood oxygen level–dependent [17,18]. A decrease in deoxyhemoglobin concentration results in increasing signal intensity on fMRI images [Fig. 2]. While the individual is performing a motor task, there is increased neuronal activity in M1, blood flow increases by as much as 45%, and oxygen extraction

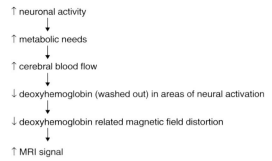

↑ neuronal activity

↓

↑ metabolic needs

↓

↑ cerebral blood flow

↓

↓ deoxyhemoglobin (washed out) in areas of neural activation

↓

↓ deoxyhemoglobin related magnetic field distortion

↓

↑ MRI signal

Fig. 2. Cortical activation and fMRI image. When performing a motor task, cortical activity increases, resulting in increases in metabolic need. The increase in metabolic need results in increased cerebral blood flow that delivers more oxygen than the tissue can consume even in its activated state. Oxyhemoglobin therefore replaces deoxyhemoglobin in the microcirculation. The signal-distorting effect of deoxyhemoglobin is hence diminished and the MRI signal increases.

increases by as much as 16% [19]. Replacement of deoxyhemoglobin by oxyhemoglobin takes place in the microcirculation, increasing the MRI signal intensity by approximately 2% [20]. fMRI can produce activation maps with high spatial resolution by comparing images obtained during resting and active states (eg, performing a motor task) [21–23]. Because the magnitude of MRI signal changes related to brain activation is small, acquisition of thousands of images in multislice studies of the brain is necessary, with multiple iterations of the resting and task cycles, before statistically significant regions of the brain can be identified. fMRI is an effective tool for assessing motor cortical plasticity.

Transcranial magnetic stimulation

TMS makes use of a brief, high-current pulse through a coil of wire to induce magnetic field lines perpendicular to the coil. An electric field is

Table 1: Comparison among positron emission tomography, magnetoencephalograpy, functional MRI, and transcranial magnetic stimulation

	PET	MEG	fMRI	TMS
Spatial resolution	Good	Fair to good	Excellent	Poor
Temporal resolution	Poor (min)	Excellent (ms)	Good (s to min)	Excellent (ms)
Measurement	Blood flow — direct	Neuronal activity	Blood flow — indirect	Neuronal excitability, inhibitory and excitatory circuits
Invasiveness	IV radioactive tracer	None	None	None

induced perpendicular to this magnetic field. When applied over the scalp, TMS currents are capable of activating underlying neural structures [**Fig. 3**]. Therefore, TMS may be used to access many indices of cortical organization and function. Most TMS studies involve the M1, because electromyographic (EMG) responses known as motor-evoked potentials (MEPs) can be easily recorded and quantified by surface EMG recording from contralateral muscles. For example, focal figure-of-eight magnetic coils are used to map muscle representations in M1 [24,25]. The center-of-gravity (COG) is a measure derived from mapping studies and is the amplitude-weighted center of the motor map. Movement of the COG indicates a shift in motor representations [26]. TMS maps have been shown to correlate with areas of cortical activation associated with hand movements in PET and fMRI studies [27,28].

Another TMS measure is the motor threshold (MT) that is related to both cortical and spinal excitability. MT refers to the minimum TMS intensity (usually expressed as percentage of stimulator output) necessary to induce a small MEP from a specific muscle. MT is increased by sodium channel blockers [29,30] and likely reflects neuronal membranes' excitability. Increased

corticospinal excitability leads to lower MT. Another measure of corticospinal excitability is MEP amplitudes. To account for the muscle mass in different muscles and different individuals, the maximum MEP evoked by TMS is often expressed as a ratio of the maximum compound muscle action potential evoked by peripheral nerve stimulation (MMax). This ratio is the percentage MMax (%MMax).

Cortical inhibition and facilitation may also be measured with paired TMS techniques [31]. One method involves pairing a subthreshold pulse that excites cortical inhibitory and excitatory circuits, followed by a suprathreshold test pulse. At short interstimulus intervals (1–4 ms), the MEP amplitude is reduced compared with test pulse alone; this is referred to as short-interval intracortical inhibition (SICI). At longer interstimulus intervals (10–15 ms), the response is larger than the test pulse alone; this is known as intracortical facilitation (ICF) [13,31]. Several studies have shown that SICI and ICF reflect excitability of inhibitory and excitatory networks in the motor cortex rather than subcortical or spinal structures [32]. Voluntary muscle activity is associated with reduction of SICI [33]. Decreased SICI has also been found in several neurologic and psychiatric disorders,

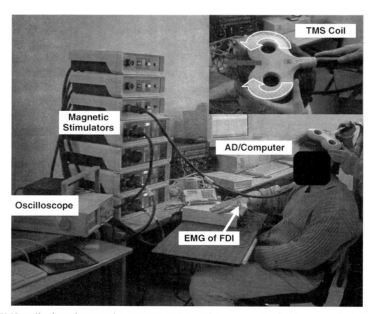

Fig. 3. TMS. The TMS coil placed over the motor cortex. The magnetic field generated stimulates that hand representation of the motor cortex. Motor evoked potential in the contralateral first dorsal interosseous (FDI) muscle is recorded with surface electromyography (EMG) electrodes. In the insert, the open arrows represent the direction of the electrical current in the coil and the filled arrow represents the direction of the induced current in the brain.

such as Parkinson's disease [34] and schizophrenia [35]. Pharmacologic studies suggested that gamma-aminobutyric acid A ($GABA_A$) receptors may be involved in mediating SICI [36–38].

Amputation-induced cortical plasticity

Primate and human research has established that the cortex can undergo plasticity following amputation. Amputation can result in expansion of the motor cortical representation of the muscle just proximal to the injury in rats [39], in primates [40,41], in humans [42–48], and specifically following human hand replantation [48].

MEG studies have shown that, following a hand amputation, an expansion of sensory representation from facial regions into the zone formally represented by the hand occurs [49,50]. fMRI amputation studies have shown the capacity of surviving motor and sensory representations to "invade" a deafferented zone [51–54]. Borsook and colleagues [55] used fMRI to study a subject 24 hours and 1 month after an arm amputation and observed that reorganization of sensory pathways developed soon after amputation. This finding indicates that cortical reorganization can occur soon after amputation.

Cortical plasticity following amputation has been demonstrated using TMS. TMS studies in humans found that M1 contralateral to the amputation becomes more excitable [42,43,45–47] with reduced intracortical inhibition [56]. In addition, TMS pulses produced greater MEP and recruited a larger percentage of the motor neuron pool for resting muscles proximal to the stump than for the same muscles in the intact extremity. Furthermore, the cortical motor maps of muscles proximal to the stump were larger than maps corresponding to the same muscles on the intact side [57]. This pattern roughly parallels the results obtained from ischemic nerve block experiments, suggesting that short-term and long-term plasticity make use of similar fundamental mechanisms. Chen and colleagues (1998) [56] have shown that the plasticity is likely due to a decrease in GABA-mediated inhibition and increased membrane excitability, because both SICI and MT are decreased on the affected side. In line with the TMS findings, an fMRI study of M1 organization after upper extremity amputation early in life [47] found an unusual, broad activation in M1 contralateral to stump movement. These findings suggest that the large activation is not only the result of disinhibition but also the consequence of aberrant physiologic differentiation and maturation. Cortical reorganization following amputation can be associated with phantom pain [58] and may be maladaptive. Thus, fMRI and MEG studies are consistent with the TMS findings of increased cortical excitability, reduced SICI, and expansion of cortical representation of adjacent motor units following amputation.

Cortical plasticity after peripheral nerve injury

Peripheral nerve lesions have immediate and longstanding effects on cortical representations [59]. Plasticity research in the primate has shown that transection of the median nerve initially results in a silent "black hole" in S1 corresponding to the sensory representations of the median nerve (ie, thumb, index, middle, and ring fingers). This silent "black hole" eventually becomes responsive to intact regions adjacent to the deafferented hand. Initial sensory input is unrefined, and the expanding territories from adjacent cortical areas are large and overlapping. With time, the cortical representation shrinks and becomes more refined, and within 2 to 3 weeks the cortical representation shows sharp boundaries between the expanding territories from adjacent cortical areas [60,61]. This primate model illustrates reorganization of S1 following a peripheral nerve lesion. Deafferentation following a median nerve lesion results in the immediate invasion of the former median nerve cortical representation by adjacent cortical areas. Thereafter, subsequent cortical plasticity is dependent on the nature of the nerve lesion and its treatment.

If the median nerve is not surgically repaired, thereby preventing nerve regeneration, the extensive reorganization of the cortical map persists, so that the cortical area previously receiving input from the median nerve remains completely occupied by expanded adjacent cortical areas. If the peripheral nerve is crushed (ie, axonotemesis) and the axons regenerate, the ensuing process is considerably different, because regenerating axons are capable of reaching most of their original sensory end organs. The resulting cortical representation of the median nerve will not be substantially different from the normal representation.

If the median nerve is transected and then surgically repaired, different reorganizational changes are seen. Because of random axonal growth, most original sensory end organs will not be reinnervated by their axons. This state will result in significant reorganizational changes in the cortex, specifically restricted to those regions where input from the median nerve is normally represented. Over a long period of observation in the primate model, the cortical representation of cutaneous areas appears to change continuously. Thus, nerve transection results in both immediate and ongoing changes in the cortical maps of a cutaneous surface.

Cortical plasticity and plastic surgery

Using fMRI and TMS, the authors' group has studied cortical plasticity following motor reconstruction and rehabilitation in patients undergoing toe transfer for thumb reconstruction and free-functioning muscle transfers for upper extremity paralysis reconstruction.

Toe transfers

Traumatic amputation of the thumb has a dramatic effect on the sensorimotor cortex (SMC). In 2002, the authors described cortical changes that occurred in a case of thumb amputation and great toe transfer [62]. In this case report, serial fMRI studies obtained pre- and postoperatively examined cortical activity in the SMC of a patient who underwent a left great toe transfer for reconstruction of the right thumb. From this study, the authors gained further insight into the cortical changes that occur following successful recovery of motor and sensory function after thumb reconstruction.

The case study's subject was a 28-year-old right-hand-dominant male who sustained a severe right hand crush injury resulting in the amputation of the index finger and thumb. The right thumb was amputated through the proximal phalanx. At 15 months post-trauma, the patient underwent a left trimmed great toe transfer [Fig. 4]. Hand therapy started at 4 weeks postoperatively, and the patient performed active range of motion exercises of the thumb interphalangeal joint (IPJ) every 2 hours over the course of the next week. Table 2 describes the sensorimotor recovery in this patient. At 14 weeks, the patient reported pins-and-needles and vibration sense (256 Hz) over the ulnar aspect of the thumb. At 102 weeks, he had opposition to the tip of the small finger with minimal effort. He performed his activities of daily living requiring grip and pinch with greater ease. Bilateral tasks that had been primarily performed with the left hand were now equally shared with the right hand. By 115 weeks, the patient returned to activities that required heavy use of his right thumb.

fMRI was performed at five time points: preoperatively and at 5, 14, 102, and 115 weeks postoperatively. The motor tasks used during fMRI included self-paced tapping of the thumb and a

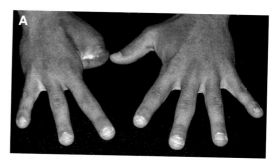
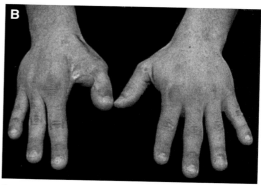

Fig. 4. Pre- and postoperative photographs of right hand. (*A*) Level of amputation of the right thumb at the proximal phalanx. A groin flap was used to provide soft tissue coverage following the initial trauma. (*B*) Right hand following transfer of the left trimmed great toe.

button-press task. The patient grasped a plastic cylindrical object with a nonmoving button at the tip. The task involved pressing the button with the thumb at a comfortable self-paced rate. The button-press task was performed for 15-second periods with intervening resting periods of 15 seconds for a total for 4 to 6 minutes. This task was performed for each thumb.

Cortical activation occurred in both the anterior and posterior banks of the central sulcus but less consistently in the SMC [Fig. 5A]. A plot of the cortical activation volume (ie, pixels) [Fig. 5B] revealed that the right thumb task produced consistently greater activation of the primary SMC contralateral to the movement than that seen with the left thumb task. For the right thumb task, a marked increase in SMC activation was observed at 5 and 14 weeks postoperatively. The activation volume then decreased below the preoperative level by 115 weeks. This pattern indicates the presence of cortical adaptation coinciding with the time of sensorimotor recovery and re-establishment of thumb function. The volume of SMC activation during the left thumb task initially decreased, com-

Table 2: Sensorimotor recovery of toe to thumb

Sensory/motor test	Postoperative week no.				
	5	14	52	102	115
Perception	Vibration	Vibration	Vibration, light touch	Vibration, light touch	Vibration, light touch
Dynamic 2-point discrimination, mm	Not tested	Not tested	>8	>8	>8
SWM, radial/ulnar	Not tested	Not tested	Not tested	4.31/4.31[a]	3.84/4.31[a]
IPJ active flexion	10	15	15	20	25
Right key pinch, kg	3.5	4.5	5.5	5.5	10
Left key pinch, kg	10	10	9	9	12

Abbreviation: SWM, Semmes Weinstein monofilament.
[a] These monofilaments are within the range of diminished protective sensation.
From Manduch M, Bezuhly M, Anastakis DJ, et al. Serial fMRI assessment of the primary motor cortex following thumb reconstruction. Neurology 2002;59(8):1279; with permission.

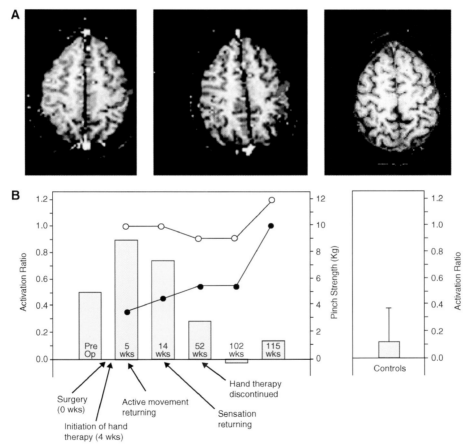

Fig. 5. Activation maps and SMC activation ratios. (*A*) Activation maps showing sequential changes (*left* = preoperative; *center* = 5 weeks postoperative; *right* = 115 weeks postoperative) in the contralateral primary somatosensory cortex during the button-press task before and after the toe-to-thumb transfer in the index case. There are well-defined clusters (*red*) of activation around the central sulcus in the cortical representation of the right upper extremity. Note the visible increase in the extent of activation in the Week 5 image (*center*). (*B*) SMC activation ratio and pinch strength in the index case at specific time points pre- and postoperatively. Right pinch strength in solid circles, left pinch strength in open circles. Mean SMC activation ratio with SE bar obtained from eight controls is shown for comparison. The early phase of recovery is characterized by increased left SMC activation coinciding with the return of active movement and sensation. During the later phase of recovery, as pinch strength normalized, SMC activation returned to control levels. (*From* Manduch M, Bezuhly M, Anastakis DJ, et al. Serial fMRI assessment of the primary motor cortex following thumb reconstruction. Neurology 2002; 59(8):1280; with permission.)

paring the preoperative and 5 weeks postoperative studies, and then consistently remained above the preoperative level. **Fig.** 5A shows that very little activation occurred in the ipsilateral SMC, suggesting a minor role for the ipsilateral cortex in motor recovery.

The trend observed in the SMC was investigated further by examining the activation ratios in the index case [see **Fig.** 5B] compared with normal controls. The ratio in the index case increased to a maximum value of 0.90 at 5 weeks postoperatively. By 52 weeks, the ratio had decreased below the preoperative level and remained there for the duration of the study. The ratios at 5 weeks and at 14 weeks represented a statistically significant increase in left SMC activation compared with the preoperative baseline study and the 1- through 2-year postoperative studies.

This study confirmed, for the first time, marked cortical plasticity observed by fMRI following a toe-to-thumb transfer over a 2-year period. The activation ratio for the SMC increased 5 to 14 weeks postoperatively and subsequently returned to the preoperative level, where it remained for the duration of the study. These changes in SMC activation correlated with specific events in the reconstruction and functional recovery of the patient's thumb, namely the return of active flexion and sensation. The ratio increase was observed 1 week following mobilization of the IPJ and the initiation of hand therapy. A number of explanations may account for this increase. It is possible that more effort was required by the recovering right hand to maintain IPJ flexion at the target pace of 1 Hz. Several investigators have demonstrated that increased activation of neurons within the SMC is necessary for an increased output to target neurons [63,64]. However, effort was likely to have played only a minor role, given that the patient reported being able to perform the motor task with minimal effort before the 5-week postoperative fMRI scan. Another possibility is that the increase in the activation ratio represents a reversal of a disuse phenomenon. Liepert and colleagues [65] reported that immobilization of the ankle resulted in reduced motor maps targeting the immobilized tibialis anterior muscle as compared with the same muscle in the active leg. The reduction in the size of the motor map correlated well with the period of immobilization and could be reversed with voluntary flexion of the immobilized joint. Zanette and colleagues [66] observed a similar finding in the upper extremity, with immobilization resulting in decreased excitability of M1. Although the muscles supplying the right thumb maintained their innervation following the trauma, they were used less preopera-

tively owing to absence of the IPJ. It may be argued that this relative disuse was subsequently reversed by the mobilization of the IPJ following the toe transfer, leading to an observed expansion of the SMC area activated with right IPJ flexion.

The increase in the activation ratio may have involved motor learning. Classen and colleagues [67] have observed that practiced movements involving a number of digits are encoded as a single cortical network and do not activate distinct networks representing each of the fingers. In this study, although the thumb may have been reconstructed, the persistent absence of the right index finger may have required that the seemingly simple motor task be effectively relearned. The observed increase in SMC activation with right IPJ flexion may thus have represented the expansion of the cortical representation of the trained sequence in motor related areas, namely those for the thumb and middle fingers. This explanation would be consistent with the initial, within-session increase in the area of SMC activation following repetition of a motor sequence that was termed "fast" learning by Karni and colleagues [68].

An elevated activation ratio was still observed at 14 weeks postoperatively. This persistent elevation of the ratio over the course of several weeks may have been the result of "slow" learning. Alternatively, the increase in the ratio may be explained by the return of vibration and pressure sensation to the transferred thumb at this time. With activation of cutaneous afferents from the thumb during task performance, a more extensive activation of the sensory neuron pool of the SMC would be expected. Because of the limited resolution of fMRI in distinguishing S1 and M1, especially as they merge indistinctly at the bottom of the central sulcus, it was not possible to segregate activation between M1 and S1. This phenomenon would have led to an apparent increase in the extent of SMC activation with the return of sensation. An alternative mechanism for the sensory involvement has been suggested by the TMS work of Rossini and colleagues [69]. They showed that the motor map of the first dorsal interosseous was reduced in size during a radial and median nerve anesthetic block that completely deprived the muscle of its cutaneous sensory information, even though it maintained its usual proprioceptive feedback and strength through the ulnar nerve. The work of Rossini and colleagues suggests that somatosensory input may be capable of modulating cortical motor outputs in humans. By extension, the elevated activation ratio observed at 14 weeks postoperatively may be the result of direct cutaneous input from the thumb modulating M1.

Motor learning offers a possible explanation for the decreased area of activation observed. With months of practice, a specific pool of neuronal connections are strengthened, leading to a reduction in the number of neurons needed to perform what was previously a complex task, not unlike the example of a piano player who practices a complex sequence of finger movements [70]. The work of Stefan and colleagues [71] has suggested a possible mechanism by which the selection of specific neuronal connections occurs during acquisition of a motor skill. In their experimental protocol, TMS of the first digital nerve was paired with stimulation of the ipsilateral abductor pollicis brevis. They found that the paired associative stimulation led to long-term potentiation of the cortical representation of the abductor pollicis brevis. This theory suggesting "network pruning" appears to agree with the authors' findings that the drop in the activation ratio to levels seen in the control group occurred following the return of sensation to the reconstructed thumb. We can therefore hypothesize that increased activation in the SMC was the result of a learning-related generalized decrease in cortical inhibition, with network recruitment associated with increased cortical excitability. As the patient's sensory perception improved and motor proficiency increased, network pruning and consolidation occurred, the learning phase was completed, and cortical excitability returned to normal. Future work studying multiple toe transfer patients with both fMRI and TMS is currently under way to assess this and other theories.

Changes in M1 contralateral to the reconstructed hand that correlated with specific events in the recovery of the reconstructed thumb were observed throughout the 2-year postoperative period [Box 1]. The results of this study suggest that somatosensory input may play an important role in the modulation of motor plasticity and thus warrants further investigation. If functional gain and motor cortical reorganization are indeed dependent on inputs such as cutaneous afferents, sensory re-education may not only be important in the recovery of protective sensation but may also play a role in optimizing gains in motor function following reconstruction of the upper extremity. The temporal pattern of activation observed in the index case may in fact represent a "signature" of good functional recovery. Reconstructive failures that occur despite physically and electrophysiologically intact neuromuscular connections in the periphery might be explainable by the lack of cortical sensorimotor network recruitment observed in this study (ie, a "central"

Box 1: Key points following toe transfer

Somatosensory input may play an important role in the modulation of motor plasticity.

Sensory re-education may also play a role in optimizing gains in motor function following reconstruction of the upper extremity.

Temporal pattern of activation observed in the index case may in fact represent a "signature" of good functional recovery.

Reconstructive failures may be due to maladaptive plasticity in which there is a lack of cortical sensorimotor network recruitment, indicating a "central" mechanism of treatment failure.

fMRI may become an important tool for assessing these failures and may eventually become useful for optimizing rehabilitation strategies.

---

mechanism of treatment failure). This work indicates that fMRI may become an important tool for assessing these failures and may eventually be used to optimize rehabilitation strategies. Confirmation of this capability will require the assessment of additional surgical successes as well as failures.

Free-functioning muscle transfers

Although motor system plasticity in response to peripheral injury has been documented, few studies have examined recovered and functioning muscles in the human. Free-functioning muscle transfer (FFMT) patients present a unique opportunity to examine motor system plasticity and recovery in functioning muscles. FFMT are able to restore motor function in selected patients with severe neuromuscular injury [72,73]. They can restore the following movements: shoulder flexion, elbow flexion, elbow extension, finger flexion, and extension. In most cases, the gracilis muscle is reinnervated using a motor nerve of the upper extremity. In cases of complete brachial plexus avulsion with no available nerves in the paralyzed upper extremity, motor nerves outside the brachial plexus may be used to innervate the transferred muscle. The most common nerves used in this situation are the intercostal nerves. Each FFMT patient has had a period of motor paralysis followed by restoration of movement. Adaptive changes in the motor system must occur after FFMT, and these changes could be related to time after surgery and motor outcome.

Table 3: **Clinical information for free-functioning muscle transfer study patients**

Patient	Age/Sex	Hand dominance	Injury	Time since surgery	Target muscle	Donor nerve	Muscle power and outcome
1	17 M	Right	C5,6,7 root avulsion	4 months	R biceps	Intercostal nerves 2, 3	M3 fair
2	42 M	Right	Crush injury[a]	17 years	L biceps	Musculocutaneous[b]	M4 successful
3	47 M	Left	Crush injury	15 years	R finger flexors	Anterior interosseous	M4 successful
4	41 M	Right	Crush injury	23 years	R finger flexors	Anterior interosseous	M4 successful
5	50 M	Right	Crush injury	15 years	L finger flexors	Anterior interosseous	M4 successful
6	30 F	Left	Crush injury	8 years	R finger flexors	Anterior interosseous	M4 successful
7	27 F	Right	Tumor resection (sarcoma)	8 years	R deltoid	Axillary	M4 successful
8	21 F	Right	Atrophic deltoid[c]	1.25 years	R deltoid	Musculocutaneous[d]	M3 fair
9	32 M	Right	Laceration/trauma	6 years	R triceps	Axillary	M4 successful

[a] Crush injury involves significant trauma to the upper extremity with functional muscle loss.
[b] Awake nerve stimulation was used to differentiate sensory from motor nerve fibers within the musculocutaneous nerve to provide motor supply for the gracilis muscle transfer.
[c] Complete deltoid paralysis — etiology idiopathic.
[d] Motor branches to the brachialis were sacrificed and dissected proximally to provide motor supply for the gracilis muscle transfer.

From Chen R, Anastakis DJ, Haywood CT, et al. Plasticity of the human motor system following muscle reconstruction: a magnetic stimulation and fMRI study. Clin Neurophysiol 2003;114(12):2435; with permission.

In a study by the authors' group, TMS and fMRI were used to study a unique group of nine patients who had upper extremity motor function restored using microneurovascular transfer of the gracilis muscle [74]. The clinical information and out-comes for the nine patients are summarized in Table 3. Changes in the primary SMC contralateral to the reconstructed limb were observed and are described in Box 2. TMS showed that the MT [Fig. 6] and SICI [Fig. 7] were reduced on the transplanted side while at rest but not during muscle activation. The difference in MT decreased with the time since surgery. MEP amplitudes were higher on the intact than on the FFMT side [Fig. 8]. TMS mapping showed no significant difference in the location and size of the representation of the reconstructed muscle in the motor cortex com-pared with the intact side or with normal subjects [Fig. 9].

The authors used TMS to study motor system reorganization following FFMT and found evi-dence of plasticity in the motor projection to func-tioning muscles. The reduced rest MT and SICI on the reconstructed side compared with the intact side is similar to the changes following lower ex-tremity amputation [56]. SICI may be enhanced by drugs that increase $GABA_A$ activity [36] and by antiglutaminergic drugs [75,76]. These finding are consistent with the hypothesis that motor cor-

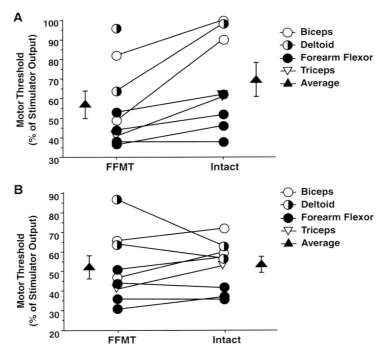

Fig. 6. Motor thresholds of FFMT. Rest and active MTs from TMS. There was a large between-subject variation, in part because the authors studied different muscles. As expected, forearm flexors tended to have lower MT than more proximal muscles. In one patient, the rest MT on the intact side was higher than maximum stimu-lator output. (*A*) The rest MT was lower on the FFMT side (56 ± 6.9%) than on the intact side (68.4 ± 8.6%) in all nine patients ($P = .001$). (*B*) However, the active MT was similar on the two sides (FFMT 51.9 ± 5.9%, intact 53.1 ± 4.1%). (*Modified from* Chen R, Anastakis DJ, Haywood CT, et al. Plasticity of the human motor system following muscle reconstruction: a magnetic stimulation and fMRI study. Clin Neurophysiol 2003;114(12):2438; with permission.)

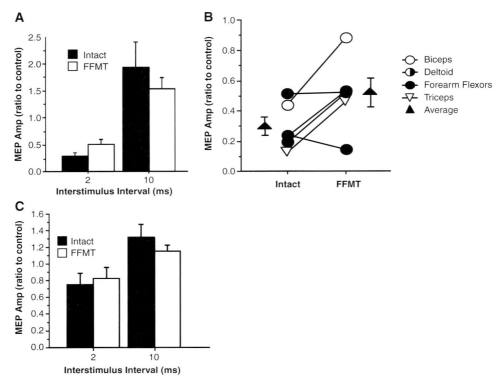

Fig. 7. SICI and ICF. Resting SICI and ICF in the six patients tested is shown in (*A*). The SICI was significantly reduced on the FFMT side (*P* = .05) (*A,B*), but the ICF did not differ significantly. SICI and ICF during voluntary contraction were tested in all nine patients (*C*). SICI and ICF were reduced compared with rest, but there was no significant difference between the FFMT and intact sides. (*From* Chen R, Anastakis DJ, Haywood CT, et al. Plasticity of the human motor system following muscle reconstruction: a magnetic stimulation and fMRI study. Clin Neurophysiol 2003;114(12):2440; with permission.)

tex plasticity may involve adjustment of balance between inhibition and facilitation in the intrinsic horizontal connections mediated by GABA-ergic and glutaminergic mechanisms [77,78]. However, other mechanisms, such as long-term potentiation [79] and axonal sprouting with formation of new synapses [80], may also contribute to cortical plasticity [77].

The authors found no change in the motor representation of the target muscle following FFMT with TMS mapping. This result indicates that alterations in the neuronal level, as demonstrated by changes in SICI and MT, are not necessarily accompanied by changes in the motor representational level. The changes following FFMT are different from the expansion and shift of motor representation following nerve injury or amputation in animals [39–41,81] and humans [42–47] and following hand replantation in humans [48]. Following peripheral nerve injury, amputation, and even hand replantation, large areas of the body are deafferentated. FFMT procedures do not lead

to significant deafferentation because the authors strived to use a predominantly motor donor nerve, although some patients had a small degree of deafferentation due to other nerve injuries. Deafferentation may be necessary for shift and expansion of motor representation to occur.

The change in MT and SICI following FFMT was evident only with the muscle relaxed and not during voluntary contraction. The need precisely to control the excitability of cortical neurons to perform specific voluntary activity may account for the absence of significant change during voluntary activation. Similar observations have been made in other settings of cortical plasticity. Reduced MT and SICI in the motor cortex may make it easier to activate corticospinal neurons to produce voluntary activity with less excitatory synaptic drive. This possibility is supported by the progressive reduction in SICI just before voluntary movement [82] and the finding that forearm deafferentation leads to faster elbow flexion movement [83].

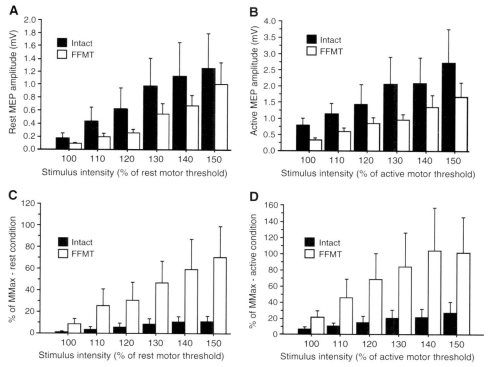

Fig. 8. MEP recruitment. (*A*) and (*B*) show the MEP amplitudes at different stimulus intensities. The effects of side (FFMT versus intact) (*P* = .04 rest, *P* = .005 active) and stimulus intensity (*P* < .0001) were significant for both the rest and active conditions, but their interaction was not significant. MEP amplitudes were higher on the intact than the FFMT side. (*C*) and (*D*) show the %MMax (MEP/MMax) recruited at different stimulus intensities. The %MMax recruited was higher for the FFMT side than the intact side. The effects of side (*P* = .0004 rest, *P* = .002 active) and stimulus intensity (*P* = .005 rest, *P* = .02 active) were significant for both the rest and active conditions, and their interaction was not significant. The %MMax was higher on the FFMT than the intact side. (*From* Chen R, Anastakis DJ, Haywood CT, et al. Plasticity of the human motor system following muscle reconstruction: a magnetic stimulation and fMRI study. Clin Neurophysiol 2003;114(12):2439; with permission.)

Although the motor outcome of FFMT improved with time, the change in rest MT diminished, suggesting that the maximum change in MT probably occurred early. Change in MT may represent one step in motor reorganization that involves various mechanisms at different times. It appears likely that the motor reorganization continues to evolve and may be modified by training and experience long after the muscle reconstruction procedure. The reduced MT may also be a compensatory mechanism for deficits in peripheral innervation that improved with time.

Although changes in MT and SICI have been demonstrated in muscles proximal to transient deafferentation or amputation, the authors' results show that these changes occur in functioning muscles. Successful outcome following FFMT probably requires adaptive changes in the central nervous system, because the movement mediated by the transferred muscle is often different from that mediated by the donor nerve and because of the random nature of axonal regeneration from the proximal stump into the distal pathways. Clinical experience suggests that a period of rehabilitation and retraining is necessary for successful outcome, and there is evidence that cortical plasticity occurs with motor learning.

The authors' result demonstrated plasticity in cortical areas projecting to functionally relevant muscles. The mechanisms may include changes in membrane excitability and reduction in intracortical inhibition. Changes in the neuronal level are not necessarily accompanied by changes in motor representation. Brain reorganization may involve multiple processes mediated by different mechanisms and continues to evolve long after a static injury.

One patient in the authors' study differed from the other eight patients because the donor intercostal nerve originally innervated truncal muscles

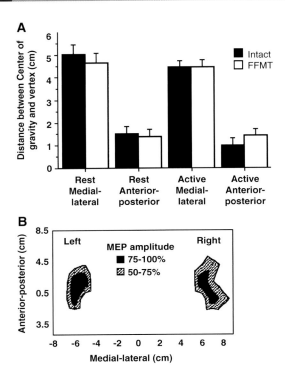

A

B

Fig. 9. TMS mapping. (*A*) TMS mapping at rest was performed in six patients and in all nine patients during voluntary contraction. The location of the center of gravity and the size of the motor map were similar on the FFMT and the intact sides. (*B*) Patient 1, who had FFMT with the right biceps muscle innervated by the intercostal nerves, also showed similar map location and size on the two sides. (*From* Chen R, Anastakis DJ, Haywood CT, et al. Plasticity of the human motor system following muscle reconstruction: a magnetic stimulation and fMRI study. Clin Neurophysiol 2003;114(12):2441; with permission.)

rather than the upper extremity muscles. Therefore, additional studies were performed in this patient. Surface EMG recordings showed rhythmic activity in the intercostal muscle and no activity in the reconstructed biceps during both normal breathing and voluntary breathing at maximum effort. With the biceps activated at maximum effort, there was no activity in the intercostal muscles. Volitional breathing before FFMT operation activated M1 medial to the upper extremity area [Fig. 10A] but not the upper extremity area. Six months after FFMT, the patient was able voluntarily to contract the reconstructed right biceps innervated by the intercostal nerves and had antigravity strength. Right elbow flexion activated the upper extremity area of the left M1 [Figs. 10B, C], similar to activation of the right M1 with movement of the intact left biceps [Figs. 10D, E].

In a finding similar to those of previous studies [84,85], volitional inspiration before the FFMT activated the M1 medial to the upper extremity area. Six months after the FFMT procedure, TMS mapping [see Fig. 9] and fMRI [see Fig. 10] showed that the control of motor neurons that originally innervated the intercostal muscles (in the T2 and T3 spinal levels) had shifted to the upper extremity area of the motor cortex. These results are similar to that of Mano and colleagues [86], who reported that, following coaptation of the musculocutaneous and intercostal nerves for treatment of cervical root avulsion, TMS mapping showed that cortical representation for the biceps was initially located in the areas of the intercostal muscles. It gradually moved laterally to the upper extremity area as the patients gained voluntary control of the biceps muscle. Thus, the adult human motor cortex is capable of large-scale reorganization.

Summary

Today's view of the adult central nervous system is that of an adaptive and responsive system. Cortical plasticity occurs in the sensorimotor cortex in response to anything from learning to use a new thumb following great toe transfer to flexing the elbow with an FFMT. At the onset of learning a new motor skill, there is an expansion of motor cortical representation. In addition, there is increased excitability and decreased intracortical inhibition. This phenomenon may represent a "priming" of the cortex to learn a new motor skill. As the patient practices the motor skill, there is an increase in the amount of cortical representation. Motor learning offers a possible explanation for the increased area of activation observed. These changes in cortical representation are correlated with specific events in the reconstruction, rehabilitation, and functional recovery. As the skill is mastered, the degrees of cortical representation and excitability decrease and approach normal levels. Repetition and practice are considered important elements in facilitating motor learning and, ultimately, the cortical plasticity seen as a skill is mastered. In addition, motor reorganization continues to evolve and may be modified by training and experience long after reconstruction. There may be inherent value in increasing the duration of therapy well beyond 2 years after reconstruction to facilitate ongoing cortical plasticity and ultimately improve functional outcome.

Studies suggest that sensory input is important in the modulation of cortical plasticity during motor learning. Ensuring optimal sensory function

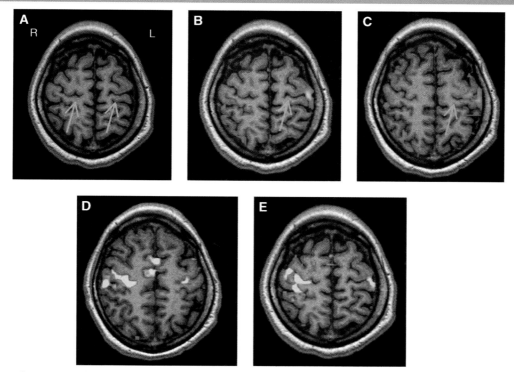

Fig. 10. fMRI studies following intercostal nerve transfer to gracilis for biceps reconstruction. fMRI color maps for Patient 1 showing areas of task-related cortical activation. (*A*) Activation (*blue arrows*) in the medial aspect of both primary motor cortices during volitional breathing. (*B,C*) Activation maps in the same patient 6 months following surgery using the right biceps muscle transfer to restore elbow flexion. The patient was performing low amplitude elbow flexion using the intercostal nerves. The cortical areas activated are located in the primary motor cortex controlling upper extremity movement. They are clearly separate from the area activated by volitional breathing seen in (*A*) (*blue arrows*). (*D,E*) Cortical activation during flexion of the normal left elbow. The areas activated are in similar locations (laterality) along the motor cortex for each extremity. (*From* Chen R, Anastakis DJ, Haywood CT, et al. Plasticity of the human motor system following muscle reconstruction: a magnetic stimulation and fMRI study. Clin Neurophysiol 2003;114(12):2443; with permission.)

before motor reconstruction may be an important aspect to consider in the reconstructive plans for patients with combined motor and sensory deficits. One may speculate that the absence of sensory input contributes to aberrant cortical plasticity during motor relearning, ultimately affecting functional outcomes. Hence, efforts should be made to restore sensory function in advance of motor reconstruction.

Plastic surgeons are familiar with less than ideal functional results following motor reconstruction. If functional gain and motor cortical reorganization are indeed dependent on inputs such as cutaneous afferents, sensory re-education may not only be important in the recovery of protective sensation but may also play a role in optimizing gains in motor function following reconstruction of the upper extremity. The temporal pattern of activation observed in the toe transfer case may in fact represent a "signature" of good functional recovery. Reconstructive failures that occur despite physically

and electrophysiologically intact neuromuscular connections in the periphery might be explainable by a lack of cortical sensorimotor network recruitment. That is, there may be a "central" mechanism of treatment failure. Absence of this signature may indicate maladaptive plasticity. At this time, these observations remain speculative. This work shows that fMRI may become an important tool for assessing these failures and may eventually become useful for optimizing rehabilitation strategies.

The primary motor cortex can allocate areas to represent the particular motor tasks that are proportionally most used. The principles governing cortical representational plasticity following manipulations of inputs, including learning, are increasingly understood to rely on the more elementary rules of synaptic plasticity. Steps have been taken toward defining the molecular mechanisms underlying these fundamental plasticity processes and their induction. Today the challenge facing investigators is to link the fields of cortical map plasticity and cortical synaptic plasticity. Although great strides have been made, many initial findings remain to be elaborated. A complete understanding of the mechanisms underlying motor cortical plasticity holds the possibility of establishing effective recovery strategies following brain injury in humans. The modulation of cortical excitability may someday be used to facilitate plasticity when it is beneficial or suppress it when it is maladaptive.

Plasticity, the brain's ability to learn a new motor skill, will become an important factor in terms of functional recovery following reconstructive surgery. Brain plasticity occurs throughout the neuraxis. In the future, surgeons may work with neuroscientists to establish a patient's ability to learn a new motor skill following reconstruction. We may see the augmentation of cortical plasticity through pharmacologic manipulation (ie, priming the brain's ability to learn a new motor skill). Further investigations into the cortical plasticity that appears during both motor and sensory recovery will affect the timing and types of rehabilitation strategies used. In the future, cortical plasticity and its manipulation may be an important contributor to functional outcome following reconstruction.

Acknowledgments

The authors acknowledge the work carried out by Ms. Camillia Matuk in the preparation of the homunculus used in this manuscript.

References

[1] Lundborg G. Brain plasticity and hand surgery: an overview. J Hand Surg [Br] 2000;25(3):242–52.

[2] Woolf CJ, Salter MW. Neuroscience—neuronal plasticity: increasing the gain in pain. Science 2000;288(5472):1765–8.

[3] Anwyl R. Metabotropic glutamate receptors: electrophysiological properties and role in plasticity. Brain Res Rev 1999;29(1):83–120.

[4] McAllister K, Katz LC, Lo DC. Neurotrophins and synaptic plasticity. Annu Rev Neurosci 1999;22: 295–318.

[5] Byrne JH. Synapses—plastic plasticity. Nature 1997;389:791–2.

[6] Pascual-Leone A, Grafman J, Hallett M. Modulation of cortical motor output maps during development of implicit and explicit knowledge. Science 1994;263:1287–9.

[7] Karni A, Meyer G, Jezzard P, et al. Functional MRI evidence for adult motor cortex plasticity during motor skill learning. Nature 1995;377:155–8.

[8] Pascual-Leone A, Nguyet D, Cohen LG, et al. Modulation of muscle responses evoked by

[9] Nudo RJ, Milliken GW, Jenkins WM, et al. Use-dependent alterations of movement representations in primary motor cortex of adult squirrel monkeys. J Neurosci 1996;16:785–807.

[10] Classen J, Liepert A, Wise SP, et al. Rapid plasticity in human cortical movement representation induced by practice. J Neurophysiol 1998; 79:1117–23.

[11] Elbert T, Pantev C, Wienbruch C, et al. Increased cortical representation of the fingers of the left hand in string players. Science 1995;270: 305–7.

[12] Pascual-Leone A, Torres F. Plasticity of the sensorimotor cortex representation of the reading finger in Braille readers. Brain 1993;116: 39–52.

[13] Hallett M. Transcranial magnetic stimulation and the human brain. Nature 2000;406:147–50.

[14] Chen R. Studies of human motor physiology with transcranial magnetic stimulation. Muscle Nerve 2000;9:S26–32.

[15] Barker AT, Jalinous R, Freeston IL. Noninvasive magnetic stimulation of human motor cortex. Lancet 1985;1:1106–7.

[16] Gevins A, Leong H, Smith ME, et al. Mapping cognitive brain function with modern high-resolution electroencephalography regional modulation of high resolution evoked potentials during verbal and non-verbal matching tasks. Trends Neurosci 1995;18:429–36.

[17] Ogawa S, Tank DW, Menon R, et al. Intrinsic signal changes accompanying sensory stimulation: functional brain mapping with magnetic resonance imaging. Proc Natl Acad Sci USA 1992; 13:5951–5.

[18] Ogawa S, Lee TM, Kay AR, et al. Brain magnetic resonance imaging with contrast dependent on blood oxygenation. Proc Natl Acad Sci USA 1990;87:9868–72.

[19] Davis TL, Kwong KK, Weissfoff RM, et al. Calibrated fMRI: mapping the dynamics of oxidative metabolism. Proc Natl Acad Sci USA 1998; 95(4):1834–9.

[20] Kwong KK, Belliveau JW, Chesler DA, et al. Dynamic MRI of human brain activity during primary sensory stimulation. Proc Natl Acad Sci USA 1992;89:5675–9.

[21] Cohen MS, Bookheimer SY. Localization of brain function using magnetic resonance imaging. Trends Neurosci 1994;17:268–76.

[22] Crease RP. Biomedicine in the age of imaging. Science 1993;261:554–61.

[23] DeYoe EA, Bandettini P, Neitz J, et al. Functional magnetic resonance imaging (fMRI) of the human brain. J Neurosci Methods 1994;54:171–87.

[24] Cohen LG, Bandinelli S, Topka HR, et al. Topographic maps of human motor cortex in normal and pathological conditions: mirror movements, amputations and spinal cord injuries. Electro-

transcranial magnetic stimulation during the acquisition of new fine motor skills. J Neurophysiol 1995;74:1037–45.

encephalogr Clin Neurophysiol 1991;43(Suppl): 36–50.

[25] Brasil-Neto JP, Cohen LG, Panizza M, et al. Optimal focal transcranial magnetic activation of the human motor cortex: effects of coil orientation, shape of the induced current pulse, and stimulus intensity. J Clin Neurophysiol 1992;9: 132–6.

[26] Cohen LG, Gerloff C, Faiz L, et al. Directional modulation of motor cortex plasticity induced by synchronicity of motor outputs in humans. Abstr Soc Neurosci 1996;22:1452.

[27] Gevins A, Brickett P, Costales B, et al. Beyond topographic mapping: towards functional-anatomical imaging with 124-channel EEGs and 3-D MRIs. Brain Topogr 1990;3:53–64.

[28] Wasserman EM, Wang W, Zeffiro TA, et al. Locating the motor cortex on the MRI with transcranial magnetic stimulation and PET. Neuroimage 1996;3:1–6.

[29] Chen R, Samii A, Caños M, et al. Effects of phenytoin on cortical excitability. Neurology 1997; 49:881–3.

[30] Mavroudakis N, Caroyer JM, Brunko E, et al. Effects of diphenylhydantoin on motor potentials evoked with magnetic stimulation. Electroencephalogr Clin Neurophysiol 1994;93:428–33.

[31] Chen R. Interactions between inhibitory and excitatory circuits in the human motor cortex. Exp Brain Res 2004;154:1–10.

[32] Kujirai T, Caramia MD, Rothwell JC, et al. Corticocortical inhibition in human motor cortex. J Physiol 1993;471:501–19.

[33] Ridding MC, Taylor JL, Rothwell JC. The effect of voluntary contraction on cortico-cortical inhibition in human motor cortex. J Physiol 1995;487: 541–8.

[34] Ridding MC, Inzelberg R, Rothwell JC. Changes in excitability of motor cortical circuitry in patients with Parkinson's disease. Ann Neurol 1995;37:181–8.

[35] Daskalakis ZJ, Christensen BK, Chen R, et al. Evidence for impaired cortical inhibition in schizophrenia using transcranial magnetic stimulation. Arch Gen Psychiatry 2002;59:347–54.

[36] Ziemann U, Lönnecker S, Steinhoff BJ, et al. Effects of antiepileptic drugs on motor cortex excitability in humans: a transcranial magnetic stimulation study. Ann Neurol 1996;40:367–78.

[37] Hanajima R, Ugawa Y, Terao Y, et al. Paired-pulse magnetic stimulation of the human motor cortex: differences among I waves. J Physiol 1998;509:607–18.

[38] Sanger TD, Garg RR, Chen R. Interactions between two different inhibitory systems in the human motor cortex. J Physiol 2001;530:307–17.

[39] Donoghue JP, Suner S, Sanes JN. Dynamic organization of primary motor cortex output to target muscles in adult rat. II. Rapid reorganization following motor nerve lesions. Exp Brain Res 1990;79:492–503.

[40] Schieber MH, Deuel RK. Primary motor cortex reorganization in a long-term monkey amputee. Somatosens Mot Res 1997;14:157–67.

[41] Wu CW, Kaas JH. Reorganization in primary motor cortex of primates with long-standing therapeutic amputations. J Neurosci 1999;19: 7679–97.

[42] Cohen LG, Bandinelli S, Findley TW, et al. Motor reorganization after upper extremity amputation in man. Brain 1991;114:615–27.

[43] Kew JJM, Ridding MC, Rothwell JC, et al. Reorganization of cortical blood flow and transcranial magnetic stimulation maps in human subjects after upper extremity amputation. J Neurophysiol 1994;72:2517–24.

[44] Pascual-Leone A, Peris M, Tormos JM, et al. Reorganization of human cortical motor output maps following traumatic forearm amputation. Neuroreport 1996;7:2068–70.

[45] Ridding MC, Rothwell JC. Stimulus/response curves as a method of measuring motor cortical excitability in man. Electroencephalogr Clin Neurophysiol 1997;105:340–4.

[46] Roricht S, Meyer BU, Niehaus L, et al. Long-term reorganization of motor cortex outputs after arm amputation. Neurology 1999;53:106–11.

[47] Dettmers C, Liepert J, Adler T, et al. Abnormal motor cortex organization contralateral to early upper extremity amputation in humans. Neurosci Lett 1999;263:41–4.

[48] Roricht S, Machetanz J, Irlbacher K, et al. Reorganization of human motor cortex after hand replantation. Ann Neurol 2001;50:240–9.

[49] Yang TT, Gallen CC, Rivlin AS, et al. Effect of duration of acute spinal cord compression in a new acute cord injury model in the rat. Surg Neurol 1978;10:39–43.

[50] Yang TT, Gallen CC, Ramachandran V, et al. Noninvasive detection of cerebral plasticity in adult human somatosensory cortex. Neuroreport 1994;5:701–4.

[51] Gilbert CD, Wiesel TN. Receptive field dynamics in adult primary visual cortex. Nature 1992;356: 150–2.

[52] Merzenich MM, Nelson RJ, Stryker MP, et al. Somatosensory cortical map changes following digital amputation in adult monkeys. J Comp Neurol 1984;224:591–605.

[53] Pons TP, Garraghty PE, Ommaya AK, et al. Massive cortical reorganization after sensory deafferentation in adult macaques. Science 1991; 252:1857–60.

[54] Rasmusson DD, Turnbull BG, Leech CK. Unexpected reorganization of somatosensory cortex in a raccoon with extensive foreextremity loss. Neurosci Lett 1985;55:167–72.

[55] Borsook D, Becerra L, Fishman S, et al. Acute plasticity in the human somatosensory cortex following amputation. Neuroreport 1998;9: 1013–7.

[56] Chen R, Corwell B, Yaseen Z, et al. Mechanisms of cortical reorganization in lower-extremity amputees. J Neurosci 1998;18:3443–50.

[57] Ridding MC, Rothwell JC. Reorganization in human motor cortex. Can J Physiol Pharmacol 1995;73:218–22.

[58] Flor H, Elbert T, Knecht S, et al. Phantom-extremity pain as a perceptual correlate of cortical reorganization following arm amputation. Nature 1995;375:482–4.

[59] Garraghty LB, Muja N. NMDA receptors and plasticity in adult primate somatosensory cortex. J Comp Neurol 1996;367:19–26.

[60] Merzenich MM, Jenkins WM. Reorganization of cortical representations of the hand following alterations of skin inputs induced by nerve injury, skin island transfers and experience. J Hand Ther 1993;6:89–104.

[61] Wall JT, Kaas JH, Sur M, et al. Functional reorganization in somatosensory cortical areas 3b and 1 of adult monkeys after median nerve repair: possible relationships to sensory recovery in humans. J Neurosci 1986;6:218–33.

[62] Manduch M, Bezuhly M, Anastakis DJ, et al. Serial fMRI assessment of the primary motor cortex following thumb reconstruction. Neurology 2002;59(8):1278–81.

[63] Schlaug G, Sanes JN, Thangaraj V, et al. Cerebral activation varies with movement rate. Neuroreport 1996;7:879–83.

[64] Wexler BE, Fulbright RK, Lacadie CM, et al. An fMRI study of the human cortical motor system response to increasing functional demands. Magn Reson Imaging 1997;15:385–96.

[65] Liepert J, Tegenthoff M, Malin JP. Changes of cortical motor area size during immobilization. Electroencephalogr Clin Neurophysiol 1995;97:382–6.

[66] Zanette G, Tinazzi M, Bonato C, et al. Reversible changes of motor cortical outputs following immobilization of the upper extremity. Electroencephalogr Clin Neurophysiol 1997;105:269–79.

[67] Classen J, Liepert A, Hallett M, et al. Use-dependent modulation of movement representation in the human motor cortex. Abstr Soc Neurosci 1996;22:1452.

[68] Karni A, Meyer G, Rey-Hipolito C, et al. The acquisition of skilled motor performance: fast and slow experience-driven changes in primary motor cortex. Proc Natl Acad Sci USA 1998;95:861–8.

[69] Rossini PM, Rossi S, Tecchio F, et al. Focal brain stimulation in healthy humans: motor map changes following partial hand sensory deprivation. Neurosci Lett 1996;214:91–5.

[70] Krings T, Topper R, Foltys H, et al. Cortical activation patterns during complex motor tasks in piano players and control subjects. A functional magnetic resonance imaging study. Neurosci Lett 2000;278:189–93.

[71] Stefan K, Kunesch E, Cohen LG, et al. Induction of plasticity in the human motor cortex by paired associative stimulation. Brain 2000;123:572–84.

[72] Manktelow RT, Zuker RM. The principles of functioning muscle transplantation: applications to the upper arm. Ann Plast Surg 1989;22:275–82.

[73] Manktelow RT, Anastakis DJ. Functioning free muscle transfer. In: Green DP, Hotchkiss RN, Pederson WC, editors. Green's operative hand surgery. New York: Churchill Livingstone; 1999. p. 1201–19.

[74] Chen R, Anastakis DJ, Haywood CT, et al. Plasticity of the human motor system following muscle reconstruction: a magnetic stimulation and fMRI study. Clin Neurophysiol 2003; 114(12):2434–46.

[75] Liepert J, Schwenkreis P, Tegenthoff M, et al. The glutamate antagonist riluzole suppresses intracortical facilitation. J Neural Transm 1997;104:1207–14.

[76] Ziemann U, Chen R, Cohen LG, et al. Dextromethorphan decreases the excitability of the human motor cortex. Neurology 1998;51:1320–4.

[77] Jacobs K, Donoghue J. Reshaping the cortical map by unmasking latent intracortical connections. Science 1991;251:944–7.

[78] Sanes JN, Donoghue JP. Plasticity and primary motor cortex. Annu Rev Neurosci 2000; 23:393–415.

[79] Hess G, Donoghue JP. Long-term potentiation of horizontal connections provides a mechanism to reorganize cortical maps. J Neurophysiol 1994;71:2543–7.

[80] Jones TA, Schallert T. Use-dependent growth of pyramidal neurons after neocortical damage. J Neurosci 1994;14:2140–52.

[81] Sanes JN, Suner S, Donoghue JP. Dynamic organization of primary motor cortex output to target muscle in adult rats. I. Long-term patterns of reorganization following motor or mixed peripheral nerve lesion. Exp Brain Res 1990;79:479–91.

[82] Reynolds C, Ashby P. Inhibition in the human motor cortex is reduced just before a voluntary contraction. Neurology 1999;53:730–5.

[83] Ziemann U, Muellbacher W, Hallett M, et al. Modulation of practice-dependent plasticity in human motor cortex. Brain 2001;124:1171–81.

[84] Colebatch JG, Adams L, Murphy K, et al. Regional cerebral blood flow during volitional breathing in man. J Physiol 1991;443:91–103.

[85] Evans KC, Shea SA, Saykin AJ. Functional MRI localisation of central nervous system regions associated with volitional inspiration in humans. J Physiol (Lond) 1999;520:383–92.

[86] Mano Y, Nakamuro T, Tamura R, et al. Central motor reorganization after anastomosis of the musculocutaneous and intercostal nerves following cervical root avulsion. Ann Neurol 1995; 38:15–20.

CLINICS IN
PLASTIC
SURGERY

Clin Plastic Surg 32 (2005) 635–641

ELSEVIER
SAUNDERS

Possible Uses of Computer Modeling of the Functioning Human Hand

Nancy H. McKee, MD[a],*, Anne M.R. Agur, PhD[a,b],
Winnie Tsang, MSc[c], Karan S. Singh, PhD[c]

- Standing on the shoulders of others
- The "helping hand": a functional three-dimensional model
- Possible uses of computer models of a functioning hand
  Gesturing: improving the understanding and ability to document deficits
  Coordination and discoordination exploration
  Injury exploration: nerve, tendon, or muscle

  Reconstructive analysis
  Therapeutic modalities of integrating muscle function
  Educational tools
  Improved understanding of the word "reconstructive"
  Contribute to science
- The future
- Acknowledgments
- References

The human hand is an awe-inspiring organ of acute sensory discrimination, dexterity, and creative expression, seamlessly capable of both gross muscular grasp and delicately fine motor control. A complete deconstruction of its development and function still awaits explication. It seems that the evolution of the hand, with its opposable thumb and lightweight, dexterous fingers, was interleaved with the move by our ancestors to bipedalism; their growing use of hand-held implements; their need to grip variably-sized objects; and the development of verbal, written, gestural, and musical communication. An exquisitely flexible, neurobiomechanical device emerged from such a multiplicity of function. As with many marvels of evolution, it is easy to ignore the importance of hands, until one sustains even the smallest injury that inhibits their form or function.

This article includes a brief description of an approach to functional limb modeling including a summary of "helping hand," a computer model created by the authors. Potential uses of three-dimensional computer modeling of hand function are presented with some illustrations relevant to clinicians.

Standing on the shoulders of others

There are many components that have been developed and incorporated into various limb-related

[a] Department of Surgery, University of Toronto, Medical Sciences Building, Room 6270, I Kings College Circle, Toronto, ON, M5S 1A8, Canada
[b] Division of Anatomy, Department of Surgery, University of Toronto, Medical Sciences Building, Room 1158, I Kings College Circle, Toronto, ON, M5S 1A8, Canada
[c] Department of Computer Science, University of Toronto, 40 St. George Street, Toronto, ON, M5S 2E4, Canada
* Corresponding author.
E-mail address: n.mckee@utoronto.ca (N.H. McKee).

doi:10.1016/j.cps.2005.07.001

models [1–5]. The challenges of creating and using accurate three-dimensional anatomic data [6,7], creating physiologically appropriate muscle contractions from detailed internal muscle architectural data [8–11], assembling muscles and tendons [5], bones and joints [12], including deformable overlying skin [13] have been tackled. Much of this can be demonstrated with Software for Interactive Musculoskeletal Modeling created by the Neuromuscular Biomechanics Laboratory at Stanford University and available through MusculoGraphics [14].

Desirable attributes for a computer model of a functioning hand include the following [15–18]:

- Forward simulation: given muscle excitations the model creates motion.
- Inverse simulation: given hand motion the model explores the possibilities of muscle excitations.
- Relevant performance ranges: explores muscles' function by controlling both neural activation and muscle contraction.
- Includes relevant physiology: models dynamic physiology (features that are time dependent) and allows relevant flexibility within interrelated functional control units (eg, for the parts of flexor digitorum profundus to the individual digits).
- Includes relevant anatomy: model incorporates in situ volumetric data of the musculotendinous components.

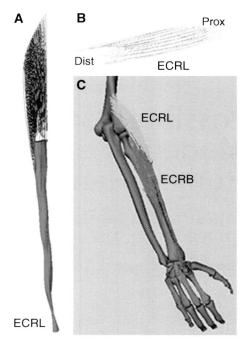

Fig. 1. Three-dimensional modelling muscle architecture. (*A*) Extensor carpi radialis longus (ECRL), posterior view. (*B*) One layer of fiber bundles in the central region of ECRL muscle belly. Prox, proximal; Dist, distal. (*C*) ECRL and ECRB (extensor carpi radialis brevis) on three-dimensional skeleton.

The "helping hand": a functional three-dimensional model

The authors have created a model with incorporation of the previously mentioned attributes [4]. The helping hand includes 42 muscles and tendons of the hand and forearm. This model can include digitized three-dimensional anatomic data from cadaveric specimens. The anatomic level of detail is unique and provides a data catalog for hand research [Figs. 1 and 2]. As currently configured the "helping hand" uses dynamic optimization to create a hand simulator [Fig. 3] that can explore hand motion with different amounts of performance of any or all of the 42 muscles [Fig. 4], and inversely to determine what muscles are used (and how vigorously) to put the fingers into specified positions [Fig. 5]. Areas of future development include incorporation of tissue properties of the musculotendinous unit, adding more aspects of muscle physiology, and verification of computer-generated muscle activation measurements by exploring muscle contractions with clinical research studies. External forces are not considered in the present model, but will be a focus of future work.

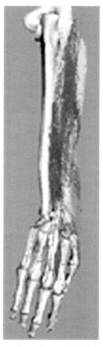

Fig. 2. Three-dimensional model of forearm extensors, posterior view. Detailed muscle fiber bundles architecture and structure tendons are included.

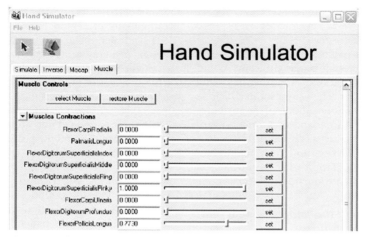

Fig. 3. Interface for keyframing musculotendinous contraction.

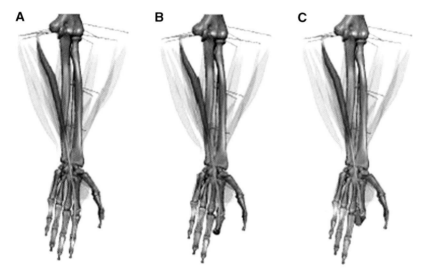

Fig. 4. (*A–C*) Helping hand model. Forward simulation sequence of contraction of the flexor digitorum superficialis of the index finger, anterior views.

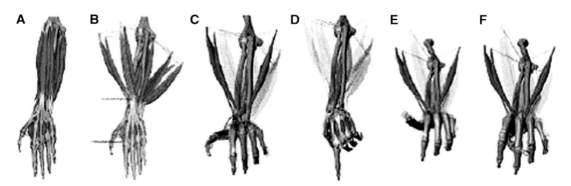

Fig. 5. Helping hand model. (*A*) Muscle in situ, posterior view. (*B*) Spreading, highlighting, and annotating selected muscles, anterior view. (*C, D*) Inverse simulation solutions to motion drills, posterior views. (*E, F*) Inverse solution to the motion capture of the letters "A" and "S" as performed in American Sign Language. A ghosted hand shows the fitting error.

Possible uses of computer models of a functioning hand

The following is an exploration of possible ways that hand surgeons and other clinicians could benefit from the capabilities of computer modeling of functional hands. The suggestions include acquiring new information about basic attributes of hands, such as gesturing and coordination; improving understanding of specific functional deficits and the reconstruction and rehabilitation of these; and the dissemination of this information created by studying hand functioning data.

Gesturing: improving the understanding and ability to document deficits

Gesturing is said to have preceded speech in the evolution of the development of communication skills [19]. The absence of spontaneous gesturing in one extremity likely stems from a change in a fundamental aspect of the human brain programming. Such an absence is usually associated with dysfunctional attempts voluntarily to use the hand. Generally, a patient is unaware of the spontaneous hand movement deficit. Gesturing could be studied by motion analysis [20] of many individuals and the data analyzed to characterize normal gesturing. Computer modeling in conjunction with clinical research tools, such as electromyogram and ultrasound, provides the necessary tools to investigate why abnormalities deviate from the normal pattern. An example of a possible hypothesis is "The inability to gesture is not just a lack of input to create a movement but frequently represents excess input to some muscles to maintain a lack of movement." In a model it is possible to simulate increased contraction of some muscles (greater than normal) that could contribute to the creation of an immobile hand that resists movement. It is also possible to increase the contraction status of some muscles (eg, extensors) and then see how much effort is needed from other muscles (eg, flexors) to create movement. Studying these possibilities through modeling could shed new light on the phrase "over-use."

Coordination and discoordination exploration

The manifestations of problems with coordination may include

- No or minimal movement
- Protective behavior of uninvolved body parts
- Extraneous muscle activity when affected part is approached or moved voluntarily
- A stiffness or rigidity where none is expected
- Jerky movement

Although dystonia is diagnosed relatively rarely, its components of central nervous system alterations [21] and peripheral manifestations are probably present in many other frustrating situations where a patient struggles excessively and abnormally to achieve a given movement. Motion analysis can help define the abnormalities and normal motion space [Fig. 6]. These specific abnormalities of positioning can be entered into an inverse simulation of a computer model and the possible combinations of muscle activations explored. Three-dimensional ultrasound could study the affected extremity in different positions and confirm which muscles are overacting. The ultrasound studies could be used to illustrate an increased level of contraction of some muscles to the patient and the computer model could then demonstrate what impact those increases have on movement and potential strategies for normalizing the movement pattern.

Injury exploration: nerve, tendon, or muscle

Motion analysis can study patients with a specific nerve injury at a specific level (eg, ulnar nerve above the elbow) and create data about the limits and range of movements with such an injury. A computer model can be set up to create lack of stimulation to the appropriate muscles and then demonstrate how specific movements of the joints might be achieved. New understandings of muscle innervation and function would result from such studies. A more precise evaluation could be made of an individual's deficits.

Reconstructive analysis

Tendon transfers [22] and free-functioning muscle operations [23] can be planned and explored on a model that mimicked the deficit of an individual patient. Actual motion analysis data can quantify the

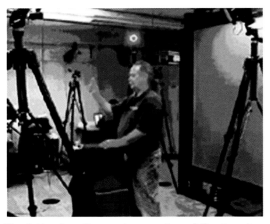

Fig. 6. Hand motion capture session of the American Sign Language.

deficits in unconstrained hand motion of a hand being considered for treatment. This can be supplemented with three-dimensional imaging providing information on which muscles can contract. Using forward simulation with this clinically acquired information as inputs, a computer model can show possible movements. Reconstructive efforts can be superimposed and then modeled to check what the planned reconstructive efforts could achieve.

Using a computer model for free-functioning muscle transfers, some questions can be individually asked and modeled. How much (bulk and length) of what sort of muscle is needed to create the desired range or excursion and the estimated needed power? Where best should the origin and the insertion be attached to achieve the desired movement? Information from anatomic three-dimensional data collection of internal nerve branching patterns and from clinical nerve bundle stimulations can contribute to the creation and use of appropriately innervated portions of a donor muscle [24].

It is understood that nonmuscle models can be used for assessing dimensions and volume of a reconstruction where that is all that is required. Volume data are also readily available with the modeling approach herein described.

Therapeutic modalities of integrating muscle function

Modeling can help therapy be better focused on an individual's clinical problems. With the addition of motion analysis [20], ultrasound of muscles [25], and three-dimensional computer modeling as new diagnostic tools, new more precise diagnoses can be made about the varied states of relaxation and contraction. The patient can demonstrate their problems, have them assessed, and then be provided with verbal and visual feedback from the assessment tools and the computer modeling.

Models can provide a framework to assess muscle function in currently minimally treated neuromuscular disorders. Those interested in hand function can then be involved in the understanding and assessment of possible therapeutic interventions. Potential applications derived from functional explorations of hand function through modeling include examination of the use of Botox in dystonia and spasticity and the creation of new training programs for athletes.

Some themes may need to be reiterated frequently and supported with these tools.

- Protection is an instinct (very fundamental)
- Vicious cycles can be disrupted
- Gesturing is a normal, essentially "hard-wired" activity" (it needs to be restored)
- Inappropriate effort is counterproductive

The possibility that showing a patient a model simulation that demonstrates how their muscles are interfering with the improvement that they would like may be a powerful way of gaining their confidence that their problem is understood and that there is hope and a definite means of monitoring progress. Such approaches avoid the false dichotomy of organic versus psychologic illness. A computer model and the use of motion analysis [see **Fig. 6**] and ultrasound studies [26] create an innovative combination of approaches that may help diagnose, inform, and improve treatment outcomes of some challenging patients.

Might such approaches help prevent the arrival of symptoms and decrease the burden of work-related upper extremity symptoms? The inverse simulation of observed hand motion gives clinicians the potential to identify and visualize muscle activity patterns that are high risk for hand injury and more generally to understand the etiology of these injuries in the future.

Educational tools

Models of the functioning hand can be used to create new visuals for teaching medical students and other health care and physical training workers, exciting new web sites available to all, new displays at science centers, and so forth. Already, refinements of hand movements of a computer-generated guitar player have been explored in a model that creates music [**Fig. 7**] [27].

Improved understanding of the word "reconstructive"

The reconstructive component is still key to so much of what is done. With a combination of the planning discussed previously in the sections on reconstructive analysis and the development of exciting education tools there is the potential

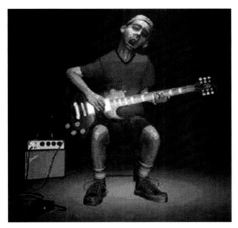

Fig. 7. Handrix: a computer-generated guitar player.

to improve the comprehension, appreciation, and visibility of this work. The meticulous planning of the field now could be supplemented and demonstrated with three-dimensional computer planning tools.

Contribute to science

Another area that is benefiting is the study of the evolution of this amazing human appendage. The thrust to explore the precise anatomy and function of the human hand can provide data for those who explore the development of this remarkable appendage [28].

The future

Functioning hand models will benefit from refinements. The challenges are many but the benefits are numerous. Creative ingenuity on many fronts is advancing the capabilities and applications of computer modeling. This list of uses of computer modeling of the hand and its function may be realized and expanded. The exploration and control of dynamic hand function, morphology, and pathology have exciting implications for medicine, anthropology, human computer interaction, art, and animation.

Acknowledgments

The authors acknowledge the ongoing support and encouragement of Eugene Fiume, PhD. Many high school students, undergraduate students, medical summer research students, project students, and graduate students have contributed to the development of three-dimensional anatomic muscle modeling. A special thanks to Victor Ng-Thow-Hing, PhD, who sought to bridge muscle physiology and computer science. Elizabeth Condliffe, MS, helped with the integration of modeling and medical material for this manuscript. The authors also thank Alias® for the use of MAYA™.

References

[1] Zajac FE, Neptune RR, Kautz SA. Biomechanics and muscle coordination of human walking. Part I: introduction to concepts, power transfer, dynamics and simulations. Gait Posture 2002;16: 215–32.

[2] Thelen DG, Anderson FC, Delp SL. Generating dynamic simulations of movement using computed muscle control. J Biomech 2003;36: 321–8.

[3] Biryukova E, Yourovskaya V. A model of hand dynamics. In: Schuind F, editor. Advances in the biomechanics of hand and wrist. New York: Plenum Press; 1994. p. 107–22.

[4] Tsang W. An anatomically accurate inverse dynamics solution for unconstrained hand motion [masters thesis]. Toronto: University of Toronto; 2005.

[5] Hoy MG, Zajac FE, Gordon ME. A musculoskeletal model of the human lower extremity: the effect of muscle, tendon, and moment arm on the moment-angle relationship of musculotendon actuators at the hip, knee, and ankle. J Biomech 1990;23:157–69.

[6] Agur AM, Ng-Thow-Hing V, Ball KA, et al. Documentation and three-dimensional modelling of human soleus muscle architecture. Clin Anat 2003;16:285–93.

[7] Agur AM. Architecture of the human soleus muscle: three-dimensional computer modelling of cadaveric muscle and ultrasonographic documentation in vivo [doctoral thesis]. Toronto: University of Toronto; 2001.

[8] Ng-Thow-Hing V. Anatomically-based models for physical and geometric reconstruction of humans and other animals [doctoral thesis]. Toronto: University of Toronto; 2001.

[9] Ng-Thow-Hing V, Agur A, McKee N. A muscle model that captures external shape, internal fibre architecture, and permits simulation of active contraction with volume preservation. Presented at the Fifth International Symposium on Computer Methods in Biomechanics and Biomedical Engineering. Rome, Italy, October 31–November 3, 2001.

[10] Ng-Thow-Hing V, Fiume E. Application-specific muscle representations. In: Proceedings Graphics Interface; 2002:107–16. Available at: http://www.graphicsinterface.org/proceedings/2002/203/.

[11] Blemker SS, Delp SL. Three-dimensional representation of complex muscle architectures and geometries. Ann Biomed Eng 2005;33:661–73.

[12] Kovler M, Lundon K, McKee N, et al. The human first carpometacarpal joint: osteoarthritic degeneration and 3-dimensional modeling. J Hand Ther 2004;17:393–400.

[13] Albrecht I, Haber J, Seidel H. Construction and animation of anatomically based human hand models. In: Proceedings of SIGGRAPH Symposium for Computer Animation. San Diego (CA): ACM Press / ACM SIGGRAPH; 2003. p. 98–102.

[14] Neuromuscular Biomechanics Laboratory. Stanford University. Available at: https://www.stanford.edu/group/nmbl/research/computational/simm.html.

[15] Anderson FC, Pandy MG. Static and dynamic optimization solutions for gait are practically equivalent. J Biomech 2001;34:153–61.

[16] Hill AV. The effect of load on the heat of shortening of muscle. Proc R Soc Lond B Biol Sci 1964;159:297–318.

[17] Brand P, Hollister A. Clinical mechanics of the hand. 3rd edition. St. Louis: Mosby-Year Book; 1999.

[18] Yamaguchi GT, Moran DW, Si J. A computationally efficient method for solving the redundant problem in biomechanics. J Biomech 1995;28: 999–1005.

[19] Wilson F. The hand. New York: Panthenon Books; 1998.

[20] Su FC, Chou YL, Yang CS, et al. Movement of finger joints induced by synergistic wrist motion. Clin Biomech (Bristol, Avon) 2005;20(5):491–7.

[21] Stinear CM, Byblow WD. Impaired modulation of intracortical inhibition in focal hand dystonia. Cereb Cortex 2004;14:555–61.

[22] Lieber RL, Friden J. Implications of muscle design on surgical reconstruction of upper extremities. Clin Orthop Relat Res 2004;419: 267–79.

[23] Manktelow RT, Zuker RM, McKee NH. Functioning free muscle transplantation. J Hand Surg [Am] 1984;91:32–9.

[24] Loh EY, Agur AM, McKee NH. Intramuscular innervation of the human soleus muscle: a 3D model. Clin Anat 2003;16:378–82.

[25] Martin DC, Medri MK, Chow RS, et al. Comparing human skeletal muscle architectural parameters of cadavers with in vivo ultrasonographic measurements. J Anat 2001;199(Pt 4): 429–34.

[26] Somani S, Mackeen LD, Morad Y, et al. Assessment of extraocular muscles position and anatomy by 3-dimensional ultrasonography: a trial in craniosynostosis patients. J AAPOS 2003;7:54–9.

[27] ElKoura G. Animating the human hand [masters thesis]. Toronto: University of Toronto; 2003.

[28] Marzke MW, Marzke RF. Evolution of the human hand: approaches to acquiring, analysing and interpreting the anatomical evidence. J Anat 2000;197(Pt 1):121–40.

CLINICS IN
PLASTIC
SURGERY

Clin Plastic Surg 32 (2005) 643–656

Cumulative Index 2005

Note: Page numbers of article titles are in **boldface** type.

doi:10.1016/S0094-1298(05)00093-3

Changing Your Address?

Make sure your subscription changes too! When you notify us of your new address, you can help make our job easier by including an exact copy of your Clinics label number with your old address (see illustration below.) This number identifies you to our computer system and will speed the processing of your address change. Please be sure this label number accompanies your old address and your corrected address—you can send an old Clinics label with your number on it or just copy it exactly and send it to the address listed below.

We appreciate your help in our attempt to give you continuous coverage. Thank you.

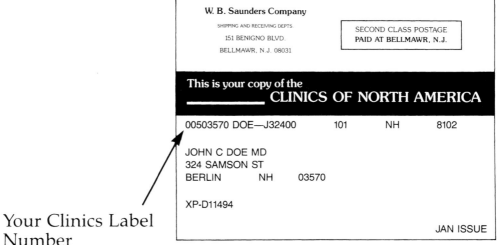

Your Clinics Label Number
Copy it exactly or send your label along with your address to:
W.B. Saunders Company, Customer Service
Orlando, FL 32887-4800
Call Toll Free 1-800-654-2452

Please allow four to six weeks for delivery of new subscriptions and for processing address changes.

United States Postal Service

Statement of Ownership, Management, and Circulation

1. Publication Title	2. Publication Number								3. Filing Date
Clinics in Plastic Surgery	0	0	4	-	1	2	9	8	9/15/05

4. Issue Frequency	5. Number of Issues Published Annually	6. Annual Subscription Price
Jan, Apr, Jul, Oct	4	$245.00

7. Complete Mailing Address of Known Office of Publication *(Not printer) (Street, city, county, state, and ZIP+4)*

Elsevier, Inc.
6277 Sea Harbor Drive
Orlando, FL 32887-4800

Contact Person
Gwen C. Campbell

Telephone
215-239-3685

8. Complete Mailing Address of Headquarters or General Business Office of Publisher *(Not printer)*

Elsevier, Inc., 360 Park Avenue South, New York, NY 10010-1710

9. Full Names and Complete Mailing Addresses of Publisher, Editor, and Managing Editor *(Do not leave blank)*

Publisher *(Name and complete mailing address)*

Tim Griswold, Elsevier, Inc., 1600 John F. Kennedy Blvd., Suite 1800, Philadelphia, PA 19103-2899

Editor *(Name and complete mailing address)*

Joe Rusko, Elsevier, Inc., 1600 John F. Kennedy Blvd., Suite 1800, Philadelphia, PA 19103-2899

Managing Editor *(Name and complete mailing address)*

Heather Cullen, Elsevier, Inc., 1600 John F. Kennedy Blvd., Suite 1800, Philadelphia, PA 19103-2899

10. Owner *(Do not leave blank. If the publication is owned by a corporation, give the name and address of the corporation immediately followed by the names and addresses of all stockholders owning or holding 1 percent or more of the total amount of stock. If not owned by a corporation, give the names and addresses of the individual owners. If owned by a partnership or other unincorporated firm, give its name and address as well as those of each individual owner. If the publication is published by a nonprofit organization, give its name and address.)*

Full Name	Complete Mailing Address
Wholly owned subsidiary of	4520 East-West Highway
Reed/Elsevier, US holdings	Bethesda, MD 20814

11. Known Bondholders, Mortgagees, and Other Security Holders Owning or Holding 1 Percent or More of Total Amount of Bonds, Mortgages, or Other Securities. If none, check box ▶ ☐ None

Full Name	Complete Mailing Address
N/A	

12. Tax Status *(For completion by nonprofit organizations authorized to mail at nonprofit rates) (Check one)*
The purpose, function, and nonprofit status of this organization and the exempt status for federal income tax purposes:
☐ Has Not Changed During Preceding 12 Months
☐ Has Changed During Preceding 12 Months *(Publisher must submit explanation of change with this statement)*

(See Instructions on Reverse)

PS Form **3526**, October 1999

13. Publication Title	14. Issue Date for Circulation Data Below
Clinics in Plastic Surgery	July 2005

15.	Extent and Nature of Circulation		Average No. Copies Each Issue During Preceding 12 Months	No. Copies of Single Issue Published Nearest to Filing Date
a.	Total Number of Copies *(Net press run)*		3550	3500
b. Paid and/or Requested Circulation	(1)	Paid/Requested Outside-County Mail Subscriptions Stated on Form 3541. *(Include advertiser's proof and exchange copies)*	1870	1849
	(2)	Paid In-County Subscriptions Stated on Form 3541 *(Include advertiser's proof and exchange copies)*		
	(3)	Sales Through Dealers and Carriers, Street Vendors, Counter Sales, and Other Non-USPS Paid Distribution	696	843
	(4)	Other Classes Mailed Through the USPS		
c.	Total Paid and/or Requested Circulation *[Sum of 15b. (1), (2), (3), and (4)]*	▲	2566	2692
d. Free Distribution by Mail *(Samples, complimentary, and other free)*	(1)	Outside-County as Stated on Form 3541	72	77
	(2)	In-County as Stated on Form 3541		
	(3)	Other Classes Mailed Through the USPS		
e.	Free Distribution Outside the Mail *(Carriers or other means)*			
f.	Total Free Distribution *(Sum of 15d. and 15e.)*	▲	72	77
g.	Total Distribution *(Sum of 15c. and 15f.)*	▲	2638	2769
h.	Copies not Distributed		912	731
i.	Total *(Sum of 15g. and h.)*	▲	3550	3500
j.	Percent Paid and/or Requested Circulation *(15c. divided by 15g. times 100)*		97%	97%

16. Publication of Statement of Ownership
☐ Publication required. Will be printed in the **October 2005** issue of this publication. ☐ Publication not required

17. Signature and Title of Editor, Publisher, Business Manager, or Owner

Janet Zimmerman — Manager of Subscription Services

Date 9/15/05

I certify that all information furnished on this form is true and complete. I understand that anyone who furnishes false or misleading information on this form or who omits material or information requested on the form may be subject to criminal sanctions (including fines and imprisonment) and/or civil sanctions (including civil penalties).

Instructions to Publishers

1. Complete and file one copy of this form with your postmaster annually on or before October 1. Keep a copy of the completed form for your records.
2. In cases where the stockholder or security holder is a trustee, include in items 10 and 11 the name of the person or corporation for whom the trustee is acting. Also include the names and addresses of individuals who are stockholders who own or hold 1 percent or more of the total amount of bonds, mortgages, or other securities of the publishing corporation. In item 11, if none, check the box. Use blank sheets if more space is required.
3. Be sure to furnish all circulation information called for in item 15. Free circulation must be shown in items 15d, e, and f.
4. Item 15h., Copies not Distributed, must include (1) newsstand copies originally stated on Form 3541, and returned to the publisher, (2) estimated returns from news agents, and (3) copies for office use, leftovers, spoiled, and all other copies not distributed.
5. If the publication had Periodicals authorization as a general or requester publication, this Statement of Ownership, Management, and Circulation must be published; it must be printed in any issue in October or, if the publication is not published during October, the first issue printed after October.
6. In item 16, indicate the date of the issue in which this Statement of Ownership will be published.
7. Item 17 must be signed.

Failure to file or publish a statement of ownership may lead to suspension of Periodicals authorization.

PS Form **3526**, October 1999 *(Reverse)*